Evaluation and Treatment of the Shoulder: *An Integration of the Guide to Physical Therapist Practice*

Evaluation and Treatment of the Shoulder: *An Integration of the Guide to Physical Therapist Practice*

Brian J. Tovin, MMSc, PT, SCS, ATC, FAAOMPT
Clinic Director
The Sports Rehabilitation Center at Georgia Tech
Director of Rehabilitation
Georgia Tech Sports Medicine
Atlanta, Georgia

Bruce H. Greenfield, MMSc, PT, OCS
Instructor
Department of Rehabilitation Medicine
Division of Physical Therapy
Emory University School of Medicine
Atlanta, Georgia

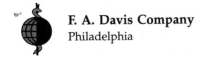

F. A. Davis Company
Philadelphia

F. A. Davis Company
1915 Arch Street
Philadelphia, PA 19103
www.fadavis.com

Copyright © 2001 by F. A. Davis Company

Printed in the United States of America

Last digit indicates print number: 10 9 8 7 6 5 4 3 2 1

Publisher: Jean Francois Vilain
Developmental Editor: Sharon Lee
Cover Designer: Louis J. Forgione

As new scientific information becomes available through basic and clinical research, recommended treatments and drug therapies undergo changes. The author(s) and publisher have done everything possible to make this book accurate, up to date, and in accord with accepted standards at the time of publication. The author(s), editors, and publisher are not responsible for errors or omissions or for consequences from application of the book, and make no warranty, expressed or implied, in regard to the contents of the book. Any practice described in this book should be applied by the reader in accordance with professional standards of care used in regard to the unique circumstances that may apply in each situation. The reader is advised always to check product information (package inserts) for changes and new information regarding dose and contraindications before administering any drug. Caution is especially urged when using new or infrequently ordered drugs.

Library of Congress Cataloging-in-Publication Data

Tovin, Brian J.
    Evaluation and treatment of the shoulder: an integration of the guide to physical therapist practice / Brian J. Tovin, Bruce H. Greenfield.
        p. cm.
    Includes bibliographical references and index.
    ISBN 0-8036-0262-6
        1. Shoulder—Diseases—Physical therapy. 2. Shoulder pain—Patients—Rehabilitation. 3. Shoulder pain—Physical therapy. I. Greenfield, Bruce H., 1953- II. Title.

RC939 .T68 2001
617.5'72062—dc21   00-065752

Dedication

This book is dedicated to my most significant others: my wife and best friend, Stacey, for making me a better person and being my b'shert; and my parents, Stefanie and Ian, for their continuous love, support, and guidance.

Brian Tovin

This book is dedicated to my wife Amy, who has provided me with unconditional love and support, and to my children, Heather, Suzanne, and Eleanor, gifts from God.

Bruce Greenfield

Foreword

As we enter the new millennium, we pause for a moment to recognize that publication of *Evaluation and Treatment of the Shoulder: An Integration of the Guide to Physical Therapist Practice* marks the 15th anniversary of the **Contemporary Perspectives in Rehabilitation** series. Throughout this time, a consistent and conscientious effort has been made to present a variety of topics to rehabilitation specialists, clinicians, and students. Our texts have received recognition for their diversity and comprehensive informational formats. In all of the volumes in the CPR series, material is critically and consistently presented using a challenging and problem-solving approach, often through the incorporation of case studies, decision trees, and comprehensive tables.

This approach was undertaken so that we could be "contemporary." Clearly, within the past decade, multiple changes in health-care policy have impacted the circumstances under which rehabilitation is provided. Opinions about these changes have varied, with most professionals showing a multitude of emotions, ranging from ambiguity to recalcitrance to anger. Yet, one undeniable fact remains—the concept of *contemporary* has changed, or at least its fabric appears manufactured from a different fiber and design. What was once labeled clinical decision making has now been transformed into evidence-based practice; and while empiricism was at one time permitted to reign as the basis for evaluation and treatment, defined guidelines that speak to documentation and evidence are now prevalent.

Against this background, the editors of this text on shoulder evaluation and treatment have brought together a unique combination of competence, skill, dedication, and friendship to carve a niche in contemporary physical therapy. This niche is embedded in the text's application of the *Guide to Physical Therapist Practice* (Physical Therapy, (11) 77, 1997) as it pertains to a musculoskeletal problem pervasive among clients ranging from young athletes to frail, older adults.

This text is more than a detailed study on evaluation, physical therapy diagnoses, treatment, and reassessment of the shoulder. Tovin and Greenfield have taken a courageous step to offer their interest in the treatment of this body segment as one of the first efforts for rethinking the way physical therapists interface and treat patients. To succeed in this task required the contributions of authors whose sense of destiny is redefining how therapists evaluate and treat parallels those of the editors. Indeed, many of the contributors to this book are well known to many orthopedic physical therapists and their students. Guccione, Davies, Binkley, McClure, Stralka, McConnell, and Snyder-Mackler can easily be classified as visionaries with the ability to sense the course that clinicians must chart to secure further growth and autonomy.

To accomplish the task, the text is divided into three major sections. The first section reviews anatomy (Greenfield) and kinesiology (Abelew) while also reviewing the fundamental constructs underlying the evolution of impairment-based diagnosis by physical therapists (Guccione) and its application to the shoulder girdle (Tovin and Greenfield). The importance of clinical examination (Davies et al.) and integration of quantified outcome measures (Binkley) complete this section. The second section addresses the preferred practice patterns. To better appreciate the thought that has made this section unique, the reader is referred to Chapter 4 of the "Guidelines." Students and clinicians are presented with a discussion of the relationship between the suggested guidelines and specific shoulder joint or girdle pathologies, along with commentary that challenges their reasoning and thought processes. Lastly, Section III describes the principles of treatment. In this section, the reader is exposed to clinical reasoning in the use of manual therapy techniques (Jones and Magarey), alternative treatment modes, such as aquatic therapy (Tovin), and the role of open versus closed kinetic chain exercises as treatment for the shoulder (Livingston). Highlighting this section is Jenny McConnell's discussion of appropriate neuromuscular re-education strategies and a presentation of the rationale underlying the orderly functional progression in therapeutic exercise plans (Chmielewski and Snyder-Mackler).

I have served as Editor-in-Chief for all of the volumes in the CPR series, but many factors make this book particularly endearing to me. Both Brian Tovin and Bruce Greenfield are past students of mine. Perhaps I have contributed a small portion to their academic accomplishments. Most of their contributors are friends or colleagues whose work I have respected for many years. As a total team, they have embarked on a venture that may some day be viewed as a model that symbolized a change in how (and why) physical therapy services are provided.

As students and therapists read this book, they should be reminded of the prudent words of the great American humorist, Mark Twain, "A man cannot be comfortable without his own approval." The time has come for us to alter our comfort level by not only approving the guidelines, but more importantly, by applying them. This book affords all of us that special opportunity. At the risk of sounding somewhat dramatic, perhaps we might consider the following:

> The dogmas of the quiet past are inadequate to the stormy present. The occasion is piled high with difficulty, and we must rise to the occasion. As our case is new, so we must think anew and act anew. We must disenthrall ourselves.

This thought is as true for the physical therapist pondering changing practice patterns as it was for Abraham Lincoln more than 140 years ago as he pondered the fate of a nation.

Steven L. Wolf, PhD, FAPTA
Series Editor

Preface

In November 1997, the American Physical Therapy Association published the *Guide to Physical Therapist Practice.* "The Guide," as it came to be known, provided the physical therapy and medical community with a comprehensive document that outlined the nature and scope of physical therapy practice. The Guide is divided into two parts: part one discusses patient/client management and explains the tests and measures that are used in patient management; part two discusses patterns of practice for selected diagnostic categories. The patterns of practice describe the components of patient management that a panel of expert clinicians deemed reasonable for a diagnostic group and include examination techniques, evaluation, diagnosis, prognosis, and intervention. The items in each diagnostic group share common impairments and functional losses that distinguish them from other groups. Diagnostic groups encompass the major body systems and include musculoskeletal, neuromuscular, cardiopulmonary, and integumentary. Up to this point, there is limited documentation that the guidelines included in the patterns of practice are superior to others. The challenge to the profession is to apply the guidelines to the treatment of patients and determine their effectiveness by gauging outcomes.

Evaluation and Treatment of the Shoulder: An Integration of the Guide to Physical Therapist Practice provides physical therapists, as well as occupational therapists, athletic trainers, and others, with a resource that integrates the musculoskeletal practice patterns in the Guide with the rehabilitation of the shoulder. This text introduces orthopedic conditions based on clustering impairments and in so doing embraces the Guide's philosophy that physical therapists and other rehabilitation specialists diagnose the consequences of disease, pathology, injury, or surgery on the musculoskeletal system. These consequences include related impairments, functional losses, and disabilities that have been and continue to be the purview of physical therapy practice.

The purpose of *Evaluation and Treatment of the Shoulder* is twofold: to serve as a model that presents shoulder conditions from an impairment-based perspective so that the Guide's preferred practice patterns outlining treatment strategies can be used and assessed for their feasibility and effectiveness. Second, the text is an excellent basic resource for the entry-level clinician for all aspects of shoulder rehabilitation. Whether or not practicing clinicians embrace the guidelines contained in the Guide, this text provides them with an excellent updated resource on the care and management of selected shoulder conditions.

Evaluation and Treatment of the Shoulder is divided into three parts. Part I discusses shoulder anatomy and kinesiology, reviews the historical basis of impairment-based practice, and extrapolates and operationally defines the impairment-based categories of the shoulder from the Guide that serve as the organizing construct for the rest of the text. Part I concludes with a review of the examination of the shoulder and functional outcome measures.

Part II presents the main body of the text—selected shoulder conditions. In keeping with a philosophy that we believe to be unique to this text, conditions are introduced based on their primary impairments, rather than on the traditional medical diagnoses. The medical diagnoses are presented as secondary concerns that guide the pace and nature of treatment, rather than direct the primary approach to evaluating and ameliorating impairments and functional losses. An example is Chapter 7, "Musculoskeletal Pattern D: Impaired Joint Mobility, Motor Function, Muscle Performance, and Range of Motion Associated with Capsular Restriction." The rehabilitation of a painful and stiff shoulder that is the result of primary adhesive capsulitis or secondary to post-surgical shoulder immobilization is consistently based on identifying, assessing, and correcting the impairments that affect function. What varies is the pace of treatment dictated by soft tissue healing and the individual's functional goals.

Finally, Part III reviews principles of rehabilitation for the shoulder. Historically, the treatment strategies and techniques for shoulder conditions have varied both in their scope and effectiveness. The challenge was to sift through the large number of treatments, tossing the irrelevant ones and exposing the "nuggets." In meeting this challenge, we were guided by our commitment and that of the **Contemporary Perspectives of Rehabilitation** series to present, whenever possible, evidence-based outcome treatments. Chapters on manual therapy strategies, neuromuscular education techniques, aquatic therapy, functional progression exercises, and closed kinetic chain exercises, all contain information rich in detail but scrupulous in scientific rigor.

Contributors were selected for their expertise, academic credentials, and professional integrity. The selection criteria are reflected in the quality of the text and the attention paid to pedagogy. Every chapter includes pedagogy designed to enhance the content. Chapter outlines give readers a quick overview of the content. Chapter introductions explain all relevant principles and operational definitions. Specific case studies within the chapters allow the reader to learn how the information is integrated into patient care.

In using this text, we anticipate that readers will apply the process method and the content to formulate treatments for their patients. We feel confident we are offering cutting-edge material aimed at influencing the future practice of physical therapy and rehabilitation in general. Since this venture is directed toward the profession's growth, we invite the reader's feedback to see if our predictions are accurate. Future editions will reflect that feedback and the dynamic changes in health care policy to effect even better and more relevant treatment assessments and approaches.

Brian Tovin
Bruce Greenfield

Acknowledgments

A professional career is not only guided by the amount of knowledge, perseverance, and motivation of that individual, but equally by the surrounding cast of people who have helped to shape, direct, and influence that individual along the way. I would like to thank those individuals who have done all of these things for me and helped contribute, both directly and indirectly, to the development of this text. To Pam Levangie for taking a chance on me by admitting me to physical therapy school at Boston University. To Lynn Snyder-Mackler, who guided me on the right track early in my career and taught me to strive for excellence. She continues to be a source of inspiration and motivation in my career. To Steve Wolf, who has patiently taught me the finer points of research, writing, and editing. Both Lynn and Steve have been friends and mentors, serving as my "professional parents" and teaching me that balancing academics and clinical practice is possible. To Geoff Maitland and Keith Kleven for teaching me that being an expert clinician not only requires advanced clinical skills, but compassion for the patient as well. They taught me that no patient cares how much you know until they know how much you care. To Mark Jones and Steve Kraus for motivating me to continually challenge myself and for helping me refine my clinical reasoning process and manual therapy skills. To Jay Shoop, who has given me the opportunity to have my "dream" job and who has taught me that "old school" is sometimes better than "new school." To my brothers Cory and Todd Tovin, and sisters-in-law Melissa and Renee Tovin, who have taught me that a family of physical therapists does not necessarily make for boring dinner conversation. To my colleagues Catherine Duncan, David Pasion, and Gina Boomershine for all that they do for our clinics. To Grace Jones for being the backbone of our office. I owe a great deal of gratitude to Dr. Angelo Galante, Dr. John Xerogeanes, and Dr. "Chip" Pendleton for their friendship and confidence in me. I would also like to thank Joelle Szendel for assisting with typing and Kelly Ramsdell, Adria Gravely, and Adam Snyder for serving as models. To Jean-Francois Vilain, Sharon Lee, and the staff at F.A. Davis for making this challenging task an unforgettable experience. Finally, to Bruce Greenfield, without whose assistance, support, patience, and friendship this book would never have happened.

Brian J. Tovin

As human beings, we have good and bad traits that result from the confluence of a number of factors, not the least of which is the influence of individuals during our personal and professional development. Hopefully, the good traits outweigh the bad, and we are able to accomplish things that make life meaningful.

The following individuals have helped to identify and nurture the attitudes, values, and habits that constitute the good in me. My greatest debt of gratitude is owed to my late mother, Eleanore Greenfield, my father, Seymour Greenfield, and my sister, Meryl Jacobs. I would like to thank my in-laws, Edward and Florence Schuman, and my brother-in-law, Andrew Jacobs, for their love and support. I would like to thank my colleagues and friends on the faculty of the Division of Physical Therapy at Emory University for their unfailing support and friendship. In particular, I would like to express my gratitude to Dr. Pamela Catlin, who allowed me to "carve out" my own professional time to work on this book. I would like to thank Steve Wolf, a friend, colleague, and role model who impressed upon me the value of rigorous scholarship. I would like to thank Marie Johanson for her friendship and support. I would also like to thank some of my colleagues who still toil in the clinic and to me are the true heroes of the profession of physical therapy: Michael Wooden, Tim McMahon, Robert Donatelli, Mark Albert, Steve Kraus, Zita Gonzales, and Greg Bennett. These people did it right in the beginning, and they continue to do it right.

All the contributors and I owe a great deal to the reviewers whose constructive criticisms were instrumental in shaping this text. My thanks to F.A. Davis for its support, particularly to Jean-Francois Vilain and Sharon Lee, both of whom helped to guide the entire project, and in the case of Sharon, she did it with a soft but steady voice.

Finally, I would like to thank Brian Tovin, friend, colleague, and co-editor, for taking on this task with me; his determination and energy provided the impetus to complete this project.

Bruce Greenfield

Contributors

Thomas Abelew, PhD
Assistant Professor
Department of Rehabilitation Medicine
Division of Physical Therapy
Emory University School of Medicine
Atlanta, Georgia

Jill Binkley, PT, MClSc, FCAMT, FAAOMPT
Assistant Professor
School of Physiotherapy
McMaster University
Hamilton, Ontario, Canada

Lori Thein Brody, MS, PT, SCS, ATC
Senior Clinical Specialist
University of Wisconsin Clinics
    Research Park
Sports Medicine and Spine Center
Madison, WI
Program Director
Rocky Mountain University of Physical
    Therapy
Provo, Utah

Kevin Cappel, MS, PT, SCS, ATC, CSCS
Director of Sports Medicine
Gunderson Lutheran Sports Medicine
Winona, Minnesota

Terese L. Chmielewski, MA, PT, SCS
Doctoral Student, Biomechanics and
    Movement Sciences Program
Department of Physical Therapy
University of Delaware
Newark, Delaware

Michael A. Clark, MS, PT, CSCS
Sports Physical Therapy and
    Performance Specialist
Physiotherapy Associates Tempe Sport
    Clinic
Director of Sports Science
Athletic Institute
Franklin, Pennsylvania

George J. Davies Med, PT, SCS, ATC, CSCS
Professor, Graduate Physical Therapy
    Program
University of Wisconsin-Lacrosse
Director, Clinical and Research Services
Gunderson Lutheran Sports Medicine
Lacrosse, Wisconsin

Todd S. Ellenbecker, MS, PT, SCS, CSCS
Clinic Director
Physiotherapy Associates
Scottsdale Sports Clinic
Scottsdale, Arizona

Bruce H. Greenfield, MMSc, PT, OCS
Instructor
Department of Rehabilitation Medicine
Division of Physical Therapy
Emory University School of Medicine
Atlanta, Georgia

Andrew A. Guccione, PhD, PT, FAPTA
Senior Vice President
Division of Practice and Research
American Physical Therapy Association
Alexandria, Virginia

Penny L. Head, PT, SCS, ATC
Director of Physical Therapy
The Campbell Clinic
Memphis, Tennessee

Mark A. Jones, BS, PT, MAppSc
Senior Lecturer, Centre for Allied
    Health Research
Coordinator, Postgraduate Programs in
    Manipulative Physiotherapy
School of Physiotherapy, Division of
    Health Sciences
University of South Australia
Adelaide, South Australia

Beven P. Livingston, MS, PT, ATC
Graduate Student, PhD Program in
    Neuroscience
Emory University
Atlanta, Georgia

**Mary M. Magarey, PhD, Grad Dip
Man Ther**
Senior Lecturer, Centre for Allied
    Health Research
Coordinator, Postgraduate Programs in
    Sports Physiotherapy
School of Physiotherapy, Division of
    Health Sciences
University of South Australia
Adelaide, South Australia

Phil McClure, PhD, PT, OCS
Associate Professor
Department of Physical Therapy
Beaver College
Glenside, Pennsylvania

**Jenny McConnell, BAppSci (Phty),
    Grad Dip Man Ther, MBiomedE**
Director, McConnell & Clements
    Physiotherapy
New South Wales, Australia

Karen J. Mohr, PT, SCS
Research Director
Kerlan-Jobe Orthopaedic Clinic
Hermosa Beach, California

Diane Radovich Schwab, MSPT
Champion Rehabilitation
San Diego, California

**Lynn Snyder-Mackler, ScD, PT, ATC,
    SCS**
Associate Professor
Department of Physical Therapy
University of Delaware
Newark, Delaware

Susan W. Stralka, MS, PT
Director, Outpatient Rehabilitation
    Services
Director, The Orthopaedic and Sports
    Medicine Institute
Baptist Memorial Healthcare
Memphis, Tennessee

**Brian J. Tovin, MMSc, PT, SCS, ATC,
    FAAOMPT**
Clinic Director
The Sports Rehabilitation Center at
    Georgia Tech
Director of Rehabilitation
Georgia Tech Sports Medicine
Atlanta, Georgia

Reviewers

Charles D. Ciccone, PhD, PT
Professor
Department of Physical Therapy
Ithaca College
Ithaca, New York

Gary Lentell, MS, PT
Professor
Department of Physical Therapy
California State University, Fresno
Fresno, California

Mark R. Wiegand, PhD, PT
Associate Professor
Department of Physical Therapy
    Program
University of Louisville Health Sciences
    Center
Louisville, Kentucky

Contents

SECTION II: Musculoskeletal Patterns of the Shoulder

Chapter 11   Musculoskeletal Pattern I: Impaired Joint Mobility, Motor Function, Muscle Performance, and Range of Motion Associated with Joint Arthroplasty

Susan W. Stralka, MS, PT
Penny L. Head, PT, SCS, ATC

Chapter 12   Musculoskeletal Pattern J: Impaired Joint Mobility, Motor Function, Muscle Performance, and Range of Motion Associated with Bony or Soft Tissue Surgical Procedures

Lori Thein Brody, MS, PT, SCS, ATC

SECTION III   Treatment Strategies

SECTION I

Introduction

CHAPTER 1

Anatomy of the Shoulder

Bruce H. Greenfield, MMSc, PT, OCS†

INTRODUCTION

Physical therapists provide services to patients experiencing impairments, functional limitations, disabilities, or changes in physical function resulting from injury or disease.[1] To be successful, physical therapists combine a clear understanding of the theories of movement science that includes a strong foundation in the basic sciences of anatomy, physiology, kinesiology, and neuroscience with clinical management skills of patient examination, evaluation, diagnosis, and prognosis and treatment intervention. For example, the ability to identify structural and physiological impairments at the shoulder for treatment planning is predicated on knowledge and understanding of normal shoulder structure and function. Therefore, functional anatomy of the shoulder provides the basis from which physical therapists begin to understand abnormal function.

This chapter reviews the anatomy of the shoulder complex and illustrates areas of particular clinical concern and significance in injury, surgery, and rehabilitation. The interrelationship and interdependency of the upper quarter of the body with the shoulder is reviewed to establish the importance of cervical and thoracic spine and related tissue impairment in shoulder pain referral and secondary areas of dysfunction contributing to shoulder movement dysfunction. This chapter serves to compliment the next chapter, which reviews the kinesiology of the shoulder complex.

COMPONENTS OF THE SHOULDER

The shoulder girdle is a multijoint complex that functions to produce movement of the upper extremity and, ultimately, to position the hand in space. Because the upper extremity literally can move in many thousands of spatial planes, with each separated by approximately 1° of motion, the shoulder is an extremely mobile structure.[2] The shoulder, particularly the glenohumeral (GH) joint, is inherently mobile. The muscles and joint proprioceptors around the shoulder must maintain

†Acknowledgment: The author thanks Robert Donatelli for the use of the fresh cadaver illustrations.

stability of its various segments for normal function. This precarious relationship of mobility and stability during normal shoulder function is a primary reason that many shoulder injuries occur during overhead shoulder activities and sports.[3]

The shoulder is described as an integrated series of links functioning harmoniously during movement of the upper extremity.[4] This concept is similar to Steindler's description of the shoulder and upper extremity as a kinematic chain.[5] The components that constitute the links or kinematic chain of the shoulder include the scapulothoracic (ST) joint or junction, the sternoclavicular (SC) and acromioclavicular (AC) joints, and the GH joint.[6] The entire arrangement is supported by the upper quarter of the body, including the occiput, cervical, and thoracic spines and related neural and soft tissue connections.[6] Thus, normal shoulder function includes stability and mobility of the upper quarter.

Scapulothoracic Joint

STRUCTURE

Mechanical analysis of the shoulder indicates two competing demands: stability between the scapula and thorax and mobility between the humerus and scapula. Stability between the scapula and thorax is satisfied through a closed kinematic chain mechanism between the scapula, the SC joint, and the AC joint, and balance and control of the various muscles that attach to the scapula.[7] A closed kinematic chain is present when segmental movement is interrelated so that isolated movement of one segment around a joint cannot occur.[5] During normal function, isolated scapular movement is impossible to achieve without concomitant movement at either the SC joint or the AC joint. Descriptive movement of the shoulder complex is described in the following chapter.

Because it does not contain a capsule or synovial tissue, the ST joint is classified as a physiologic joint rather than a synovial joint.[5] The scapula is encapsulated by numerous soft tissue attachments with the sole bony attachment to the axial skeleton via the sternoclavicular joint (Fig. 1–1). This soft tissue arrangement stabilizes the scapula firmly against the posterior surface of the thorax. According to Steindler,[5] a primary stabilizing force holding the scapula to the thorax is atmospheric pressure. The arrangement of the scapular, SC joint, and AC joint is intimately related so that movement of the scapula in any plane always produces concurrent motion in the other two related joints.[5,6] The clinical importance of this arrangement will be addressed later in the text when restricted range of motion in any one of these joints results in limited movement of the other two joints.

According to Culham and Peat,[8] during erect standing the scapulae should be positioned over ribs two through seven and between T2 and T8. Also, the spine of the scapulae should be level with the spinous process of T3. The vertebral border should lie about 5 cm from the midline, with the scapula oriented 30° to 45° anterior to the frontal plane[9,10,11,12] (Fig. 1–2).

KINETICS AND THE AXIOSCAPULAR MUSCLES

Various muscles attach to both the thorax and scapula, maintaining contact between these surfaces while producing movement of the scapula. Saha[13] classifies

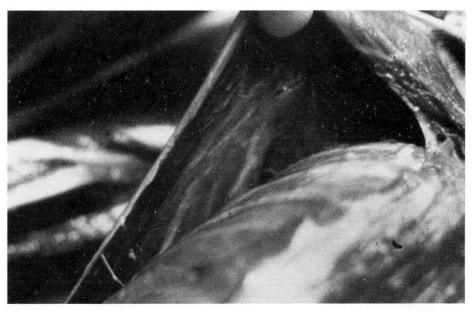

FIGURE 1–1. Fresh cadaver specimen showing the scapula from an inferior view with the broad attachment of the serratus anterior muscle. Manual distraction of the scapula indicates the firm soft tissue attachments to the scapula.

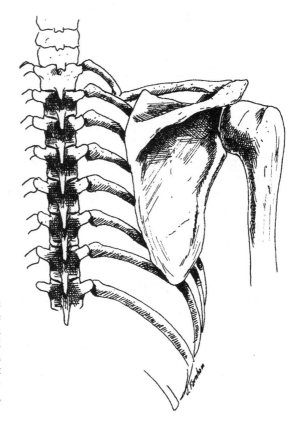

FIGURE 1–2. Resting position of the scapula on the thorax. Changes from the normal resting position could indicate an underlying impairment in the structural arrangements around the scapula. (From Norkin, CC, and Levangie, PK: Joint Structure and Function: A Comprehensive Analysis, ed 2. FA Davis, Philadelphia, 1992, p 210, with permission.)

TABLE 1–1 Classification of Shoulder Muscles

Axioscapular Muscles	*Upper, Middle, and Lower Trapezius*
	Levator Scapula Muscles
	Rhomboid (major and minor)
	Muscles
	Serratus Anterior
	Pectoralis Minor
	Omohyoid
	Subclavius
Scapulohumeral Muscles	*Deltoid*
	Triceps Brachii
	Biceps Brachii
	Subscapularis
	Infraspinatus
	Teres Minor
	Teres Major
Axiohumeral Muscles	Latissmus Dorsi
	Pectoralis Major

these muscles, which are listed in Table 1–1 as axioscapular muscles. Functions of these muscles are described in Chapter 2. During upper extremity movement, the axioscapular muscles work together to produce a smooth synchronous scapular motion.[13,14] Balance of these muscles is therefore of paramount importance to normal scapulohumeral function. Impairment resulting in weakness and tightness in these muscles can result in altered movement patterns and injury.

FUNCTION OF SCAPULA

The scapula functions as a stable base of support for rotation of the humerus during elevation of the extremity. Upward rotation and elevation of the scapula, occurring during humeral elevation, maintains normal orientation of the glenoid fossa, allows the scapulohumeral muscles to maintain an adequate length-tension relationship permitting continued rotation and elevation of the humerus, and keeps the acromion adequately elevated to allow clearance of the humeral head.[2,7,14] The ultimate effect of normal scapular movement is to provide additional range to overall shoulder motion without overstressing the GH joint. When the scapula functions well, overall upper extremity motion is enhanced, and the system is capable of high levels of performance.

Sternoclavicular Joint

STRUCTURE

The SC joint is described as a modified synovial sellar joint.[6,11] The proximal articulating surface of the clavicle is convex in a superior to inferior direction and concave anterior to posterior. The relationship of the articulating surface of the clavicle with the sternum is incongruous; the bulbous end of the clavicle extends considerably

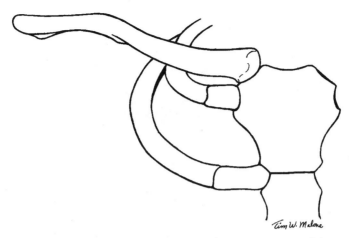

FIGURE 1–3. The sternoclavicular articulation. Note the incongruency of the sternal end of the clavicle overriding the corresponding articulating surface of the sternal notch of the manubrium. (From Norkin, CC, and Levangie, PK: Joint Structure and Function: A Comprehensive Analysis, ed 2. FA Davis, Philadelphia, 1992, p 211, with permission.)

over the sternal notch to produce an unstable osseous joint (Fig. 1–3). A fibrocartilage disc enhances stability of the SC joint. The upper portion of the disc is attached to the superior clavicle; the lower portion is attached to the manubrium and first costal cartilage (Fig. 1–4). In this way, the disc actually divides the SC joint into two joint cavities and acts as a hinge during clavicular movement.[11] The disc also acts as a shock absorber for SC joint compression that causes considerable stress during shoulder function. In addition to the disc, strong anterior and posterior ligaments, an interclavicular ligament, and a costoclavicular ligament also stabilize the SC joint (Fig. 1–5). The anterior and posterior SC joint ligaments reinforce the SC joint capsule, primarily serving to check anterior and posterior movement of the proximal end of the clavicle.[11] The costoclavicular ligament serves as the site of the axis, or fulcrum, for

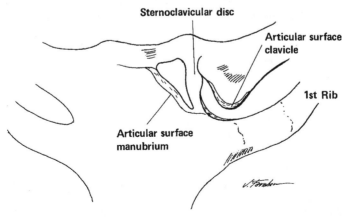

FIGURE 1–4. The SC joint shown with the clavicle elevated to view the articulation of the manubrium, the medial clavicle, and the interposed SC disc. (From Norkin, CC, and Levangie, PK: Joint Structure and Function: A Comprehensive Analysis, ed 2. FA Davis, Philadelphia, 1992, p 213, with permission.)

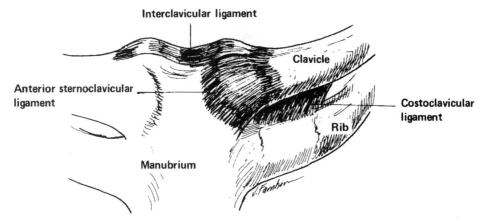

FIGURE 1–5. The SC joint ligaments. (From Norkin, CC, and Levangie, PK: Joint Structure and Function: A Comprehensive Analysis, ed 2. FA Davis, Philadelphia, 1992, p 214, with permission.)

elevation and depression and protraction and retraction. Because of its strong tensile properties, this ligament limits the amount of clavicular elevation and superior glide of the clavicle.[6,11] The costoclavicular ligament is supported by the subclavius muscle, which attaches from the first rib to the undersurface of the clavicle. The interclavicular ligament checks excessive depression or downward glide of the clavicle, which is critical to protecting structures like the brachial plexus and subclavian artery, which pass between the clavicle and the first rib below it.[6] Therefore, in spite of its inherent osseous incongruity, the SC joint, because of its soft tissue attachments, is relatively stable and accounts for less than 1% of all joint dislocations.[15]

ARTICULAR NEUROLOGY AND VASCULAR SUPPLY

Innervation is supplied by spinal nerves C5 and C6 via the supraclavicular and the nerve to the subclavius.[6] Therefore, injury to the SC joint often refers pain to other tissues sharing the same segmental innervation of C5 and C6. The SC joint receives its blood supply from the internal thoracic and suprascapular arteries.

Acromioclavicular Joint

STRUCTURE

The AC joint is classified as a plane synovial joint formed by the articulation of a relatively flat acromial process and slightly convex distal clavicle[6,11] (Fig. 1–6). The presence of an articular disc is variable in both size and shape. The disc has been found to degenerate with age and no longer be functional by the fourth decade of life.[16] Capsular ligaments around the AC joint include the capsule and superior and inferior AC joint ligaments (Fig. 1–7). The superior AC joint ligament is particularly strong partly because of aponeurotic expansions of the deltoid and upper trapezius muscles. The AC joint ligaments provide horizontal stability of the joint. The extrinsic ligaments of the AC joint are the coracoclavicular ligaments. These can be further subdivided as the laterally placed trapezoid and the more medial conoid

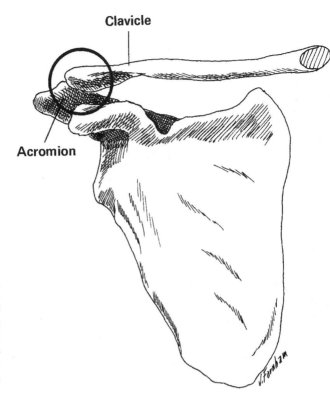

FIGURE 1–6. The AC joint. Articulation between the acromion of the scapula and the lateral clavicle is shown. (From Norkin, CC, and Levangie, PK: Joint Structure and Function: A Comprehensive Analysis, ed 2. FA Davis, Philadelphia, 1992, p 215, with permission.)

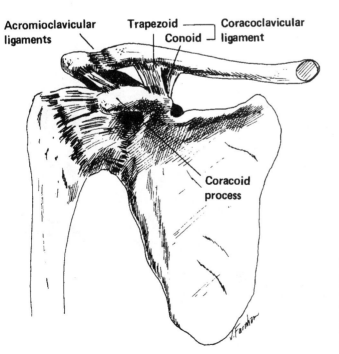

FIGURE 1–7. The AC ligament. (From Norkin, CC, and Levangie, PK: Joint Structure and Function: A Comprehensive Analysis, ed 2. FA Davis, Philadelphia, 1992, p 217, with permission.)

ligaments (Fig. 1–7). Both ligaments, which attach to the undersurface of the distal clavicle, provide a passive tensile or tractive force to the distal clavicle after 100° of humeral elevation. In addition, tension in these ligaments during outward rotation of the scapula produces additional clavicular rotation necessary for full overhead humeral elevation (see Chap. 2).[7,11] Therefore, no muscles act directly on the AC joint; motion is produced in passive response to active scapula motion.

ARTICULAR NEUROLOGY AND VASCULAR SUPPLY

The innervation to the AC joint is primarily from the anterior primary ramus of spinal nerve C4 supplied by the suprascapular and lateral pectoral nerves.[6] Therefore, unlike the SC joint, injury or disease of the AC joint does not commonly refer pain around the shoulder girdle. The arterial supply to the AC joint includes the suprascapular and thoracoacromial arteries.

Glenohumeral Joint

BONY ANATOMY

The GH joint is formed by the articulation between the head of the humerus and the glenoid fossa. Because the humeral head can move freely and to some extent in isolation of the scapula, the GH joint is considered by some as an open kinetic chain.[5,7] The humeral head is a spherical, or convex, structure that articulates with a concave or relatively flat glenoid fossa. The articulating surface of the humeral head is approximately 3 to 4 times the size of the glenoid fossa, resulting in an osseous unstable joint[17] (Fig. 1–8). The humeral head is oriented in a superior, medial position

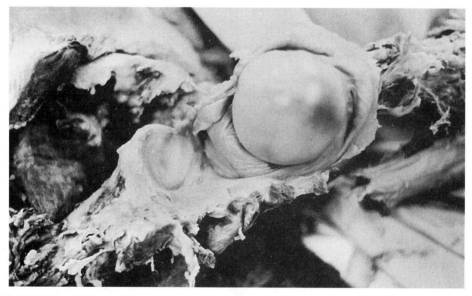

FIGURE 1–8. Cadaver specimen showing the relative size difference between the humeral head and the glenoid.

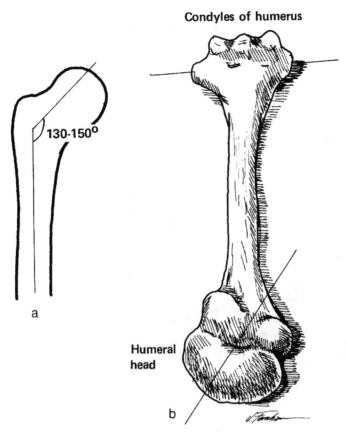

FIGURE 1–9. The humeral head in the transverse plane is commonly angled posteriorly with respect to an axis through the humeral epicondyles (retroversion). (From Norkin, CC, and Levangie, PK: Joint Structure and Function: A Comprehensive Analysis, ed 2. FA Davis, Philadelphia, 1992, p 219, with permission.)

and is slightly retroverted, whereas the glenoid fossa is superior, lateral, and slightly retroverted[7,11] (Fig. 1–9). The retroversion of both the humeral head and glenoid fossa is thought by some to offer some anterior osseous stability to the joint.[17] A labrum attaches around the rim of the glenoid and is composed of both fibrous and fibrocartilage tissue. The inner fibrocartilage surface of the labrum is attached to the glenoid rim, and the outer surface of fibrous tissue is continuous with the capsule of the GH joint, including the glenohumeral ligaments. The tendons of the long head of the biceps brachii and the triceps brachii contribute to the structure and reinforcement of the labrum.[18] The labrum is better developed along the anterior and inferior aspects of the glenoid as compared to the posterior portion, but the entire labrum is designed to deepen the glenoid socket (Fig. 1–10).

CAPSULE STRUCTURE

The GH joint capsule is a thin structure that attaches around the surgical neck of the humerus.[6] The capsule is lax and allows approximately 1 cm of distraction with manual force between the articulating surface of the glenoid and humeral head. The capsule forms a vacuum and provides a negative pressure between the articulating

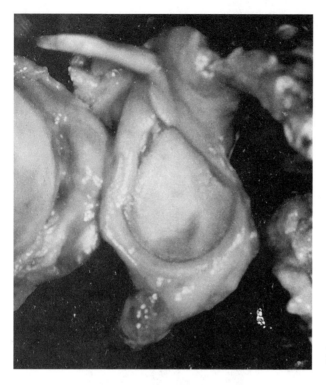

FIGURE 1–10. The glenoid labrum.

surfaces.[19] The negative pressure provides a suction effect to help hold the humeral head to the glenoid.

The anterior aspect of the capsule contains a small cleft or opening thinly veiled with fibrofatty, synovial tissue. This cleft is known anatomically as the rotator cuff interval because it is present between the tendons of the supraspinatus and subscapularis.[20,21] The rotator cuff interval is significant because surgeons often enter the shoulder capsule through it to minimize tissue damage. Additionally, and in some cases, if larger than normal, this interval is a source of instability requiring plication to stabilize the GH joint.[21]

BURSAE

Numerous bursae are present around the GH joint.[6] The subacromial bursa is located between the deltoid muscle and the joint capsule. The bursa extends under the acromion and coracoacromial ligament (Fig. 1–11) and over the supraspinatus muscle, and may communicate with the joint in the presence of a rotator cuff tear.[19] The subscapularis bursa is located between the subscapularis tendon and the neck of the scapula and may communicate with the GH joint cavity between the superior and middle glenohumeral ligament in the rotator cuff interval (Fig. 1–12).

The bursae, which allow free gliding of tissues, are particularly susceptible to inflammation (bursitis) with repetitive friction. Other bursae associated with the GH joint structures, but of less clinical significance, are located between the infraspinatus muscles and the capsule, on the superior surface of the acromion, between the coracoid process and the capsule, under the coracobrachialis muscle, between the teres major and the long head of the triceps, and in front and behind the tendon of the latissimus dorsi muscles.[6]

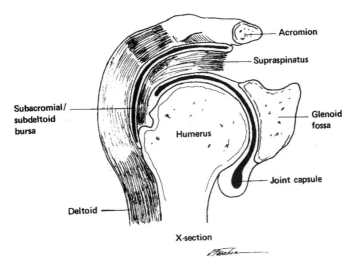

FIGURE 1–11. Subacromial bursa is contiguous and allows smooth gliding of the supraspinatus muscle and the humeral head under the deltoid muscle and the acromion. (From Norkin, CC, and Levangie, PK: Joint Structure and Function: A Comprehensive Analysis, ed 2. FA Davis, Philadelphia, 1992, p 221, with permission.)

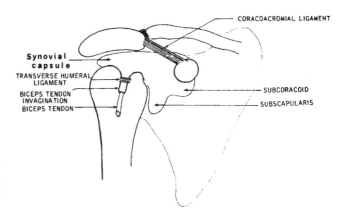

FIGURE 1–12. The subscapularis bursa. (From Calliet, R: Shoulder Pain, ed 3. FA Davis, Philadelphia, 1991, p 13, with permission.)

LIGAMENT STRUCTURE AND FUNCTION

The intrinsic ligaments of the GH joint, which include the superior, middle, and inferior glenohumeral ligaments, are described as thickening of the capsule.[22,23] The superior glenohumeral ligament is a small, thin ligament that covers the long head of the biceps muscle. It attaches from the labrum of the glenoid to the inferior tuberosity of the humeral head. The middle glenohumeral ligament has a wide attachment and lies under the subscapularis tendon. The points of attachment include the middle labrum and along the inferior facet of the inferior tuberosity of the humerus. Both the superior and middle glenohumeral ligaments form the floor of the rotator cuff interval. The inferior glenohumeral ligament, also known as the axillary pouch, has recently been investigated by O'Brien[24] and found to have three distinct portions: anterior, posterior, and inferior bands (see Fig. 8–4). The inferior glenohumeral ligament complex (IGHLC) functions like a hammock during overhead elevation. For example, the anterior band of the IGHLC becomes taut with humeral abduction and

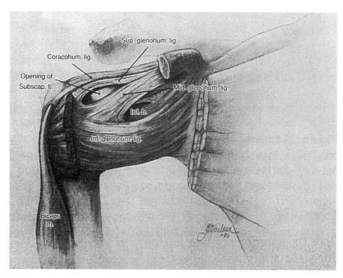

FIGURE 1–13. The glenohumeral ligaments make a Z configuration in approximately 88% of shoulders. Note the position of the coracohumeral ligament above the superior glenohumeral ligament. (Adapted from Ferrari, DA: Capsular ligament of the shoulder: anatomical and functional study of the anterior superior capsule. Am J Sports Med 18:20, 1990, p 21, with permission.)

external rotation, while the posterior band relaxes. Conversely, the posterior band becomes taut with humeral internal rotation and adduction, while the anterior band relaxes. The inferior band of the IGHLC helps support the humeral head within the glenoid and prevents inferior subluxation. Laxity in this ligament leads to instability of the GH joint. Tearing of the ligament occurs with traumatic anterior dislocation. Because the anterior band attaches to the inferior labrum and glenoid, a tear of the anterior band of the IGHLC results in a concomitant tear of this area of the labrum and is known as a Bankhart lesion.[24]

The glenohumeral ligaments form a distinct Z pattern (Fig. 1–13) in 88% of the population.[25] The coracohumeral ligament attaches from the coracoid process into the greater and lesser tuberosities of the humerus.[10] The ligament creates a tunnel through which the biceps tendon passes.

Twelve percent of the population exhibits variability in the shape and presence of the middle glenohumeral ligament (Fig. 1–14A and B). This group is particularly predisposed to anterior subluxations and dislocations. The functions of the glenohumeral ligaments are listed in Table 1–2.

TABLE 1–2 Anterior Restraints to External Rotation

Position	Ligament
Neutral or Adducted Position	Superior glenohumeral ligament; coracohumeral ligament and subscapularis muscle
Approximately 45° abduction	Middle glenohumeral ligament
90° abduction	Anterior band of inferior glenohumeral ligament

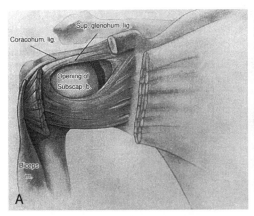
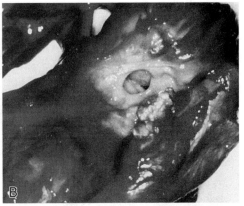

FIGURE 1–14. *(A)* Schematic shows the absence of the middle glenohumeral ligament. (From Ferrari, DA: Capsular ligament of the shoulder: anatomical and functional study of the anterior superior capsule. Am J Sports Med 18:20, 1990, p 22, with permission.) *(B)* Fresh cadaver dissection shows the absence of the middle glenohumeral ligament. Note the humeral head and glenoid fossa that are visible within the capsular opening.

MUSCLE ATTACHMENTS

Rotator Cuff

A distinguishing feature of the scapulohumeral muscles and to a lesser extent the axiohumeral muscles (Table 1–1) are their intimate connection to the glenohumeral capsule. The blending of the rotator cuff muscles to the capsule provides a dynamic capsuloligamentous structure that serves to alter the stiffness in the joint during contraction of the muscles.[26] In cadaver studies, Cain found that experimental tightening of the infraspinatus and teres minor muscle resulted in reduced anterior humeral translation.[27]

Figure 1–15 and Figure 1–16 illustrate the primary rotator cuff muscles and attachments at the GH joint. The specific functions of the muscles are reviewed in the following chapter. The subscapularis attaches along the anterior capsule into the lesser tuberosity. The supraspinatus, infraspinatus, and teres minor muscles attach along

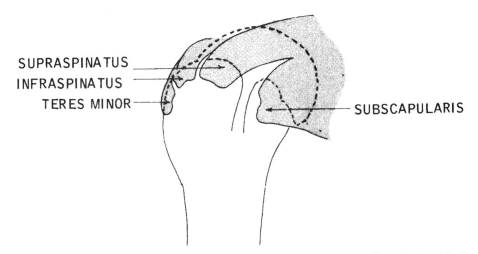

FIGURE 1–15. The attachment sites of the rotator cuff muscles. (From Calliet, R: Shoulder Pain, ed 3. FA Davis, Philadelphia, 1991, p 24, with permission.)

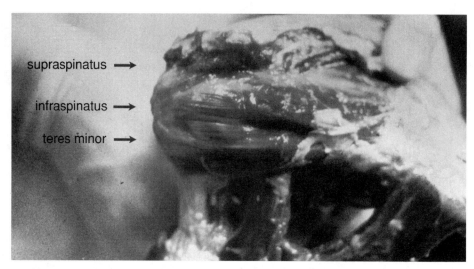

supraspinatus →

infraspinatus →

teres minor →

FIGURE 1–16. Fresh cadaver section of the posterior aspect of the GH joint and showing the posterior rotator cuff muscles including the supraspinatus, infraspinatus, and teres minor muscles.

the superior and posterior humeral head onto the facets of the greater tuberosity. Ligaments and muscles on both sides of the glenohumeral joint provide static and dynamic stability so that shoulder stability can be thought of as a dynamic circle concept.[28] The circle concept indicates that structures on all sides of the joint provide either primary or secondary restraint of humeral head movement in any one direction. For example, for a shoulder to dislocate anteriorly, both the anterior and posterior structures must be damaged; that is, the anterior capsule is the primary restraint to anterior dislocation, and the posterior capsule is the secondary restraint.

Tightening or active contraction of the rotator cuff muscles has the additional effects of centering the humeral head in the glenoid and providing increased joint compression during elevation of the limb.[29,30] Poppen and Walker[31] found that the movement of instantaneous axis of rotation of the humeral head was limited to approximately 3 mm in a superior direction along the glenoid during active shoulder elevation. This limited arthrokinematic motion was controlled by the contraction of the rotator cuff muscles to offset the strong elevatory contraction of the deltoid muscles. Saha[17] appropriately refers to the rotator cuff muscles as *steerers* of the humeral head. Interestingly, Poppen and Walker found increased superior humeral head translation greater than the normal 3 mm in patients with rotator cuff disease. An in-depth review of both the kinematics and kinetics of the GH joint is presented in Chapter 2.

Biceps Brachii Mechanism

The long head of the biceps runs superiorly from the anterior shaft of the humerus through the bicipital groove between the greater and lesser tuberosities to attach to the supraglenoid tubercle above the glenoid fossa, and blend in the superior labrum.[6,11] The tendon exits the joint capsule but, within, the capsule remains extrasynovial. However, a synovial sheath and a transverse bicipital ligament along its course within the bicipital groove cover the tendon (Fig. 1–17). The ligament adds additional support to the rotator cuff muscles to stabilize the GH joint.[32] This is particularly evident during the cocking phase of baseball pitching, when the biceps tendon concentrically contracts to compress the humeral head inferiorly within the glenoid.[33] The attachment of the biceps tendon to the labrum can result in a traction

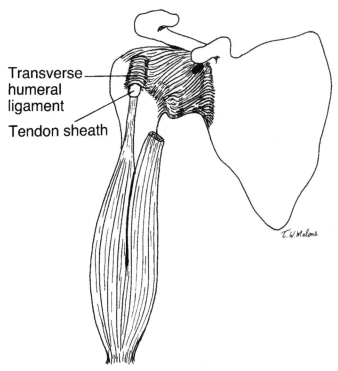

Transverse humeral ligament

Tendon sheath

FIGURE 1–17. The long head of the biceps brachii passes through a fibro-osseous tunnel formed by the bicipital groove and the transverse-humeral ligament. It is produced within the tunnel by a tendon sheath. (From Norkin, CC, and Levangie, PK: Joint Structure and Function: A Comprehensive Analysis, ed 2. FA Davis, Philadelphia, 1992, p 228, with permission.)

injury during repetitive overhead throwing with a tendonitis and labrum tear, known as a S.L.A.P. (superior labrum anterior and posterior) tear.[34]

ARTICULAR NEUROLOGY

The innervation of the GH joint is derived from spinal nerves C5 and C6, with a minor contribution from C4.[6] The AC joint has an isolated innervation from C4. The peripheral nerves supplying the glenohumeral capsule, ligaments, synovial membrane, and rotator cuff tendons are the axillary, suprascapular, subscapular, and musculocutaneous.

Afferent receptors from these nerves are listed in Table 1–3. The Ruffini endings and Golgi tendon organs are slowly adapting receptors and contribute primarily to position sense and awareness.[6] The Pacinian corpuscles are rapidly adapting receptors that sense sudden motion and contribute to awareness of joint motion (kinesthesia). Stimulation can cause muscle contraction (protective reflex) of the rotator cuff muscles, which are assisted by various afferent muscle spindles.[26] The protective reflex modulating protective reflexes at the shoulder is considered polysynaptic.[26] Strong evidence exists that illustrates the importance of these joint receptors to provide stability and position sense to the shoulder. Smith and Brunolli found kinesthetic deficits in patients with anterior shoulder dislocations when compared with healthy-matched subjects.[35]

TABLE 1–3 Joint Receptor

Type	Action	Function
Ruffini endings	Numerous in superficial joints Slow adaptation Low threshold stimulation	Provides joint position sense
Pacinian corpuscles	Numerous in deep capsule Rapid adaptation Low threshold to stimulation	Provides information concerning rapid change in motion Adjusts muscle tone
Golgi end organs	Intrinsic and extrinsic ligaments Slow adaptation High threshold to stimulation	Produces reflex effect on muscle tone
Free nerve endings	Location in most tissues No adaptation High threshold for stimulation	Produces tonic muscle contraction

VASCULAR SUPPLY

The vascular supply to the rotator cuff comes from the posterior humeral circumflex and the suprascapular arteries.[36] These arteries principally supply the infraspinatus and teres minor muscle areas of the tendinous cuff. The anterior aspect of the glenohumeral capsule is supplied by the anterior humeral circumflex artery and the thoracoacromial, suprahumeral, and subscapularis arteries. Superiorly, the thoracoacromial artery supplies the supraspinature. Of clinical importance, the supraspinatus tendon has an area of low vascularity approximately 1 cm proximal to its humeral insertion on the greater tuberosity.[36] Codman[37] referred to this area as the *critical zone* in the rotator cuff, because of the high incidence of degeneration. Rothman and Parke[36] found that this area of vascularity decreased with age. Rathbun and McNab noted that the critical zone of the rotator cuff had an adequate blood supply when the vessels were injected with the arm in the abducted position. However, this area was hypovascular when the injection was given with the arm in the adducted position.[38] The authors hypothesize that an area of transient hypovascularity occurs in the critical zone as a result of vessels being stretched across the humeral head when the upper extremity is fully adducted. This phenomenon is known as the "wringing-out" effect of the rotator cuff tendon blood vessels.[37]

CORACOACROMIAL ARCH

Figure 1–18 illustrates the coracoacromial arch. The arch, also known as the supraspinatus outlet, forms the roof for the underlying subacromial tissues including the rotator cuff tendon, subacromial bursa, and long head of the biceps brachii.[39] The tough and sharp-edged coracoacromial ligament encloses the arch. The ligament is thought to help prevent superior traumatic dislocation of the humeral head.[6]

The coracoacromial arch is a significant site for potential dysfunction and injury. The arch space enclosing the subacromial tissues is normally, approximately 9 to 10 mm.[40] This small space allows the subacromial tissues to glide freely during humeral elevation, but leaves very little margin of error for free gliding. In fact, some low-level impingement of these tissues invariably occurs during humeral elevation.[39] During dysfunction, such as rotator cuff muscle weakness, the subacromial impingement force increases, resulting in mechanical impingement syndrome and inflammation of

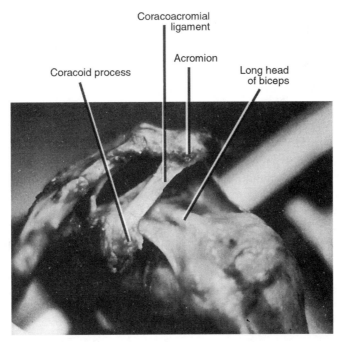

Coracoacromial ligament

Acromion

Coracoid process

Long head of biceps

FIGURE 1–18. Fresh cadaver view of the coracohumeral arch. Note the coracohumeral ligament and the long head of the biceps tendon.

these tissues. In some cases, the shape of the anterior acromion is slightly hooked or curved. This results in a less inherent subacromial space, predisposing to impingement syndrome in the presence of overuse injury.[41]

SUMMARY OF FACTORS THAT RELATE TO GLENOHUMERAL JOINT STABILITY

The factors that influence the normally tenuous stability of the GH joint are listed in Table 1–4. These factors are delineated dynamic or static stabilizers. The physical therapist's identification of the dynamic factors amenable to rehabilitation guides decision making.

Dynamic stabilizers include rotator cuff muscle strength, parascapular muscle strength, and proprioception. Static factors include the shape and size of the articulating surface, soft tissue configurations including the labrum, the presence and status of the middle glenohumeral ligament, the size of the rotator cuff interval, or the

TABLE 1–4 Factors Affecting Glenohumeral Joint Stability

Stability Factors	Type of Stabilizer
Adequate glenoid size	Static stabilizer
Posterior tilt glenoid and humeral head	Static stabilizer
Intact capsule and labrum	Static stabilizer
Axioscapular muscle control and balance (See Chap. 2)	Dynamic stabilizer
Rotator cuff muscle control and balance (See Chap. 2)	Dynamic stabilizer
Intact proprioception and neuromuscular control	Dynamic stabilizer

laxity of the IGHLC. These factors are beyond the control of the rehabilitation specialist. When shoulder symptoms are present, if one or more static factors is compromised and not accessible to rehabilitation, then additional medical and/or surgical management is necessary.

STRUCTURAL RELATIONSHIPS AND INTERDEPENDENCE OF UPPER QUARTER FUNCTION

Any discussion of shoulder anatomy should include a review of some of the structures in the upper one-quarter of the body because of the close relationship in function between many of these structures (Box 1–1). Many conditions affecting the shoulder can originate in other tissue and structures within the upper quarter. For example, postural changes with muscle imbalances can result in aberrant movement patterns affecting normal scapulohumeral rhythm (see Chap. 2) subsequently leading to subacromial impingement and tissue pathology. (See Chap. 9.) Referred pain from tissues that share the same segmental spinal innervation as the shoulder must be ruled out. (See Chap. 10.) Clearly, a thorough clinical evaluation for shoulder pain and impairments should include a screening assessment of related structures and knowledge of upper quarter structure and function. (See Chap. 5.)

Functional Anatomy

The information that follows is extrapolated from Donatelli and Wooden.[42] The upper quarter includes the occiput, the cervical spine, the shoulder girdle, the upper extremities, associated soft tissues, and related nerves and blood vessels.

The shoulder girdle is attached to the axial skeleton by the SC joint. Numerous soft tissue and muscular attachments join the occiput, mandible, cervical spine, and shoulder girdle. The superficial and deep fibers of the cervical fascia join the superior nuchal line of the occipital bone, the mastoid process, and the base of the mandible above to the acromion, clavicle, and manubrium sterni below. Muscles partly responsible for scapular movement, namely the upper fibers of the trapezius and the levator scapulae, connect the occiput and cervical spine to the superior lateral and superior medial borders of the scapula, respectively. Anteriorly, the sternocleidomastoid muscle attaches from the mastoid process of the cranium to the sternum and clavicle (Fig. 1–19).

BOX 1–1 HABITUAL CERVICAL MOTION

An excellent illustration of the interdependency of function in the upper quarter is observed during limb elevation. Unilateral limb elevation produces side-bending of the upper thoracic and mid-cervical spines to the ipsilateral side and counter rotation of the atlanto-axial joint to the contralateral side. Bilateral limb elevation results in flexion of the upper thoracic spine, extension of the mid-cervical spine and the atlanto-occipital joint.[46] These coupled movements were termed habitual cervical motion, in an article by Lee[47] and illustrate the importance for normal mobility and soft tissue function in the upper quarter to allow full overhead shoulder motion.

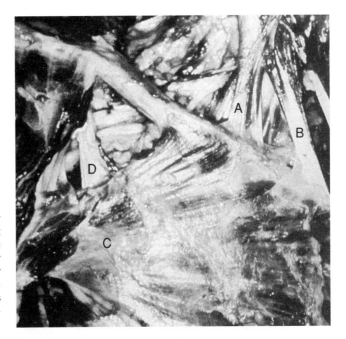

FIGURE 1–19. Fresh cadaver section showing the multiple soft tissue attachments around the thoracic outlet area of the upper quarter of the body. *(A)* Anterior scalene muscle. *(B)* Sternocleido-mastoid muscle. *(C)* Pectoralis major muscle. *(D)* Pectoralis minor muscle.

Multiple soft tissue connections are present between the cranium, mandible, hyoid bone, cervical spine, and shoulder girdle.[43] The temporalis and masseter muscles join the cranium and the mandible. The mandible is joined to the hyoid bone by the suprahyoid muscles, including the digastric, stylohyoid, mylohyoid, and geniohyoid. The infrahyoid muscles connect the hyoid bone to the shoulder girdle, and indirectly, through soft tissue connections to the cervical spine. These muscles include the sternohyoid, sternothyroid, thyrohyoid, and omohyoid. Specifically, the hyoid bone is joined to the scapula by the omohyoid muscle and to the sternum and clavicle by the sternohyoid muscle[44] (Fig. 1–20).

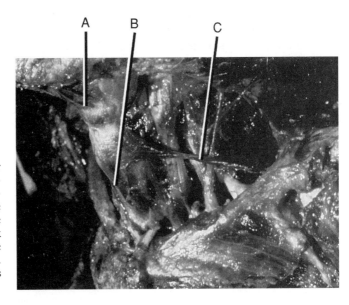

FIGURE 1–20. Fresh cadaver dissection showing the *(A)* su-prahyoid muscle; *(B)* infrahyoid muscles; *(C)* course of the omohyoid muscle along the posterior triangle of the neck from the hyoid bone to the superior border of the scapula. Note that the scalene muscles have been removed.

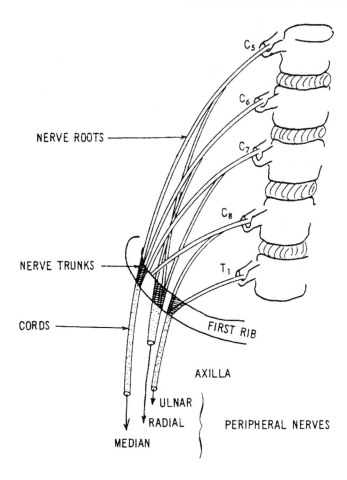

NERVE ROOTS

NERVE TRUNKS

CORDS

FIRST RIB

AXILLA

ULNAR
RADIAL   PERIPHERAL NERVES
MEDIAN

FIGURE 1–21. The Brachial plexus. The brachial plexus is composed of the anterior primary rami of segments C5 through TA. The roots emerge from the vertebral foramina through the scalene muscles. The roots merge into the trunks in the region of the first rib. The trunks via divisions become cords that divide into perpendicular nerves of the upper extremities. (From Calliet, R: Shoulder Pain, ed 3. FA Davis, Philadelphia, 1991, p 170, with permission.)

Brachial Plexus

The brachial plexus (Fig. 1–21) is derived from the anterior primary rami of C4 through T1 and supplies the innervation to the tissues and structures in the upper limb, including the shoulder.[6] The proximal part of the brachial plexus passes through the anterior and medial scalene muscles, the middle portion between the clavicle and first ribs, and the distal portion passed under the pectoralis minor tendon attachment at the coracoid process (Fig. 1–19). The plexus gives rise to the peripheral nerves that innervate the shoulder, including the scapula. Specific nerves such as the dorsal scapula nerve, the supraspinatus nerve, and the axillary nerve, are highly prone to soft tissue impingement or traction injury, particularly in the presence of trauma of postural changes.[45] Some of these conditions are presented in Chapter 10.

CHAPTER SUMMARY

The study of anatomy of the shoulder presented in this chapter includes all the relevant joints, soft tissue, and neural structures to provide a foundation for understanding the kinesiology discussed in Chapter 2 and the clinical information presented in the remainder of the text. The microanatomy and histology of certain tissues, such as the labrum, are gaining clinical importance related to potential pathology and healing/surgical factors. However, this information is not presented. That is not to diminish the importance of such information; this information was determined to be beyond the scope of this chapter. Readers are encouraged to read other sources that present this information.[48] The separation of the anatomy with the subsequent information of kinesiology was done purposefully to add refinement and scope to both chapters and a logical progression for understanding the relationship between structure and function.

The shoulder presents an anatomically complex series of joints that challenges the rehabilitation specialist to understand the individual components and to integrate overall structure and function. The approach to the study of anatomy and function of the shoulder is presented to coincide with the manner of evaluation and treatment, that is, from specific to a general consideration and analysis. An additional appreciation of the interrelationship of upper quarter structure and function of the shoulder provides the background and functional foundation for Chapter 10, "Referred Pain Syndromes of the Shoulder," and is requisite for a thorough evaluation of shoulder conditions.

REFERENCES

1. Guide to Physical Therapist Practice: Phys Ther 77:11, 1997.
2. Moseley, JB, et al: EMG analysis of the scapular muscles during a shoulder rehabilitation program. Am J Sport Med 20:128, 1992.
3. Jobe, FW, and Pink, M: Classification and treatment of shoulder dysfunction in the overhead athlete. J Orthop Sports Phys Ther 18:427, 1993.
4. Dempster, WT: Mechanisms of shoulder movement. Arch Phys Med Rehab 146A:49, 1965.
5. Steindler, A: Kinesiology of Human Body Under Normal and Pathological Conditions. Charles C. Thomas, Springfield, Ill., 1955.
6. Warwick, R, and Williams, P (eds): Gray's Anatomy, ed 35. WB Saunders, Philadelphia, 1973.
7. Calliet, R: Shoulder Pain, ed 3. FA Davis, Philadelphia, 1991.
8. Culham, E, and Peat, M: Functional anatomy of the shoulder complex. J Orthop Sport Phys Ther 18:342, 1993.
9. Johnston, TB: Movements of the shoulder joint: "plea for use of plane of the scapula" as plane of reference for movements occurring at humeroscapula joint. Br J Surg 25:252, 1937.
10. Kondo, M, et al: Changes of the tilting angle of the scapula following elevation of the arm. In Gateman, JE, and Welsh, RP (eds): Surgery of the Shoulder, CV Mosby, Philadelphia, 1984.
11. Norkin, CC, and Levangie, PK: Joint Structure and Function: A Comprehensive Analysis, ed 2. FA Davis, Philadelphia, 1992.
12. Wadsworth, W: Manual Examination and Treatment of the Spine and Extremities. Williams and Wilkins, Baltimore, 1988.
13. Saha, AK: Mechanics of elevation of glenohumeral joint. Acta Scand 44:6688, 1973.
14. Inman, VT, et al: Observations of the function of the shoulder joint. J Bone Joint Surg 726:1, 1944.
15. Sadr, B, and Swann, M: Spontaneous dislocation of the sterno-clavicular joint. Acta Orthop Scand 50:269, 1979.
16. Petersson, CJ: Degeneration of the acromio-clavicular joint. Acta Orthop Scand 54:434, 1983.
17. Saha, AK: Dynamic stability of the glenohumeral joint. Acta Orthop Scand 42:491, 1971.
18. Moseley, HP, and Overgaard, B: The anterior capsular mechanism in recurrent anterior dislocations of the shoulder: morphological and clinical studies with special reference to the glenoid labrum and glenohumeral ligaments. J Bone Joint Surg 44B:913, 1962.
19. Kummell, BM: Spectrum of lesions of the anterior capsular mechanism of the shoulder. A J Sports Med 7:111, 1979.
20. Nobuhara, K, and Ikeda, H: Rotator interval lesion. Clin Orthop 223:44, 1987.
21. Harryman, DT, et al: The role of rotator interval capsule in passive motion and stability of the shoulder. J Bone Joint Surg 74A:53, 1992.
22. Turke, SJ, et al: Stabilizing mechanism preventing anterior dislocation of the glenohumeral joint. J Bone Joint Surg 63A:1208, 1981.

23. Warner, JJ, et al: Static capsuloligamentous restraints to superior–inferior translation of the glenohumeral joint. Am J Sports Med 20:675, 1992.
24. O'Brien, SJ, et al: The anatomy and histology of the inferior glenohumeral ligament complex of the shoulder. Am J Sports Med 18:449, 1993.
25. Ferrari, DA: Capsular ligament of the shoulder: anatomical and functional study of the anterior superior capsule. Am J Sports Med 18:20, 1990.
26. Guanche, et al: The synergistic action of the capsule and the shoulder muscles. Am J Sports Med 23, 1995.
27. Hawkins, RJ, et al: The assessment of glenohumeral translation using manual and fluoroscopic techniques. Orthop Trans 12:727, 1988.
28. Cain, PR, et al: Anterior stability of the glenohumeral joint: A dynamic model. Am J Sports Med 15:144, 1987.
29. Himeno, S, and Tsumura, H: The role of the rotator cuff as a stabilizing mechanism of the shoulder. In Bateman, S, Welch, P (eds): Surgery of the Shoulder. CV Mosby, St. Louis, 1984.
30. Sharkey, NA, and Marder, RA: The rotator cuff opposes superior translation of the humeral head. Am J Sports Med 23:270, 1995.
31. Poppen, NK, and Walker, PS: Normal and abnormal motion of the shoulder. J Bone Joint Surg 58A:195, 1976.
32. Rodosky, MW, et al: The role of the long head of the biceps muscle and superior glenoid labrum in anterior stability of the shoulder. Am J Sports Med 22:121, 1994.
33. Jobe, FW, et al: An EMG analysis of the shoulder in throwing and pitching: a preliminary report. Am J Sports Med 11:3, 1983.
34. Andrews, JR, et al: Glenoid labrum tears related to the long head of the biceps. Am J Sports Med 13:337, 1985.
35. Smith, RL, and Brunolli, BS: Shoulder kinesthesia after anterior glenohumeral joint dislocation. J Orthop Sports Phys Ther 11:11, 1990.
36. Rothman, RH, and Parke, WW: The vascular anatomy of the rotator cuff. Clin Orthop 41:1965.
37. Codman, EA: The Shoulder. Thomas Dodd, Boston, 1934.
38. Rathbun, JB, and MacNab, I: The microvascular pattern of the rotator cuff. J Bone Joint Surg 52B: 540, 1970.
39. Petersson, CJ, and Redland-Johnell, I: The subacromial space in normal shoulder radiographs. Acta Orthop Scand 55:57, 1984.
40. Flatow, EL, et al: Excursions of the rotator cuff under the acromion: patterns of subacromial contact. Am J Sports Med 22: 779, 1994.
41. Morrison, DS, and Bigliani, LU: The clinical significance of variations in acromial morphology. Orthop Trans 11:234, 1987.
42. Greenfield, BH: Upper Quarter evaluation: Structural relationships and interdependence. In Donatelli, R, and Wooden, M (eds) : Orthopedic Physical Therapy, ed 2. Churchill Livingstone, New York, 1994.
43. Brodie, AG: Anatomy and physiology of head and neck musculature. Am J Orthod 36: 831, 1950.
44. Rocabado, M: Biomechanical relationship of the cranial, cervical, and hyoid regions. J Craniomandib Pract 11: 3, 1983.
45. Kopell, HP, and Thompson WAL: Peripheral Entrapment Neuropathies, ed 2. Robert E Kreiger, NY, 1976.
46. Kanpandji, IA: The Physiology of Joints, ed 2, Vol 3. Churchill Livingstone, NY, 1974.
47. Lee, D: Tennis elbow: A manual therapist's perspective. J Orthop Sport Phys Ther 8:3, 1986.
48. Prodromos, CC, et al: Histological studies of the glenoid labrum from fetal life to old age. J Bone Joint Surg 72A: 1344, 1990.

CHAPTER 2

Kinesiology of the Shoulder

Thomas Abelew, PhD

INTRODUCTION

The shoulder is a complex joint consisting of multiple bones (humerus, scapula, clavicle) connected at multiple joints (glenohumeral, acromioclavicular, sternoclavicular, and scapulothoracic). Whereas each individual joint has its own unique mechanical properties resulting in varying degrees of movement and different load-bearing capabilities, it is the combined interaction that results in the normal function of the complex referred to as the shoulder. Because of the closed mechanical system formed by the components of the shoulder "girdle," proper function of all components is required before normal upper extremity motion can be achieved.

KINEMATICS

Normal qualitative kinematics (that is, descriptions of limb displacements) of the shoulder can be understood by beginning with the traditional view of the system as a closed kinematic chain. In such a system, movement of one of the "links" must be followed by movement of each of the other links in the system. Applied to the shoulder, this phenomenon has been referred to as *scapulohumeral* rhythm, where humeral motion occurs with simultaneous scapular and clavicular motion. Thus, "simple" humeral elevation in any direction involves all joints of the shoulder complex. Therefore, dysfunction with one impairs motion of the entire complex. Multiple degrees of freedom exist in the linkage, resulting in a highly mobile joint complex that allows for a virtually unlimited number of upper limb movements.[1]

Shoulder Complex Kinematics

Traditionally, shoulder kinematics have been described from anatomical position using a right-handed Cartesian coordinate system (Fig. 2–1). The basic shoulder

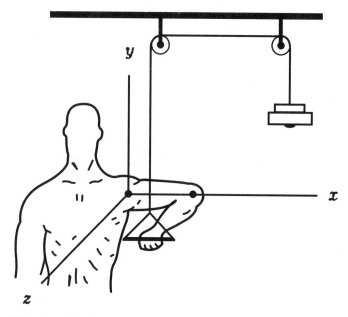

FIGURE 2–1. Right handed Cartesian coordinate system with the origin at the glenohumeral joint center. Positive rotations established using the right hand rule. With the right hand, place the thumb pointing in the direction of the axis of interest. Curl the fingers into a fist. The direction in which the fingers move is positive rotation about that axis. (From Ozkaya, N, and Nordin, M: Fundamentals of Biomechanics: Equilibrium, Motion and Deformation. Van Nostrand Reinhold, New York, 1991, with permission.)

movements described from anatomical position are summarized in Table 2–1. These movements are classified as rotations in each of the mutually orthogonal anatomical planes of motion. Rotations about the x axis (a horizontal axis) correspond to sagittal plane movements (flexion-extension-hyperextension); y axis (vertical) rotations correspond to transverse plane movements (axial rotation and horizontal abduction-adduction); and z axis (anterior-posterior axis) rotations correspond to frontal plane movements (abduction-adduction). Circumduction, also possible, is a combination of rotations about the x, y, and sometimes z axes. This planar description of motion, while helpful to visualize many of the basic motions, is an oversimplification, and may be of limited clinical use because few natural movements occur exclusively in these planes.[1,2,3]

Ranges of motion among individuals will vary with limb position and measurement methodologies. Typical values for active shoulder ranges of motion from anatomical position are summarized in Table 2–2.

TABLE 2–1 Shoulder Complex Motions

Coordinate Axis	Positive Rotation	Negative Rotation
x axis rotation	Extension Hyperextension	Flexion
z axis rotation	Abduction	Adduction
y axis rotation	Lateral axial rotation, horizontal abduction*	Medial axial rotation, horizontal adduction*

*Vertical axis rotation with shoulder abducted 90°

TABLE 2–2 Average Active Shoulder Range of Motion

Movement	Range (Degrees)
Flexion	160-180
Hyperextension	50-60
Abduction	170-180
Medial Rotation	60-100
Lateral Rotation	80-90
Horizontal Adduction #*+	130
Horizontal Abduction #*+	45

also referred to as horizontal flexion
* also referred to as horizontal extension
+ movement is initiated from 90° of abduction
(From Magee, DJ: Orthopedic Physical Assessment. WB Saunders, Philadelphia, 1987.)

Segmental Kinematics

SCAPULA

The scapula, which is partially responsible for maintaining the connection between the humerus and the thorax, serves as the site of attachment of numerous muscles. Normal scapular motion, critical for normal shoulder function, requires simultaneous movement at the scapulothoracic (ST), sternoclavicular (SC), and acromioclavicular (AC) joints.

Scapular motion consists of two translations and three rotations. (See Fig. 2–2A.) Vertical translation superiorly (elevation) and inferiorly (depression) occur along with medial and lateral translation, commonly known as retraction (adduction) and protraction (abduction), respectively. The rotational motion with the greatest range occurs around an axis of rotation projecting anteriorly and posteriorly through the body of the scapula. (The location of the axis of rotation varies throughout shoulder movement and will be discussed later.) Displacement of the inferior angle of the scapula laterally and superiorly is described as upward rotation, whereas the reverse motion is downward rotation. The normal range of scapular rotation is 60°, whereas ranges of elevation-depression and protraction-retraction have not been reported.[4,5,6]

The two remaining rotational motions of the scapula are winging and tipping.[7,5] (Winging is used to refer to a pathological condition involving excessive rotation about a vertical axis of rotation, although some rotation in this plane is considered normal and essential to proper shoulder motion.) Both of these motions, resulting from the geometry of the scapula and thorax, will occur in conjunction with elevation-depression, protraction-retraction, and upward-downward rotation as the scapula maintains its connection to the thorax. Winging is a rotation of the scapula about a vertical axis of rotation that pierces the AC joint. Tipping is a rotation about a horizontal (medial to lateral) axis of rotation that extends through the AC joint. Normal ranges of winging and tipping during humeral elevation have been reported as 40° and 20°, respectively.[5]

CLAVICLE

The clavicle connects the scapula to the sternum and has three rotational degrees of freedom due to the combined movement at the AC and SC joints (Fig. 2–2B). Protraction, anterior movement of the acromial end of the clavicle, and retraction,

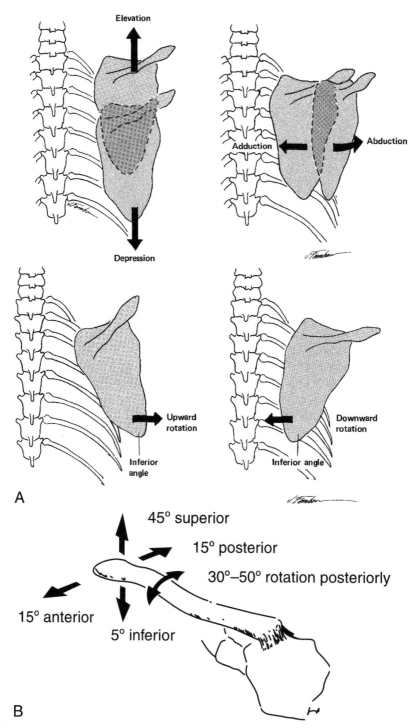

FIGURE 2–2. *(A)* Scapular motions occurring at the scapulothoracic and acromioclavicular joints (From Norkin, CC, and Levangie, PK: Joint Structure and Function. A Comprehensive Approach. FA Davis, Philadelphia, 1992, with permission.) *(B)* Clavicular motions occurring at the sternocla-vicular and acromioclavicular joints (From Soderberg, GL: Kinesiology. Application to pathological motion. Williams and Wilkins, Baltimore, 1997.)

posterior motion of the acromial end, occur around a vertical axis of rotation through the costoclavicular ligament. Anterior and posterior axial rotation occur about a longitudinal axis of rotation extending laterally along the long axis of the clavicle and projecting through the AC and SC joints. With anterior rotation, the superior surface of the clavicle rotates to face anteriorly. Posterior rotation is the reverse motion. Elevation and depression occur around an axis with an anterior-posterior orientation. Superior movement of the acromial end of the clavicle is called elevation, whereas inferior movement is clavicular depression. Figure 2–2B illustrates the motions of the clavicle and the generally accepted range of motion.[8]

MOTION COUPLING BETWEEN SCAPULA AND CLAVICLE

Because of the mechanical connections that exist between the clavicle and scapula, all movements of one bone will be coupled to movements of the other. Elevation and depression of the clavicle, for example, must be coupled to elevation and depression of the scapula, respectively. Scapular upward rotation will also occur during clavicular elevation. Protraction of the clavicle is coupled to scapular protraction and some winging, whereas clavicular retraction is coupled to scapular retraction. The function of this shoulder "girdle" allows the opposing needs of stability and mobility to be met and, in turn, allows for normal shoulder complex motion.[4,6]

Whereas the shoulder complex has been described as a closed chain, Dvir and Berme[4] suggested an alternative view. The complex as a whole can be viewed as an open chain if one considers a free distal endpoint (that is, the hand). The interdependence of motion is seen, however, when the relationship between the scapula and clavicle is examined. These bones are mechanically coupled and cannot move independently. Dvir and Berme,[4] therefore, classified the shoulder complex as a combination of both a closed chain mechanism (scapula, clavicle, and thorax) and an open chain mechanism (scapula and humerus) working together to achieve normal upper limb motion. The concept of the "continuous controlled skid bed," introduced by Dvir and Berme,[4] refers to the interaction between the glenoid fossa and humeral head. The glenoid surface serves as a "skid bed" that, while it moves, allows the humeral head to roll and translate on its articular surface. The moving "bed" allows the required changes in articular geometry to help maintain a more optimum muscle length and velocity necessary for full range of motion, while simultaneously maintaining glenohumeral (GH) joint surface congruency. Through this mechanism, both requirements of mobility and stability of the shoulder complex can be achieved.

HUMERUS

The humerus is the primary segment in the shoulder complex because upper limb motion is defined by the humeral connections to the forearm and hand. The humerus also has the largest range of motion when compared to that of the scapula and clavicle. Humeral kinematics are centered on the area where the GH joint connects the humerus to the scapula (Fig. 2–1). The movements of the humerus at the GH joint are *qualitatively* the same as those defined as shoulder complex movements (that is, flexion-extension, abduction-adduction, and axial rotation medially and laterally) However, the range of humeral motion is considerably less when the AC, SC, and ST joints are constrained.[5]

SCAPULOHUMERAL RHYTHM

During elevation of the humerus (for example, frontal plane abduction), a pattern of scapular upward rotation with concurrent clavicular elevation and axial rotation are consistently observed.[7,4,6] In the initial phases of humeral flexion or abduction, little to no scapular or clavicular motion occurs. At approximately 20° of humeral elevation, however, upward rotation of the scapula with concurrent clavicular elevation begins.[6] At approximately 90° of humeral elevation, clavicular elevation stops due to tension in the costoclavicular ligament.[5] Continued elevation of the humerus requires continued upward rotation of the scapula, which has rotated through a range of approximately 30° (for humeral elevation to 90°). The axis of rotation for the scapular rotation is located at the base of the scapular spine and extends anteriorly through the SC joint.[4]

For additional scapular motion to take place, posterior axial rotation of the clavicle must occur. The trapezius and serratus anterior muscles will continue to generate forces that tend to upwardly rotate the scapula. These muscular forces applied to the scapula are transferred to the clavicle through the coracoclavicular ligaments. As a result, the clavicle rotates posteriorly to allow the scapula to continue to rotate upward another 30°.[5] A resultant shift in the location of the axis for scapular upward rotation from the base of the scapular spine to the AC joint occurs.[4] The range of clavicular elevation is approximately 30°-36° and the posterior rotation is approximately 30°-40°.[6]

This quantitative kinematic relationship between the humerus and scapula varies throughout the normal range of humeral elevation and is dependent on shoulder load and the level of fatigue.[9,10] The average ratio for humeral elevation to scapular upward rotation across the entire range of elevation has been reported as 2:1.[5,3,8] Freedman and Monro[11] found that although the relationship between the humerus and scapula was linearly related, the ratio of humeral to scapular motion was 3:2. Poppen and Walker[7] suggested that the ratio was not linear, finding that during the initial phases of abduction (up to 30°) the humerus to scapula ratio was 4.3:1, after which it dropped to 1.25:1. Investigations examining the scapulohumeral relationship have employed different methodologies and different subject populations. Different ranges of motion, different movements (passive or active), different methods for calculation of the scapulohumeral ratios, and the use of live subjects as opposed to cadavers may all have influenced the results.

Most of the studies performed have suggested that the scapular contribution to shoulder elevation increased with the increasing elevation angle (that is, decreasing the ratio). McQuade and Smith[9] measured scapulohumeral rhythm using a magnetic tracking device in human subjects performing scapular plane elevation. Comparing passive humeral elevation, elevation under light loads, and elevation under heavy loads, tests indicated that scapulohumeral rhythm was nonlinear and varied with activity, load, and the degree of humeral elevation. During passive conditions, for example, the contribution of the scapula increased with increasing humeral elevation. In both loaded conditions, however, the scapular contribution decreased as the humeral angle increased. This finding is consistent with data reported by Doody et al.[12] Studying 25 women, Doody et al.[12] found that scapulohumeral rhythm was nonlinear and varied significantly between individual subjects. The scapular contribution to humeral elevation was observed to peak between 90° and 140° and then decrease as the humerus was elevated beyond 140°. Under loaded conditions, the scapular contribution began earlier and decreased in overall magnitude.

Whereas variations in the magnitude of scapulohumeral rhythm have been reported, it is likely that the relationship between scapular and humeral motion is not constant throughout the full range of humeral elevation.[4,7,11,12] Therefore, from a clinical standpoint, closely considering the plane of motion, the activity level (active or passive), and the load applied to the upper limb are important when assessing the status of scapulohumeral rhythm in a patient.

ARTHROKINEMATICS

Segmental motions of the scapula, clavicle, and humerus occur as a result of a specific joint structure that includes the bony configuration of the articular surfaces and the ligamentous and capsular restraints. Patterns of motion of the articular surfaces have been described as *arthrokinematic* patterns.[5] In general, these motions are a combination of rolling, sliding (translation), and spinning. The degree to which each occurs is based on the articular anatomy (Fig. 2–3). These motions result in the

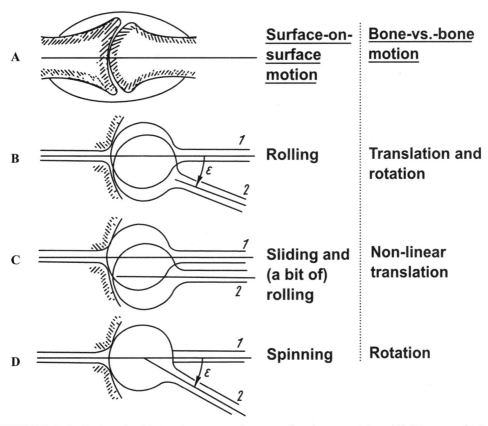

FIGURE 2–3. Basic arthrokinematic patterns that can take place at a joint. *(A)* Diagram of joint surfaces. *(B)* Rolling consisting of translation and rotation. *(C)* Primarily sliding (translational motion). *(D)* Spinning consisting of pure rotational motion. (From Zatsiorsky, VM: Kinematics of Human Motion. Human Kinetics, Champaign, 1998, with permission.)

segmental kinematic patterns that have been previously discussed and are referred to as *osteokinematics*.[5]

Sternoclavicular Joint

The arthrokinematics of the SC joint are heavily influenced by the presence of the articular disc as well as the costoclavicular ligament. The disc divides the SC joint into two distinct cavities with different movement potential.

During elevation-depression, upward movement of the lateral end of the clavicle results in a downward sliding and rolling of the medial end. The axis of rotation for elevation-depression is thought to be centered at the costoclavicular ligament and is generally considered to be oriented in an anterior-posterior direction.[5,13] However, some disagreement exists on this issue.[5,13,14] Norkin and Levangie[5] have suggested a different pattern of joint surface motion for clavicular protraction and retraction. Noting the concavity of the clavicular surface in the anterior-posterior direction, it has been suggested that the medial end of the clavicle slides and rolls in the same direction as the lateral end such that protraction of the clavicle results in anterior motion of its medial end.

Some conflicting views on the exact orientation and location of the axes of rotation for elevation-depression and protraction-retraction exists.[2,14] This inconsistency is likely a reflection of the investigators' difficulty in accurately tracking the movements of each bony segment. Differences in frame of reference may also play a significant role in divergent qualitative descriptions of axes of rotation. When describing an axis with an anterior-posterior orientation, for example, it must be specified whether this is relative to the whole body or to the clavicle.

Axial rotation of the clavicle occurs with a spinning of the medial end of the clavicle on the manubrial surface without any rolling or translational motion.

Acromioclavicular Joint

Similar to the SC joint, the AC joint allows varying degrees of sliding, rolling, and spinning that are quite significant though the range of motion is relatively small. The fibrocartilage disc allows additional movement that the bony surfaces alone would not allow. Considerable anatomical variability has been observed, resulting in arthrokinematic patterns that have yet to be clearly characterized.[5]

Glenohumeral Joint

Because of the shape and size of the humeral head in comparison to the glenoid fossa of the scapula, the bony fit at the GH joint is not symmetric. The humeral head, which has a different radius of curvature, is considerably larger than that of the glenoid fossa. The reported ratio of radii of curvature of the humeral head to glenoid fossa is approximately 0.89:1.09.[15] This measurement reflects a variation in shape between the two surfaces. The resulting lack of articular surface symmetry causes a decrease in the congruency of the surfaces.[15] The result during humeral elevation is a pattern of humeral rolling combined with translation relative to the glenoid fossa.

Numerous studies have been undertaken to quantify the arthrokinematics of the GH joint.[7,16,17] Typically, the motions are described as rolling and sliding (that is, translation) with the common pattern described as one involving initial superior rolling coupled with an inferior translation during humeral elevation.[5] Poppen and Walker[7] found small amounts of upward translation early in the range (less than 60°) during active scapular plane elevation. Average displacement of the humeral head relative to the glenoid fossa was typically less than 3 mm superiorly. Above 60°, average humeral head displacement in subjects without shoulder pathology was approximately 1 mm up or down for every 30° of elevation up to 150°. Several of the subjects with histories of dislocation, pain, or rotator cuff tear had displacements that were significantly greater.

Harryman et al.[17] examined humeral head translations during passive manipulation of cadaver shoulders. They found that translations were greatest during flexion and extension, averaging 4 to 5 mm anteriorly, during flexion, and posteriorly during extension. Translation occurred at joint angles beyond 55° during flexion and 35° during extension. The magnitude of the translations during all movements tested in this study (flexion, extension, axial rotation, and cross-body movements) was dramatically increased when the joint capsule was operatively tightened. Capsular venting with an 18 gauge needle resulted in slight increases in translational motion. The joint capsule and ligamentous structures and the intra-articular pressure of the GH joint, therefore, play a significant role in controlling translational motion of the humerus.

During active GH motions in the horizontal (transverse) plane, Howell et al.[16] showed that translational motion of the humeral head was small except at a position of maximum "extension" (actually horizontal abduction in their study) when combined with external rotation in the presence of documented anterior instability. In the extended and externally rotated position, a position similar to the cocking phase of throwing, the humeral head translated an average of 4 mm posteriorly.

In contrast to the findings of Howell et al.,[16] Wuelker et al.[18,19] developed a dynamic shoulder model consisting of hydrodynamic actuators simulating deltoid and individual rotator cuff muscle forces applied to a fresh cadaver upper limb *in vitro*. Their findings indicated that significant superior and anterior translation occurred during humeral elevation in the scapular plane. Average superior displacement across all subjects ranged from 4.4[18] to 9 mm,[19] whereas anterior displacement averaged 2.8 mm[18] and 4.6 mm[19] during humeral elevation from 20° to 90°. When muscle forces were reduced or the capsule was vented, translational displacement increased. The lack of known physiological muscle activity patterns in shoulder muscles, however, may partially explain the differences in humeral translation in the Wuelker et al.[19] studies, which speculated that variations in muscle activity *in vivo* might result in reduced humeral translation.

While the magnitude of translational motion is not consistent across investigations, the data are in agreement on several things. First, under normal physiological conditions, active elevation of the humerus results in less translational motion than with passive elevation of the humerus. Second, a decrease in the GH joint intra-articular pressure by venting the capsule resulted in increased humeral translation. Third, surgical tightening of portions of the capsule increased translation and/or changed the direction of the translation. Fourth, under passive manipulation of the relaxed shoulder, translational motion was extensive, suggesting that the musculature is critical for normal arthrokinematic motion. Speculation is that the presence of translation, or extensive translation, during active motions likely represents a pathological condition.[16,18]

KINETICS

Joint Reaction Forces

Newton's third law states that the forces of action and reaction between contacting surfaces are equal in magnitude, opposite in direction, and collinear. Articular surfaces, therefore, are subject to these contact forces, called *joint reaction forces*. Measurement of the forces transmitted to the joint surfaces of the shoulder complex is problematic. Multiple muscles crossing multiple joints makes estimating joint reaction forces quite difficult without making a significant number of simplifying assumptions.[20,21]

Whereas the shoulder is not considered a "weight bearing limb," substantial loads are necessary to move the upper limb against gravity. Relatively short muscle moment arms for shoulder muscles (on the order of 1 to 4 cm) must be used to balance or overcome moments produced by the much longer moment arm of gravity (25 to 40 cm) acting through the center of mass of an upper limb in 90° of shoulder flexion. Inman et al.[22] estimated the muscle forces required to hold the upper limb at 90° of abduction to be approximately 8.2 times that of the limb's weight. Using a similar analysis, Zuckerman and Matsen[21] estimated the GH joint reaction force to be approximately 0.5 times body weight while maintaining a position of 90° of shoulder abduction. Adding a mass of 2.5% body weight doubled the shoulder reaction force to equal body weight. This highlights the significant contribution that muscle forces can make to the overall load applied to a joint when counterbalancing the torques (moments) generated by external loads. (Although technically, moment and torque should not be used interchangeably; for most purposes these terms simply quantify the rotational load about an axis.)

To perform the analyses described previously, the authors had to assume that only one muscle acted at any one time and that this muscle was responsible for bearing the entire load. Although this is a significant oversimplification, this assumption enables one to approximate the loads that can be exerted on the upper limb and, hence, the shoulder. More elaborate models can result in estimations of load that are even higher.

Poppen and Walker[7] developed a model of the shoulder and calculated relative muscle forces under static conditions based on the cross sectional area of individual muscles and relative activation level as measured by electromyography (EMG). They reported static glenohumeral reaction forces that peaked at 0.89 times body weight at 90° during unloaded shoulder abduction and shearing forces as high as 42% body weight at 60° of shoulder abduction.

Using a detailed finite element model of the shoulder complex, Van Der Helm[23] reported three-dimensional joint reaction forces for GH, AC, SC, and ST joints. In a finite element analysis, the entire shoulder complex is modeled using component "elements," each with known mechanical characteristics. The elements are then linked into a comprehensive model that can be studied under experimental conditions.

At the GH joint, peak vertical forces exceeded 200 N during loaded abduction whereas compressive forces were approximately 500 N during loaded flexion. The load used in this simulation was 750 grams (7.5 N). Peak AC forces ranged from approximately 200 N in compression to 50 N in the vertical shear. Maximum SC loads were generally smaller than GH and AC, peaking around 75 N in anterior-posterior shear. Compression forces at the ST joint were also simulated and found to peak at approximately 90° of humeral elevation, reaching values of approximately 100 to 200 N.

These data clearly demonstrate the shoulder's potential for bearing significant loads during activities in which small loads are manipulated in the environment (that is, carrying or lifting objects). Clinical assessments, therefore, must consider the magnitude and orientation of the forces being exerted on the upper limb and the subsequent translation of those forces into shoulder loads.

Joint Moments

Although forces were considered in the previous section, examining kinetics of a joint must also include examining the moments or torques that are generated. The estimation of joint moments has been used to quantify the rotational requirements necessary to control the motion about a joint.[24,25] The term *joint moment* refers to the resultant, comprehensive effect, both active and passive, of all muscles, ligaments, and periarticular tissue acting around a joint during a particular movement condition.[26] Thus, a flexion moment calculated at the shoulder joint implies that the musculature generated a *net* flexion moment to counterbalance the extension moment resulting from all external forces and moments applied to that limb. Therefore, joint moments are a quantitative means for *estimating* the *net* muscular requirement at a joint.[27]

Joint moments are generated under all conditions of movement, whether the activity is isometric, concentric, or eccentric. Joint moments can be calculated under static and dynamic conditions and during specialized conditions such as isokinetic testing.

Joint moments for GH elevation and axial rotation are highly variable and dependent on the activity, the speed of the motion, position, age, and fitness level. Maximal joint moment data have been published for a variety of isometric and isokinetic conditions. Soderberg[8] published a detailed compilation of these data, with results being highly dependent on position of the upper limb and the angular velocity of the limb.

Interpretation of joint moment data must be done cautiously while keeping in mind precise measurement and movement conditions. Joint moments represent the resultant muscle moment at a given joint. In many circumstances, a good representation of the muscular response at a joint is provided. Care must be taken, however, when making inferences about individual muscle behavior based on joint moment calculations. For example, cocontracting musculature will confound the interpretation because the joint moment will represent *all muscle and ligamentous moment sources.* Cocontraction, therefore, may result in an underestimation of the moments produced by a muscle group, or individual muscle, because antagonistic musculature generating opposing moments will be included in the calculation. A 50 Nm (Newton meter) shoulder flexion moment, for example, does not suggest that the flexors are necessarily producing a moment of 50 Nm. Given the likelihood of some cocontraction, the flexor moment to be produced by the flexor muscles must be greater than 50 Nm to overcome any extensor moment from the cocontracting muscles.

MUSCLE FUNCTION

Muscles of the shoulder have been characterized and classified in several ways. Saha[6] grouped muscles into axioscapular, scapulohumeral, and axiohumeral groups. (See Chap. 1, Table 1–1.) Difficulty in directly recording force from any of the shoulder muscles, or their tendons, has resulted in a reliance on measures of muscle activity (EMG), on models that relate activity to architectural characteristics[20] or on more complicated models involving optimization and/or finite element analysis.[23] Table 2–3 summarizes the putative actions of the shoulder musculature. The data in this table were gathered from published works on shoulder muscle function.[5,13,28]

Muscle Synergy

The term *synergist* is perhaps one of the most highly variable terms used in kinesiology because what is included in this definition of "helping muscles" varies considerably from author to author. Enoka[29] defines synergy as "A group of muscles that are constrained to act as a unit for a specific task." Norkin and Levangie[5] refer to synergists as muscles that ". . . . help the agonist to perform a desired action. . .". Exact contributions of muscles that could be considered synergists for a particular movement are not clear during most tasks. Whereas Table 2–3 suggests some very straightforward functions for each muscle, most of these muscles have been shown to be active during some portion of many different shoulder movements.[20,28] Muscle

TABLE 2–3 Actions of Major Muscles of the Shoulder Complex

Humeral Movements		*Scapular Movements*	
Extension	**Flexion**	**Elevation**	**Depression**
Post. Deltoid	Ant. Deltoid	Levator Scapulae	Pectoralis Major
Latissimus Dorsi	Coracobrachialis	Rhomboids	Pectoralis Minor
Pect. Major	Pect Major	Trapezius (upper)	Trapezius (lower)
(sternal hd)	(clavicular hd)	Serratus Anterior	Serratus Anterior
Teres Major	Biceps Brachii	(upper)	(lower)
Triceps Brachii			
Abduction	**Adduction**	**Protraction**	**Retraction**
Supraspinatus	Latissimus Dorsi	Pectoralis Major	Rhomboids
Middle Deltoid	Teres Major	(clavicular hd)	Trapezius
	Post. Deltoid	Pectoralis Minor	
	Pectoralis Major	Serratus Anterior	
	(sternal hd)		
	Coracobrachialis		
M. Rotation	**L. Rotation**	**Up. Rotation**	**Dn. Rotation**
Ant. Deltoid	Post. Deltoid	Trapezius	Latissimus Dorsi
Latissimus Dorsi	Supraspinatus	(upper/lower)	Pectoralis Minor
Teres Major	Infraspinatus	Serratus Anterior	Rhomboids
Pectoralis Major	Teres Minor		Levator Scapulae
Subscapularis			

synergy has included a broad spectrum of intermuscular relationships often being described by a variety of terms.

Labels that have been used to describe these functional interactions are based on their proposed actions, such as agonist, prime mover, antagonist, synergist, stabilizer, and neutralizer. *Agonists* generally refer to muscles that share common functions. *Antagonists* are muscles that oppose each other, and *prime movers* are often considered the same as agonists, although the number of joints crossed by a particular agonist introduces the idea that the contribution of a muscle changes as limb position changes. This notion leads one to question whether all agonists are actually contributing equally to a given movement. *Stabilizers* are muscles considered to maintain the position of a bone to allow other muscles to act, whereas *neutralizers* are muscles thought to counter the unwanted action(s) of another muscle(s).

This terminology does not adequately reflect the dynamic relationship existing between muscles or groups of muscles. Muscles that are prime movers in one circumstance may contribute minimally as limb position changes. A muscle cannot simultaneously produce maximal force and full range of motion at all joints that it crosses. Active shortening of the muscle at one joint will limit any further active contribution to other joints that it crosses because of its instability to shorten any further. This phenomenon is referred to as *active insufficiency,* a common phenomenon in multi-articular muscles.[5]

A typical example of this behavior is the relationship between biceps brachii and the anterior deltoid during shoulder flexion. Independent of elbow and forearm position, the anterior deltoid contributes significantly to shoulder flexion. The biceps brachii, however, is sensitive to changes in elbow and radioulnar position. The length change of the biceps caused by the change in elbow and/or radioulnar joint angle reduces its ability to contribute to shoulder flexion. Therefore, a distinction must be made between agonists and prime movers based on limb position and the number of joints crossed by a muscle. One muscle (anterior deltoid in the previous example) will be the prime mover or, more accurately, the prime moment producer even though several agonists will be involved in producing the movement. Some authors have used the term *secondary movers* to refer to those muscles acting as agonists in some limb positions but not in others.[13]

The lack of specificity of these terms is further exemplified when considering all the functions of a given muscle, the influence of changes in limb position, and the influence of dynamic limb interactions.[30,31] An example of the dynamic interactions can be seen in the *task dependent* and *task independent* functions that have been suggested by Zajac.[31]

Zajac and Gordon[30] have suggested that during standing, for example, the angular acceleration that tends to cause knee extension exerted by the uniarticular soleus muscle is, at times, twice the angular acceleration that tends to cause plantar flexion at the ankle joint. The resulting interactions between limb segments are only evident when dynamical equations are formulated and used in the analysis. The equations quantify the direct effect that a muscle will have on the joint that it crosses and explicitly quantify the effects resulting from the dynamic or intersegmental interactions possibly unique to a person performing a specific movement. Based on its anatomy, the soleus only can directly generate plantar flexion moments at the ankle. This is a *task independent* function existing whenever the soleus is active. The knee extension potential of this muscle arises from its tendency to rotate the tibia, which in

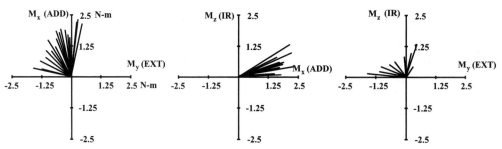

FIGURE 2–4. Three-dimensional moments produced by stimulation of the anterior deltoid muscle in one human subject. Add = adduction moment, Ext = Extension moment, IR = internal rotation moment. Note that the reference frame does not correspond to that presented in Figure 2–1. (From Buneo, CA, et al: Postural dependence of muscle actions: Implications for neural control. J Neurosci 7:2128, 1997, with permission.)

turn affects the femur. This phenomenon is highly dependent on limb position and is the *task dependent* function that can emerge under specific movement circumstances.

Only limited analyses examining these dynamic effects at the shoulder have been performed,[32] so specific conclusions regarding shoulder function cannot be made at this time. Future work examining these interactions in the upper limb is essential for a better understanding of shoulder muscle function and for optimizing rehabilitation of the shoulder following injury. Terminology regarding muscle synergy also is not standardized throughout the literature. Many of the definitions of the commonly used terms must be stated explicitly to minimize confusion.

Muscle Function in 3D

A majority of the data surrounding shoulder muscle function have been obtained using two-dimensional analyses. In 1997, however, Buneo et al.[33] recorded three-dimensional shoulder muscle moments during stimulation of selected muscles in human subjects. The position of the shoulder was varied in three-dimensional space, and isometric moments were measured for each muscle. The results demonstrated that all of the muscles generated significant moments about all three orthogonal (mutually perpendicular) axes. Figure 2–4 shows moments produced by the anterior deltoid muscle of one subject. Each line represents a moment vector at a different shoulder position, indicating a change in magnitude and direction of the moment with alterations in position. The proportion of flexion and adduction, for example, changed with each change in shoulder position indicating that the muscle may become more of a flexor or adductor depending on position.

These authors also noted that the middle deltoid contributed to flexion, abduction, and internal rotation, whereas the posterior deltoid contributed to extension, abduction, and internal rotation. These muscles are agonists in abduction and antagonists in flexion-extension and axial rotation. The contribution of each muscle varied each of these motions depending on position. This suggests that the combined effect of simultaneous activation of these muscles varies with limb position, resulting in a variable synergistic relationship.

Combining the findings of Zajac[31] and Buneo et al.,[33] some difficulty arises in describing the precise synergistic contributions of all of the muscles of the shoulder.[13] The three-dimensional functions of individual muscles and their changing con-

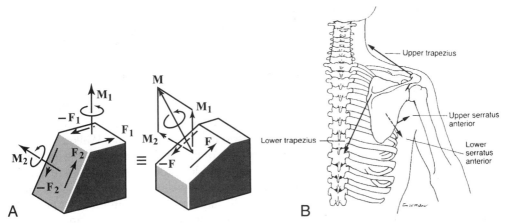

FIGURE 2–5. *(A)* Diagram showing the generation of force couples. Force pairs F, F1, and F2 create the couples M, M1, and M2, respectively. (From Meriam, JL, and Kraige, LG: Engineering Mechanics, Vol 1: Statics. John Wiley & Sons, New York, 1986, with permission.) *(B)* Diagrammatic representation of the muscular force couple created by the trapezius and serratus anterior muscles that result in upward rotation of the scapula. (From Norkin, CC, and Levangie, PK: Joint Structure and Function. A Comprehensive Approach. FA Davis, Philadelphia, 1992, with permission.)

tributions to a movement must be considered when making decisions about the appropriate rehabilitation of shoulder musculature.

Scapular Force Couple

Scapular rotation, required during humeral elevation, is a well accepted synergistic relationship occurring at the shoulder. The upper and lower trapezius muscles, in conjunction with the serratus anterior, are responsible for upward rotation of the scapula through the generation of a force couple.[4,5,6] A force couple causing rotation is created when two forces equal in magnitude and not collinear act in opposite directions. Figure 2–5A shows examples of moments created by two forces acting on a block. In a similar fashion, muscles acting on bones also can create couples.

Figure 2–5B shows how the resultant pull of the trapezius and serratus anterior can initiate upward rotation of the scapula. With the axis of rotation at the base of the scapular spine, components of the resultants will act in parallel to rotate the scapula in the same direction. As the axis shifts locations, fibers from the lower trapezius provide additional torque to ensure the appropriate scapular rotation required for humeral elevation is achieved. This demonstrates the balance that must exist between creating a stable base of support for the scapulohumeral muscles to act on the humerus and the requirement for a mobile scapula.[4]

Muscle Activity

While multiple muscles are active to varying degrees during elevation of the humerus in any plane, differences in muscle recruitment associated with changes in shoulder posture have been documented.[34] Comparing elevation in the frontal plane with elevation in the plane of the scapula (the plane in which the scapula lies in anatomical position, orientation approximately 30° anterior to the frontal plane resulting in the glenoid fossa facing slightly anteriorly), Ringleberg[34] found that both middle and posterior deltoid muscles showed significantly less activity during elevation in the plane of the scapula. The anterior deltoid showed little variation in activity between the two elevation conditions, whereas the infraspinatus muscle showed its highest activity during elevation in the scapular plane. The clavicular head of the pectoralis major showed little to no activity during elevation in either plane.

All four muscles showed a linear increase in activity with increasing humeral elevation up to 90°. Comparing these data to those of Poppen and Walker[20] reveals some conflicting findings. For elevation in the plane of the scapula, the posterior deltoid was observed to be inactive below 60° of elevation. It steadily increased its activity as the joint angle increased. However, it consistently remained at a lower relative activation level than both the middle and anterior deltoids. Poppen and Walker[20] also reported that the infraspinatus was inactive for humeral angles below 120° of elevation.

Saha[35] presented a third view, showing the infraspinatus active from 30° of abduction through 180°. However, EMG results presented by Saha[35] were absolute values of activity and, therefore, difficult to compare with other findings.

Supraspinatus has been shown to peak in activity between 60° and 120° of elevation depending on the plane of humeral elevation.[20,35] The subscapularis and teres minor muscles were shown to be active early in frontal plane elevation, progressively increasing their activity to moderate levels between 150° and 180°.[35] In scapular plane abduction, no activity was observed in the subscapularis muscles below 90° of elevation, with peak activity reached at 150°.[20]

Data from Saha,[35] Ringleberg,[34] Poppen and Walker,[20] and Buneo et al.[33] indicate that upper limb posture appears to influence observed muscle output significantly. In addition, the variation in findings across investigations illustrates the difficulty in standardizing measurements of muscle activity across subjects and experimental preparations. Interpretation of EMG findings, which requires careful comparisons, must include the circumstances under which the data were collected. Strengths and weaknesses of EMG measurements also must be understood fully to obtain accurate insight into basic mechanisms of movement or to be a useful tool for clinical assessment. Whereas additional information on individual muscle output (activity, force, and moment) is required, despite the variable findings, limb position, as well as whole body position, must be addressed when evaluating the condition of the shoulder.[8]

Rotator Cuff

The rotator cuff muscle group has received a great deal of attention by numerous investigators because of its significance in normal shoulder function.[18,20,35-38] The exact role of these muscles, however, is not entirely clear. Saha[35] stated that the rotator cuff muscle group, consisting of the supraspinatus, infraspinatus, subscapularis, and teres minor muscles, serves as a dynamic stabilization unit responsible for the rolling of the humerus and its "steering" on the glenoid fossa in both the horizontal and vertical directions. Bechtol[36] concluded that the supraspinatus and deltoid muscles contribute significantly to abduction, but the loss of the supraspinatus muscle resulted in decline in moment production that became quite dramatic with increasing angles of humeral abduction. Loss of the deltoid resulted in a constant 50% decrease in the moment throughout the full range of shoulder abduction. These results suggest that differential roles for each muscle exist and that perhaps, as suggested by Saha[35] and Norkin and Levangie,[5] the supraspinatus has a steering role that contributes significantly to the stability and normal arthrokinematics of the GH joint.

Sharkey and Marder[38] concluded that the rotator cuff's combined effect was humeral head stabilization. Using cadavers and simulated muscle loading, they found that abduction without the infraspinatus, teres minor, and subscapularis muscles resulted in significant superior translation of the humeral head. With the entire cuff intact, the superior translation was minimized to an average of 1.5 mm at 120° of abduction.

Wuekler and colleagues,[18] using cadaver shoulders and simulated muscle forces, concluded that humeral translations were increased dramatically with reduced rotator cuff activity when a displacing load was applied to the humerus during motion from 0° to 90°. These findings support the steering postulations of Saha[35] by showing that without adequate muscle force in the rotator cuff muscles, the translational motion of the humerus increases in the direction of the displacing force.

Otis et al.[37] estimated the infraspinatus moment arm and concluded that it could serve as a significant humeral abductor during the first 60° of abduction in the scapular plane. These investigators point out, however, that the wires implanted to simulate portions of the individual muscles being studied reflected the extreme edges of the muscles and were not representative of the central fibers. The combined effect, therefore, of the entire muscle or of combinations of different portions of the muscle (with different fiber orientations) could have a profoundly different effect on the humerus than the group of fibers that were analyzed.

The rotator cuff is currently viewed as playing its most substantial role in directing the humeral head and helping to maintain a normal arthrokinematic pattern. This helps ensure a stable relationship between humerus and scapula throughout the range of motion. This in turn allows for normal force and moment output.

Individual Muscle Moments

When the movement producing capability of a muscle is considered, some knowledge about force and *moment arm* for each individual muscle is important. A moment of force results in a tendency to rotate an object (for example, a bone). The moment produced by a muscle, (M), can be obtained by multiplying the magnitude of the force, (F), by the magnitude of the moment arm, (r), (that is, M = rxF). The moment arm for a muscle force can be defined as the shortest distance (perpendicular) from the line of application of the force to the axis of rotation.[29] Thus, the moment produced by a muscle will be dependent on both force and moment arm, which both change with joint angle changes. Several methods for measuring moment arms in human subjects have been suggested, though no standard methodology for their assessment has been established.[39,40] Several studies have been undertaken to estimate the moment arms for muscles of the shoulder.

Poppen and Walker[20] measured abduction moment arms on human cadavers at multiple angles of elevation in the scapular plane. Their findings are summarized in Figure 2–6 and are combined with relative activation levels for subjects performing isometric elevation. Otis et al.[37] presented abduction and adduction moment arms as a

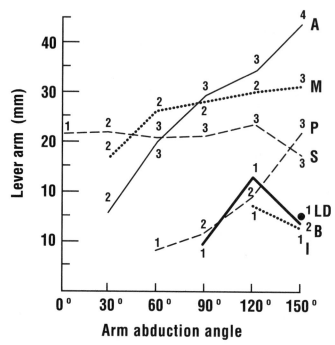

FIGURE 2–6. Moment arm (lever arm) lengths for selected shoulder muscles estimated on human cadavers as a function of humeral (arm) abduction angle. Numbers indicate relative isometric EMG levels for each muscle (1 = lowest, 4 = highest) measured in a different subject group. A = anterior deltoid, M = middle deltoid, P = posterior deltoid, S = supraspinatus, LD = latissimus dorsi, B = subscapularis, I = infraspinatus. (From Poppen, NK, and Walker, PS: Forces at the glenohumeral joint in abduction. Clin Orthop 135:165, 1978, with permission.)

function of changes in scapular plane abduction-adduction angle and axial rotation angle. Using cadaver specimens, Otis et al. implanted wires representing the average fiber orientation of portions of subscapularis, infraspinatus, supraspinatus, teres minor, and the deltoid. They measured the length change and joint angle change and calculated the resulting moment arm for each muscle. Findings indicated that changes in axial rotation of the humerus can significantly alter the abduction-adduction moment arms for each muscle. The parts of the supraspinatus were shown to work in a complimentary fashion. Anterior and posterior parts working as abductors alter their abduction moment arms as the humerus externally rotates. The moment arm for the anterior fibers increased although the moment arm for the posterior fibers decreased. Proportional changes in both parts were approximately equal resulting in a relatively consistent abduction moment arm independent of axial rotation. In addition, the moment arm for the infraspinatus was found to be of a sufficient length to act as a functional abductor, especially when the humerus was internally rotated.

Kuechle et al.[41] investigated moment arms for individual rotator cuff muscles and the three parts of the deltoid in cadaver shoulders. Moment arm lengths varied widely, depending on the plane of elevation. The infraspinatus, subscapularis, and posterior deltoid reversed their moment arms part way through the elevation.

When compared across studies, the data from Poppen and Walker[20] and Otis et al.[37] are in general agreement. However, Otis et al. limited their analysis to the first 60° of elevation. Kuechle et al.[41] differed significantly from Poppen and Walker[20] in their assessment of the supraspinatus moment arm. Poppen and Walker show a relatively constant supraspinatus moment arm throughout the full range of elevation. Kuechle et al.[41] report a significant reduction in the moment arm for this muscle, indicating that its role in scapular plane abduction beyond 25° is minimal. Kuechle et al. limited their range to 100°, whereas Poppen and Walker used measurements up through 150° of motion. Therefore, direct comparison throughout the entire range of elevation is not possible.

Methodologies in these three studies were quite different. Thus, distinguishing physiological differences from those due to differences in data collection methods is difficult. Individual muscle moments are conceptually straightforward to calculate. However, in actuality, they are quite difficult to assess because valid measurements of moment arms are very difficult to obtain. The moment producing capability of individual muscles, however, must be considered essential knowledge for a complete understanding of shoulder function. As new technologies develop, more controlled studies will be undertaken so that complete moment arm data will be obtained.

CHAPTER SUMMARY

Normal arthrokinematic patterns for each joint of the shoulder complex have been discussed and their mutual dependency, known as scapulohumeral rhythm, has been emphasized. A review of some basic kinetic analyses of the shoulder have shown that, although not a "weight bearing joint," the GH joint has reaction forces that can reach values ranging from 50% to 89% of body weight. Muscle synergies, reflected in patterns of activation and moment, have been reviewed and discussed in light of recent information on the three-dimensional nature of the muscles of the shoulder. These synergistic patterns have also been shown to be highly dependent on the dynamic qualities of the multisegment upper limb during upper limb tasks.

To provide the best rehabilitation for shoulder dysfunction, an accurate and detailed understanding of shoulder kinematics, kinetics, and muscle function must be obtained. Future research must emphasize the three-dimensional nature of shoulder muscles, the position-dependent function of shoulder muscles and their synergies, as well as the mechanisms of load transfer between the joints of the shoulder.

REFERENCES

1. Perry, J: Normal upper extremity kinesiology. Phys Ther 58:265, 1978.
2. Steindler, A: Kinesiology of the Human Body under Normal and Pathological Conditions. Charles C. Thomas, Springfield, Ill, 1955.
3. Zatsiorsky, VM: Kinematics of Human Motion. Human Kinetics, Champaign, 1998.
4. Dvir, Z, and Berme, N: The shoulder complex in elevation of the arm. A mechanism approach. J Biomech 1:219, 1978.
5. Norkin, CC, and Levangie, PK: Joint Structure and Function. A Comprehensive Approach. FA Davis, Philadelphia, 1992.
6. Saha, AK: Mechanism of shoulder movements and a plea for the recognition of the "zero position" of glenohumeral joint. Clin Orthop 173:3, 1983.
7. Poppen, NK, and Walker, PS: Normal and abnormal motion of the shoulder. J Bone and Joint Surg 58-A:195, 1976.
8. Soderberg, GL: Kinesiology. Application to pathological motion. Williams and Wilkins, Baltimore, 1997.
9. McQuade, KJ, and Smidt, GL: Dynamic scapulohumeral rhythm: The effects of external resistance during elevation of the arm in the scapular plane. J Orthopedic and Sports Phys Ther 27:125, 1998.

10. McQuade, KJ, et al: Scapulothoracic muscle fatigue associated with alterations in scapulohumeral rhythm kinematics during maximum resistive shoulder elevation. J Orthopedic and Sports Phys Ther 28:74, 1998.
11. Freedman, L, and Monroe, RR: Abduction of the arm in the scapular plane: Scapular and glenohumeral movements. J Bone and Joint Surg 48A:1503, 1966.
12. Doody, SG, et al: Shoulder movements during abduction in the scapular plane. Arch Phys Med Rehabil 51:595, 1970.
13. Schenkman, M, and Rugo De Cartaya, V: Kinesiology of the Shoulder Complex. In Andrews, JR, and Wilk, KE (eds): The Athletes Shoulder. Churchill Livingstone, New York, 1994, p 15.
14. Lehmkuhl, LD and Smith, LK: Brunnstrom's Clinical Kinesiology. FA Davis, Philadelphia, 1983.
15. Zatsiorsky, VM, and Aktov, AV: Biomechanics of highly precise movements: Movement Control: An Interdisciplinary Forum. VU University Press, Amsterdam, 1991, p51.
16. Howell, SM, et al: Normal and abnormal mechanics of the glenohumeral joint in the horizontal plane. J Bone and Joint Surg 70-A:227, 1988.
17. Harryman, DT, et al: Translation of the humeral head on the glenoid with passive glenohumeral motion. J Bone and Joint Surg 72-A: 1334, 1990.
18. Wuelker, N, et al: Dynamic glenohumeral joint stability. J Shoulder Elbow Surg 7:43, 1998.
19. Wuelker, N, et al: Translation of the glenohumeral joint with simulated active elevation. Clin Orthop 309:193, 1994.
20. Poppen, NK, and Walker, PS: Forces at the glenohumeral joint in abduction. Clin Orthop 135:165, 1978.
21. Zuckerman, JD, and Matsen, FA: Biomechanics of the shoulder. In Nordin, M, and Frankel, VH (eds): Basic Biomechanics of the Musculoskeletal System. Lea and Febiger, Philadelphia, 1989, p 225.
22. Inman, VT, et al: Observations on the function of the shoulder joint. J Bone and Joint Surg 26:1, 1944.
23. Van Der Helm, FCT: Analysis of the kinematic and dynamic behavior of the shoulder mechanism. J Biomech. 27:527, 1994.
24. Elftman, H: Forces and energy changes in the leg during walking. Am J Physiol 125:339, 1939.
25. Brester, B, and Frankel, JP: The forces and moments in the leg during level walking. Transactions of the American Society of Mechanical Engineers 72:27, 1950.
26. Zemicke, RF and Smith, JL: Biomechanical insights into neural control of movement. In Rowell, LB, and Shepard, JT (eds): Handbook of Physiology. Section 12. Exercise: Regulation and integration of multiple systems. Oxford, New York, 1996, p 293.
27. Winter, DA: Biomechanics and Motor Control of Human Movement. John Wiley & Sons, New York, 1990.
28. Basmajian, JV, and DeLuca, CJ: Muscles Alive. Their Functions Revealed by Electromyography. Williams and Wilkins, Baltimore, 1985.
29. Enoka, RM: Neuromechanical Basis of Kinesiology. Human Kinetics, Champaign, 1988.
30. Zajac, FE, and Gordon, ME: Determining muscle's force and action in multi-articular movement. In Pandolf, KB (ed): Exer Sports Sci Rev. Williams and Wilkins, Baltimore, 1989, p 187.
31. Zajac, FE: Muscle coordination in movement: A perspective. J Biomech 26:109, 1993.
32. Sainburg, RL, et al: Control of limb dynamics in normal subjects and patients without proprioception. J Neurophysiol 73:820, 1995.
33. Buneo, CA, et al: Postural dependence of muscle actions: Implications for neural control. J Neurosci 7:2128, 1997.
34. Ringleberg, JA: EMG and force production of some human shoulder muscles during isometric abduction. J Biomech 18:939, 1985.
35. Saha, AK: Dynamic stability of the glenohumeral joint. Acta Orthop Scand 42:491, 1971.
36. Bechtol, CO: Biomechanics of the shoulder. Clin Orthop Related Res 146:37, 1980.
37. Otis, JC, et al: Changes in the moment arms of the rotator cuff and deltoid muscles with abduction and rotation. J Bone and Joint Surg 76-A:667, 1994.
38. Sharkey, NA, and Marder, RA: The rotator cuff opposes superior translation of the humeral head. Am J Sports Med 23:270,1995.
39. An, KN, et al: Determination of muscle orientations and moment arms. Transactions of the ASME 106:280, 1984.
40. An, KN, et al: Tendon excursion and moment arms of index finger muscles. J Biomech 16:419, 1983.
41. Kuechle, DK, et al: Shoulder muscle moment arms during horizontal flexion and elevation. J Shoulder Elbow Surg 6:429, 1997.

CHAPTER 3

Diagnosis by Physical Therapists: Impairment-Based Model Versus Medical Model

Andrew A. Guccione, PhD, PT, FAPTA

INTRODUCTION

Modern physical therapy did not exist at the beginning of the 20th century. However, as we enter the millennium, it is remarkable to observe how physical therapy has gained prominence, emerging as a scientific profession that serves as a point of entry into the health-care system. In the last 5 years alone, the following three events have distinguished physical therapy prominence as a health profession: (1) community recognition (both internal and external to physical therapy) of diagnosis by physical therapists, (2) identification of the process of disablement as an overarching framework for physical therapist and patient/client management, and (3) elaboration of a model of physical therapist and patient/client management in the *Guide to Physical Therapist Practice.*[1] This chapter describes the evolution of diagnosis in physical therapy and the integration of the disablement model into its scope and practice.

THE EVOLUTION OF DIAGNOSIS BY PHYSICAL THERAPISTS

Diagnosis identifies the primary dysfunction toward which the physical therapist directs treatment. The dysfunction is identified by the physical therapist based on the information obtained from the history, signs, symptoms, examination, and tests that the therapist performs or requests.[2]

Rose's[3] initial thoughts about diagnosis were considered revolutionary and visionary. However, emerging responsibilities for determining treatment and manage-

45

ment strategies today dictate that physical therapists make diagnoses, whether in direct access or evaluate-and-treat modes of practice.[3]

Physical therapists engage in a diagnostic process each and every time they initially examine a patient. Identifying problems to be addressed in a physical therapy plan of care involves a diagnostic process. However, to many inside and outside of the profession, this notion was not intuitively apparent a decade ago. Sahrmann[2] provided one of the earliest formulations of diagnosis by physical therapists and showed the need for a classification scheme that would be clinically useful to physical therapists.

During the process of developing a model for physical therapy diagnosis, care was taken by the American Physical Therapy Association to ensure that the kind of problem identification or "diagnosis" made by a physical therapist was different from the type of diagnosis made by a physician. Another important consideration was to ensure that the physical therapist's use of the diagnostic process did not challenge the physician's responsibility for the diagnosis of disease.[3,4] Despite the similarities in process, the object of a physician's diagnosis and the methods to ascertain the diagnosis are quite different from the object of a physical therapist's diagnosis.

In general, physicians use medical assessment procedures to classify clinical phenomena into categories and apply diagnostic labels to these categories specifying a disease. These clinical data are recorded at the level of the cell, tissue, organ, or system. The overall goal is to facilitate the cure of disease. The traditional medical model places an emphasis on the characteristics of disease (etiology, pathology, and clinical manifestations), often ignoring the equally important psychological, social, and behavioral dimensions associated with the illness. Thus, physical therapists are also attuned to identifying problems at the level of the person and society and classifying their impact on function. By helping the individual with a disease to function optimally, the physical therapist also gains insight the person's illness.

In response to these concerns, early discussions surrounding the appropriateness of diagnosis by physical therapists centered on legal differences between professions. Three primary characteristics of diagnosis by nonphysician health professionals and discipline-specific classification schema were identified. First, the overall classification scheme applied by the professional had to be consistent within the boundaries of a profession's focus. Legal accountability for applying certain diagnostic labels and society's approval to treat specific kinds of problems and conditions were used as guidelines. Second, the tests and measures necessary to validate a particular application of a diagnostic label were to fall within the legal purview of the profession. Finally, the particular label used to categorize the patient's condition must have described the problem to imply or direct treatment procedures within the legal purview of the profession.

All of these elements are evident in the position on diagnosis that is adopted, and periodically amended, by the House of Delegates of the American Physical Therapy Association:

DIAGNOSIS BY PHYSICAL THERAPISTS HOD 06-97-06-19 [Amended HOD 06-95-12-07; HOD 06-94-22-35, Initial HOD 06-84-19-78]

1. Physical therapists shall establish a diagnosis for each patient.
2. Prior to making a patient management decision, physical therapists shall

utilize the diagnostic process in order to establish a diagnosis for the specific conditions in need of the physical therapist's attention.

3. A diagnosis is a label encompassing a cluster of signs and symptoms commonly associated with a disorder or syndrome or category of impairment, functional limitation, or disability. It is the decision reached as a result of the diagnostic process, which is the evaluation of information obtained from the patient examination. The purpose of the diagnosis is to guide the physical therapist in determining the most appropriate intervention strategy for each patient. In the event the diagnostic process does not yield an identifiable cluster, disorder, syndrome or category, intervention may be directed toward the alleviation of symptoms and remediation of impairment, functional limitation, or disability.

4. The diagnostic process includes the following: obtaining relevant history, performing systems review, selecting and administering specific tests and measures, organizing and interpreting all data.

5. In performing the diagnostic process, physical therapists may need to obtain additional information (including diagnostic labels) from other health professionals. In addition, as the diagnostic process continues, physical therapists may identify findings that should be shared with other health professionals, including referral sources, to ensure optimal patient care. When the patient is referred with a previously established diagnosis, the physical therapist should determine that the clinical findings are consistent with that diagnosis. If the diagnostic process reveals findings that are outside the scope of the physical therapist's knowledge, experience, or expertise, the physical therapist should then refer the patient to an appropriate practitioner.[5]

Because majority opinion agreed with the need for diagnosis by physical therapists, the debate on the appropriateness of engaging in the process of diagnosis ended relatively quickly. However, considerable time was spent determining a clinically useful classification scheme in keeping with the framework of physical therapy practice in the larger context of health care. The specific concern was choosing a classification scheme that adequately captured the clinical phenomena that were the object of diagnosis by a physical therapist and labeling them in a way that suggested intervention by the physical therapist. Thus, the Process of Disablement model emerged as a conceptual framework to address areas of physical therapy intervention.

THE PROCESS OF DISABLEMENT

A broad framework is necessary to understand the concept of health and its relationship to functional disability. The World Health Organization (WHO) defined *health* as a state of complete physical, psychological, and social well-being, and not merely the absence of disease or infirmity.[6] According to this definition, *health* is best understood as an end point that considers the psychological and social domains and physical state of human existence. Although such global definitions are useful as philosophic statements, they lack the precision necessary for a clinician or researcher. Nagi has been particularly influential in developing a model that explicates health status and the relationship among the various terms used to describe health status.[7,8,9,10] This model presents four distinct components of health status that evolve sequentially as an individual loses well-being. Collectively referred to as the *disablement model,* the components include disease or active pathology, impairments, functional limitations, and disability. These concepts describe the essential elements of a model that serve as an overall framework for the five steps of the physical therapist and patient/client management model: examination, evaluation, diagnosis, prognosis, and intervention.[1] Nagi's conceptual model is used in this chapter to capture the concept of health status.

Disease or Active Pathology

Disease or active pathology, the first step in the model, is defined by abnormal physical signs and symptoms indicating the body's attempt to cope with the impact on normal function. Nagi's concept of disease, which is rooted in the principle of homeostasis, emphasizes two features: (1) an active threat to the organism's normal state, and (2) an active response internally by the organism to that threat, which may be aided externally by therapeutic interventions. Disease may be the result of infection, trauma, metabolic imbalance, degenerative processes, or other causes.

Although the definition of disease implies an active condition, many of the physical signs and symptoms important to diagnosis and intervention by a physical therapist are not associated with single active or ongoing medical conditions. Numerous medical conditions may affect an individual's ability to function that are not related to a single active pathologic condition. Some medical conditions are not labels for a single pathologic entity. Rather they are clusters of signs and symptoms designating a syndrome. For example, osteoarthritis, which is neither active nor progressive in all cases, is a medical condition that is best understood as a cluster of pathologic processes rather than as a single disease entity. Overuse syndromes of the upper extremity, such as impingement syndrome, are good examples of sign and symptom clusters known to physical therapists.

Physical therapists also examine individuals whose medical diagnoses involve surgical procedures, which identify previous insults to a body part or organ. These procedures may lead to impairments and dysfunction not presently associated with any active processes. For example, a patient seen following surgical repair of a rotator cuff tear is an individual with a medical diagnosis that is no longer associated with any ongoing pathologic process. Therefore, Nagi's original model can be expanded to include threats to health also leading to impairment, such as syndromes and lesions, that are not considered active pathology.

Impairments

According to Nagi's model, impairments evolve as a consequence of pathologic conditions or disease. Impairments are defined as any alteration or deviation from normal in anatomical, physiological, or psychological structures or functions. For example, the partial or complete loss of a limb or an organ, or any disturbance in body part, organ, or system function are examples of impairments. Physical impairments, such as pain and decreased range of motion in the shoulder, may be manifestations (or symptoms and signs) of either temporary or permanent disease or pathologic processes. Physical therapists are primarily concerned with impairments of the musculoskeletal, neuromuscular, cardiopulmonary, and integumentary systems, which may involve the loss of range of motion, strength, aerobic capacity, or scar formation.

In some cases, impairments may be temporary or permanent manifestations of a disease or a pathologic state. In other cases, the sources of some impairments can often be unclear. For example, poor posture is neither a disease nor a pathologic state, but the resultant muscle shortening and capsular tightness may present as major impairments in a clinical examination. Furthermore, some impairments are attributed to other impairments. A patient with a stiff shoulder joint may eventually develop muscle weakness in those muscles surrounding the joint. In this case, impaired muscle strength would be the result of impaired joint mobility, rather than a specific disease or pathological process. Schenkman and Butler have proposed that impairments can be classified in two ways.[11,12] First, some impairments are *direct* effects of a disease, syndrome, or lesion and are relatively confined to a single system. The authors note that decreased muscle performance can be classified as a neuromuscular impairment that is a direct effect of a peripheral motor neuropathy in the upper extremity. Second, simultaneous impairments may occur in other systems. These can be regarded as the *indirect* effects of the peripheral neuropathy. For example, attempts to use an upper extremity with a peripheral motor neuropathy for functional activities such as reaching overhead may put unnecessary strain on joints and ligaments, which possibly may be detected with a clinical examination as musculoskeletal impairments. The combination of weakness and ligamentous strain possibly leading to impairments of pain and limited ROM, demonstrates the sequela of the original impairment and a composite effect of indirect or secondary impairments.

Categorizing clinical signs and symptoms into impairments that are direct, indirect, or the composite effects of both can help integrate medical history data and clinical examination findings into a cohesive relationship. Piecing clinical data together in this fashion allows the therapist to uncover the interrelationships among a patient's neuropathy, limited range of motion (ROM), loss of joint integrity, diminished muscle performance, and pain. By using a system that categorizes clinical data based on impairments, the therapist can better understand potential sources for a patient's symptoms and how to address each impairment in a comprehensive manner. For example, intervention consisting of therapeutic exercise to strengthen the shoulder musculature alone would be inappropriate. The therapist must also address the loss of joint ROM and teach the patient to compensate for the limited ROM to achieve optimal function.

Functional Limitations

A functional limitation refers to an individual's inability to perform an action or activity in the manner performed by most people. Nagi proposed that functional limitations were the result of impairments and consisted of an individual's inability to perform the tasks and roles constituting that person's usual activities. For example, function may be characterized by the ability to reach for something, the ability to reach for something on an overhead shelf, or being able to put on a shirt without assistance. Function is a measure of behaviors, not an anatomic or physiologic condition. Limitations in functional status should not be confused with diseases or impairments that encompass aberrations in specific organs or present clinically as the patient's signs and symptoms.

Accurate judgment about the relationship between impairments and functional limitations is the key to a physical therapist's examination, evaluation, diagnosis, prognosis, and intervention.[1,13] The following three main categories of function have been delineated: physical function, psychological function, and social function.

PHYSICAL FUNCTION

Physical function refers to those sensory-motor skills necessary for the performance of usual daily activities, such as getting out of bed, transferring, walking, and climbing. Physical therapists are traditionally most involved with this category of functional assessment and intervention. For example, reaching is a functional limitation that is frequently associated with problems of the shoulder. Tasks concerned with daily self-care such as feeding, dressing, hygiene, and physical mobility are called basic *activities of daily living* (ADL). Advanced skills considered vital to an individual's independent living in the community are termed *instrumental activities of daily living* (IADL). These include a wide range of high-level skills such as managing personal affairs, cooking and shopping, home chores, and driving. Shoulder impairments can have a critical impact on upper extremity skills that underlie numerous functional activities.

PSYCHOLOGICAL FUNCTION

Psychological function has two components, mental and affective. Mental function, the intellectual or cognitive abilities of an individual, contains components such as initiative, attention, concentration, memory, problem solving, and judgment. Affective function refers to the affective skills and coping strategies needed to deal with everyday "hassles" as well as with the more traumatic and stressful events each person encounters over the course of a lifetime. Factors such as self-esteem, attitude toward body image, anxiety, depression, and the ability to cope with change are examples of affective functions.

SOCIAL FUNCTION

Social function refers to an individual's performance of social roles and obligations. Categories of roles and activities relevant to assessing an individual's social function include social activity, such as participation in recreational activities and clubs; social interaction, such as telephoning or visiting relatives or friends; and social roles created and sustained through interpersonal relationships specific to one's personal life and occupation.

Although physical therapists are primarily concerned with physical functional activities, individuals typically conceive their personal identities in terms of specific social roles: worker, parent, spouse, recreational athlete, community volunteer. All of these roles demand a certain degree of physical ability, as many opportunities for social interaction occur around sports, leisure, and recreational activities. Therefore, the positive effects of a physical therapist's intervention may not be strictly limited to improvement in physical functional status. Improved social functioning also may accompany changes in physical ability. Although a therapist might appreciate the impact of shoulder impairments on physical functional activities more quickly, a comprehensive approach to the patient must also capture the impact that losing the ability to pitch a softball and subsequent restrictions on recreation and social pursuits may have on a particular individual's well-being.

One cannot assume that an individual will be unable to perform the tasks and roles of usual daily living by virtue of having an impairment alone. For example, an elderly individual with osteoarthritis (disease) may exhibit loss of range of motion (impairment) and experience great difficulty in combing hair (function). However, another individual with equal loss of ROM may use a method that allows combing of the hair without difficulty, perhaps by using available joint motion to the best advantage or by using assistive devices. Sometimes patients will overcome multiple, and even permanent, impairments by the sheer force of their motivation.

Disability

When an individual experiences a limitation in a number of functional activities and is unable to engage in critical social roles (such as worker, student, or spouse), this person may be regarded as "disabled," as conceptualized within the Nagi model. *Disability* is characterized by a discordance between the actual performance of an individual in a particular role and the expectations of the community regarding what is "normal" for an adult. Nagi reserved the term *disability* for functional limitations emerging over long periods of time that are accompanied by specific patterns of behavior. These patterns developed to such a degree that they could not be overcome to create some semblance of "normal" overall role and task performance.

Although each of the terms that have been presented involves some consensus about what is "normal," the concept of a *disability* is socially constructed. The term, *disabled,* connotes a particular status in society. Labeling a person as "disabled" requires a judgment, usually by a professional, that an individual's behaviors are somehow inadequate. This judgment is based on the professional's understanding of the expectations that the activity should be accomplished in ways that are typical for that person's age, sex, and cultural and social environment. Thus, *disability* has a meaning that is based on the community in which the individual lives and the criteria for "normal" within that social group.

Many factors can influence the relationship among disease, impairment, and function. Patients with the same disease and the same impairments may not always have the same functional limitations because of individual responses to treatment. Furthermore, although an individual may perform functional activities in a manner different than "normal," this person may successfully accomplish expected social roles and escape the label of being "disabled." Physical therapists most often think of "normal" adulthood in terms of independence in self-care activities, competence and autonomy in decision making, and productivity. In some cultural subgroups, social expectations may be quite different, particularly if the individual has certain impairments or functional limitations. Physical therapists should account for the effects of culture and social expectations in determining what is "normal" function for an individual, especially when the therapist and the patient do not share the same social or cultural backgrounds.

Disability depends on the individual's capacities and the expectations imposed on the individual by those in the immediate social environment, most often the patient's family and caregivers. Physical therapists who apply a health status perspective to patient assessment draw on a broad appreciation of a patient as a person, with individual characteristics, living in a particular social context. Changing the expectations of a social context, such as explaining to a plant manager what level of reduced work is appropriate to an injured worker, may help to diminish disability equally as supplying the patient with an assistive device or increasing the physical ability to use it.

Although deficits in behavioral or motor skills or limitations in function typically might exist in certain disease categories, the exact empirical relationship between a particular set of impairments and a specific functional disability is not yet known. The "cause-and-effect" relationship between an impairment and a functional limitation is most often inferred in the clinic from empirical evidence. For example, physical therapists may assume that the reason a patient cannot reach overhead is causally linked to the patient's loss of enough range of motion at the glenohumeral joint. The return of function following remediation of the impairment of joint mobility is then considered clinical evidence of a causal relationship between the impairment and the functional limitation. In the event that restoration of glenohumeral motion does not improve the ability to reach, then the therapist must look for other possible causes such as dysfunctional scapulohumeral rhythm. To be clinically useful, functional assessment must be linked to all the other tests and measures used by a physical therapist to examine a patient.

PHYSICAL THERAPIST AND PATIENT/CLIENT MANAGEMENT

Nagi's model describes the major concepts of a classification scheme that is potentially useful in a diagnostic process to plan and direct intervention.[13] The *Guide to Physical Therapist Practice*[1] details 34 practice patterns, 11 of which concern the impacts of musculoskeletal impairments on function. Each practice pattern is the result of an intensive effort by clinically expert physical therapists to identify the impairment clusters that name the pattern, the likely tests and measures to be applied during initial examination, the anticipated goals for intervention, and the likely interventions to be implemented. The guiding principles used to structure these patterns drew heavily from the process of disablement model discussed previously.

Some readers of the *Guide to Physical Therapist Practice* might find it odd that the organization of the musculoskeletal practice patterns is not based on regional anatomy, unlike many orthopedic textbooks. When the Musculoskeletal Panel that developed the preferred practice patterns was convened, the initial approach was to organize by regional anatomy. However, it became apparent during the 2-year developmental period that a set of diagnostic labels based on anatomical terminology was deficient in two respects. First, it would fail to describe the problem as it could be addressed by a physical therapist. Physical therapists do not examine a shoulder or knee to apply the label of *shoulder* or *knee.* They do, however, examine specific joints to identify problems in structure or function, expressed clinically as impairments of joint integrity and mobility, range of motion, muscle performance, and pain. On the other hand, the labels *impaired joint mobility, impaired range of motion,* and *impaired muscle strength* immediately conjure up images of physical therapy interventions, even for the neophyte physical therapist. Second, organizing the musculoskeletal patterns exclusively by joint would have masked the commonalities of intervention within and across the spectrum of physical therapist practice.

The developers of the preferred practice patterns settled on a schema primarily organized on two levels. The first level of organization is the impairment cluster identifying the impairments to be addressed by physical therapy intervention. The second level of organization occurs with the identification of a condition (such as localized inflammation or fracture) or a procedure (such as lower extremity amputation) that gives the impairment cluster its special character, suggesting important differences in how the physical therapist approaches treatment of the impairment cluster precisely because of that condition or procedure.

Further classification within a preferred practice pattern by joint is certainly possible, but its justification would have to be derived from the fact that there was something inherently different among the treatment of various joints exhibiting the same cluster of impairments. One musculoskeletal pattern, however, does deviate from the general organizational schema by characterizing the impairment cluster by an anatomical reference, "Impaired joint mobility, motor function, muscle performance, range of motion or reflex integrity." This pattern, similar to the neuromuscular patterns that reference the central or peripheral nervous systems, suggests that the presence of these impairments in a specific region of the musculoskeletal system requires treatment intrinsically different from other patterns, precisely because of the region affected.

Although additional research is necessary to elaborate the relationship between impairments and function, the domain of the physical therapist's expertise is based on the ability to identify cardiopulmonary, integumentary, musculoskeletal, and neuromuscular impairments underlying physical functional limitations (Fig. 3–1). To provide physical therapy interventions to achieve the goal of restoring or improving function, the physical therapist must know more than the patient's signs and symptoms, the expressions of the individual's disease and impairments. The clinician must also attempt to discern which impairments affect the patient's ability to function.

Physical therapy is a complex clinical art and science. The primary question of the discipline during examination is simple and twofold: What is the patient's current level of function and which impairments contribute to the patient's functional limitations? The answer to this question can direct treatment when the therapist's attention turns toward developing the plan of care. Specifically, the key consideration

PHYSICAL THERAPIST SCOPE OF PRACTICE

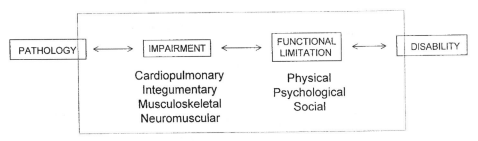

FIGURE 3–1. Physical therapist scope of practice. (Adapted from Guccione, AA: Physical Therapy Diagnosis and the relationship between impairments and function. Phys Ther 71:499, 1991.)

in evaluation and diagnosis is to establish which of the impairments related to the patient's functional limitations can also be remediated by physical therapist intervention. Subsequently, if the patient's impairments cannot be remedied, the physical therapist poses the following additional questions: (1) how can the patient use remaining abilities to compensate for unremediable impairments? and, (2) how can the task or activity be adapted to the individual's abilities?

CHAPTER SUMMARY

The challenge for orthopedic physical therapy in the years ahead will be to continue to refine the musculoskeletal patterns as they currently exist and to explore their relationships with the other cardiopulmonary, integumentary, and neuromuscular patterns.[14] The success of this effort will move the profession of physical therapy far beyond treatment of a joint and into providing intervention to restore human function at the level experienced by the individual.

REFERENCES

1. Guide to Physical Therapist Practice. Phys Ther 77:1163, 1997.
2. Sahrmann, SA: Diagnosis by the physical therapist—Prerequisite for treatment. Phys Ther 68:1703, 1988.
3. Rose, SJ: Musing on diagnosis. Phys Ther 68:1665, 1988.
4. Jette, AM: Diagnosis and classification by physical therapists: A special communication. Phys Ther 69:967, 1989.
5. House of Delegates Standards, Policies, Positions and Guidelines. Alexandria VA, American Physical Therapy Association, 1998.
6. World Health Organization: The First Ten Years of the World Health Organization. Geneva, World Health Organization, 1958.
7. Nagi, S: Disability concepts revisited. In Pope, AM, and Tarlov, AR (eds): Disability in America: Toward a national agenda for prevention. National Academy Press, Washington DC, 1991, p 309.
8. Nagi, S: Disability and Rehabilitation. Ohio State University Press, Columbus, Ohio, 1969.
9. Nagi, S: Some conceptual issues in disability and rehabilitation. In Sussman, M: Sociology and Rehabilitation, Ohio State University Press, Columbus, Ohio, 1965, p 100.
10. Nagi, S: An epidemiology of disability among adults in the United States. Milbank Q 54:439, 1976.
11. Schenkman, M, and Butler, RB: A model for multisystem evaluation, interpretation, and treatment of individuals with neurologic dysfunction. Phys Ther 69:538, 1989.
12. Schenkman, M, and Butler, RB: A model for multisystem evaluation and treatment of individuals with Parkinson's disease. Phys Ther 69:932, 1989.
13. Guccione, AA: Physical therapy diagnosis and the relationship between impairments and function. Phys Ther 71:499, 1991.
14. Delitto, A, and Snyder-Mackler, L: The diagnostic process: Examples in orthopedic physical therapy. Phys Ther 75:203, 1995.

CHAPTER 4

Impairment-Based Diagnosis for the Shoulder Girdle

Brian J. Tovin, MMSc, PT, SCS, ATC, FAAOMPT
Bruce H. Greenfield, MMSc, PT, OCS

INTRODUCTION

Physical therapy is a dynamic profession with an established theoretical base and widespread clinical applications in the preservation, development, and restoration of optimal function.[1] As clinicians, physical therapists engage in an examination process that includes taking the history, conducting a systems review, and administering tests and measures. The overall goal of this examination process is to identify potential and existing impairments, functional limitations, and disability,[2] thus enabling the clinician to formulate a diagnosis, prognosis, and an intervention.[3] These terms will be defined later in this chapter. Physical therapy examination based on the medical model focuses on differential diagnosis of disease and tissue pathology. However, the medical model has been criticized for not providing physical therapists adequate guidelines to identify impairments for treatment and to optimize function.[2-6] Recently, the American Physical Therapy Association (APTA) has advocated the use practice guidelines to direct evaluation and treatment.[1]

This chapter serves to: (1) review the evolution of diagnosis by physical therapists from the traditional medical model, (2) discuss the process of disablement as it pertains to physical therapy practice patterns, and (3) present an impairment-based classification scheme for the shoulder, incorporating preferred practice patterns of the APTA.[1]

HISTORICAL DEVELOPMENT OF THE IMPAIRMENT-BASED TREATMENT OF THE SHOULDER

Early Work

Much of the work on differential diagnosis of the shoulder was introduced by Codman[7] in the 1930s. His approach focused on the effect of pathology on shoulder function. His system of diagnosis associated clinical signs and symptoms with tissue pathology to help physicians gain a broader perspective in tissue pathology and treatment. Codman indicated that physicians should make a clinical diagnosis based on clustering signs and symptoms. He stated, ". . . pathologic entities and clinical entities are not the same. Clinical problems are the practical working diagnoses on which rational treatment may be based."[7] Many of the clinical entities that he related to complete rupture of the supraspinatus tendon would be classified as present day impairments under the International Classification of Impairments, Disabilities and Handicaps (ICIDH) or Nagi systems[8,9] (see Chap. 3). These findings include loss of active muscle power and faulty scapulohumeral rhythm with compensatory, early scapular elevation and outward rotation. The list that follows includes signs and symptoms indicative of complete rupture of the supraspinatus tendon and is adapted from Codman, with impairments identified in bold.

1. Occupation: labor
2. Age: more than 40 years old
3. No shoulder symptoms prior to injury
4. Adequate injury: usually a fall
5. **Immediate sharp, brief pain**
6. Severe pain on following night
7. **Loss of power in elevation of arm**
8. Negative x-ray
9. Little, if any, restriction when stooping
10. **Faulty scapulohumeral rhythm**
11. **Tender point, sulcus, and eminence at insertion of supraspinatus**
12. **Pain, catching, hitching, and crepitus with elevation**

One of the first comprehensive classifications for shoulder overuse injury was introduced by Neer,[10] who labeled conditions as *primary* or *mechanical impingement*. Mechanical impingement results from compression of subacromial tissues, such as the rotator cuff muscle tendons, tendon of the long head of the biceps, or subacromial bursa, underneath the anterior inferior acromial process. Table 4–1 identifies Neer's classification as a continuum of three stages of pathology. Each stage is correlated with a distinct group of impairments. The listing of impairments provides the clinician with treatment guidelines that are consistent with the philosophy of physical therapy to optimize function by identifying and correcting impairments.[1] The relationship between impairments and pathology was further developed by sports medicine physicians involved in treating shoulder pathology related to "overhead sports."[11,12]

Later Work

Currently, classifications of shoulder conditions often contain hybrids of both pathologic features and impairments. Newer classification systems were developed in response to the unique stresses and strains imparted on the shoulder complex by the athlete involved in overhead sports, such as throwing and swimming, and the resulting orthopedic injuries.[11,12] These sports involve movement patterns of glenohumeral elevation more than 90° combined with extreme internal-external rotation and

TABLE 4-1 Neer Stages of Impingement

Stages	Clinical Presentation (Impairments)	Treatment Principles
Stage I Age: Less than 25 years old Pathology: Edema and hemorrhage	Subacromial pain/tenderness Painful arc (+) Impingement/Neer test Resisted abduction and external rotation strong and painful	Reduce/eliminate inflammation Educate patient Restore proximal control: parascapular muscular control
Stage II Age: 25-40 years old Pathology: Bursitis/bursitis and fibrosis	Capsular pattern of restriction at glenohumeral joint	Re-establish glenohumeral capsular mobility
Stage III Age: More than 40 years old Pathology: Bone spurs and tendon disruption	Weakness of abduction and external rotation, "squaring" of acromion	Depends on size of tear

Adapted from Neer,[10] 1973. See Chapter 9 for definitions.

horizontal abduction-adduction. Additionally, many of these overhead sports require quick acceleration-deceleration muscle activity. The neuromuscular and biomechanical demands of these activities are different from those placed on the shoulder by the pedestrian athlete and by sedentary individuals.[13]

A biomechanical analysis of throwing illustrates how impairments lead to tissue pathology. During throwing, the glenohumeral joint accelerates in excess of 7000° per second. To enhance limb acceleration during throwing, excessive anterior glenohumeral (GH) joint laxity is required to allow the arm to achieve maximum external rotation.[12] Maximum external rotation provides a prestretch to the anterior shoulder musculature and activates muscle spindles, enhancing the concentric contraction. Athletes involved in throwing often exhibit 125° to 140° of external rotation. Excessive motion requires fine motor control to provide dynamic glenohumeral joint stability. Dynamic stability is accomplished through the combined efforts of the rotator cuff musculature, the deltoid, and long head of the biceps. Thus, the thrower is continuously balancing the necessary capsular laxity required to throw with the neuromuscular control and strength of the surrounding musculature to provide dynamic joint stability. Injuries may occur because of impairments of muscle imbalance, altered ROM, or poor motor control.[12]

A common finding in competitive swimmers and baseball pitchers with musculoskeletal shoulder injuries is instability.[11,12,13] *Instability* is defined as excessive glenohumeral mobility resulting in pain and altered motion during function.[13] The essential treatment element in patients who develop shoulder impingement in the presence of instability is to correct the instability.[14] Excessive translation of the humeral head within the glenoid fossa during a throwing motion results in a greater than normal demand for the rotator cuff muscles to provide dynamic stability.[15] Fatigue of these muscles often results in tissue overload and strain to the rotator cuff tendons with secondary subacromial impingement.[11] Specific pathophysiology of instability will be discussed in Chapter 8.

TABLE 4–2 Jobe's Classification of Shoulder Dysfunction

Group	Physical Findings	Tissue Pathology
Group I Isolated impingement without instability Age: Older, recreational athlete	(See Chapters 8 and 9 for definition of tests) (+) Impingement sign	Rotator cuff lesions of the bursal surface Subacromial spurs
Group II Instability with impingement due to overuse microtrauma Age: Young overhead athletes	(+) Impingement sign (+) Relocation test Excessive translation of the humeral head	Microtrauma to the posterior labrum, anterior capsule, and ligaments Deterioration on the posterior aspect of the humeral head Glenohumeral ligamentous laxity Tears in undersurface of supraspinatus and infraspinatus
Group III Instability due to ligamentous laxity Age: Young overhead athlete	Generalized ligamentous laxity (+) Relocation test Excessive translation of the humeral head	Humeral head, rotator cuff, and labral lesions
Group IV Singular traumatic event Instability without impingement Partial dislocations	Possibly (-) apprehension or relocation test	Bankart lesion Erosion of the posterior humeral head

Adapted from Jobe and Pink,[11] 1993.

Jobe's classification of shoulder dysfunction (Table 4–2) describes the instability-impingement relationship, and can be represented by the following scheme:

Instability ——— Subluxation ——— Impingement ——— Rotator Cuff Tear[11]

Instability is the central theme of this classification. In the young athlete, participation in overhead sports, such as throwing, swimming, tennis, and volleyball, requires large ranges, forces, and repetitions. This increased stress to the shoulder girdle can result in acquired laxity and weakness in the static (capsule) and dynamic structures (muscles), possibly leading to instability and impingement of subacromial tissues or muscle strains. Although instability with impingement occurs principally in athletes performing overhead sports, individuals may present with the same complex findings resulting from work-related activity. Repetitive overhead hammering or other construction activities produce similar loads to the shoulder as swimming and throwing do. The underlying impairments must be assessed and corrected within the context of the presenting signs and symptoms. Correction of the impairments is significantly important to physical therapists because authorities such as Jobe and Pink conclude that approximately 95% of patients with *instability-impingement* will respond to conservative treatment.[11]

The relationship between impairments and pathology was also described by Andrews.[12] Similar to Jobe's classification, Andrews distinguishes between primary compressive disease (impingement) and tensile overload and secondary compressive

TABLE 4–3 Andrews' Classification of Rotator Cuff Disease

Type	Classification
I	Primary compressive disease
II	Instability with secondary compressive disease
III	Primary tensile overload failure
IV	Tensile overload failure secondary to capsular instability
V	Macro-traumatic failure

Adapted from Meister and Andrews,[12] 1993.

disease and tensile overload (Table 4–3). Primary compressive disease and tensile overload of the rotator cuff tendons occurs during repetitive overhead movements such as throwing. Primary tensile overload results from eccentric contraction of the infraspinatus and teres minor, which occurs during deceleration of the humeral head in the follow-through phase of throwing. Primary compressive disease results from mechanical impingement of the rotator cuff tendons or long head of the biceps underneath the acromion. These conditions are referred to as types I and III in Table 4–3. According to Andrews, both type I and type III rotator cuff disease usually result from fatigue of the rotator cuff muscles and decrease the efficiency required to decelerate the throwing arm adequately. Mechanical impingement is discussed in detail in Chapter 9.

Secondary compressive disease and secondary tensile overload (types II and IV, respectively) (Table 4–3) occur in the presence of primary glenohumeral instability. The increased demand of the rotator cuff muscles to stabilize the humeral head in the glenoid fossa in the presence of capsular laxity is the primary cause of the muscle-tendon failure. Patients with types I and III rotator cuff disease present with a positive impingement sign, although patients with types II and IV present with a positive impingement sign and positive apprehension and relocation tests.[12]

Current Work

The work of both Jobe and Andrews provided the groundwork for later studies that examined impairments related to faulty posture or alignment of the upper thoracic and cervical spine, scapular position, muscle balance and performance, and motor control as measured by electromyography.[15–22] For example, Gowan et al.[15] conducted a study to determine whether muscle recruitment of professional pitchers was significantly different from that of amateur pitchers. During the acceleration phase of throwing, professional pitchers recorded increased activity of the pectoralis major, latissimus dorsi, and serratus anterior muscles, with decreased activity of the supraspinatus, infraspinatus, and teres minor muscles. These findings indicated increased efficiency during throwing motion with good proximal control of the scapula. Throwing athletes with glenohumeral instability were compared to healthy athletes in a similar manner by Glousman et al.[16] This study tested the activity of the biceps, middle deltoid, supraspinatus, infraspinatus, pectoralis major, subscapularis, latissimus dorsi, and serratus anterior muscles. Differences were noted in every muscle group except the deltoid. The authors suggest that the increased activity of the biceps and supraspinatus compensated for the instability present in the anterior capsule. The serratus anterior showed decreased activity, resulting in less control of the scapula and placing the glenoid in a compromising position during the late cocking phase. Decreased scapular control results in more stress on the labrum and anterior capsule.

Muscle imbalances around the shoulder girdle have been assessed in many studies using isokinetic dynamometry.[17–22] For example, McMaster et al.[17] found that swimmers had 52% greater concentric peak torque in shoulder internal rotation and 43% greater concentric peak torque for adduction compared to nonswimmers. In a similar study, Alderink and Kuck[18] found that baseball players had 50% greater concentric peak torque for adduction than nonthrowers. Both Chandler et al.[19] and Brown et al.[20] found higher external to internal concentric peak torque ratios in the nondominant sides of tennis and baseball players compared to the dominant sides. These differences have been referred to as athletic torque ratio shifts,[21] which are training induced changes that create disproportionate increases in concentric peak torque for internal rotators and adductors without concomitant increases in peak torque for external rotation or abduction. The resulting muscle imbalance may predispose the shoulder to injury, possibly explaining why some overhead athletes develop functional instability. These findings are supported by similar research in swimmers presenting with impingement secondary to instability.[22] Concentric peak torque values for external to internal rotation were consistently less than 50%.

The relationship between posture and tissue pathology in the shoulder has been studied by Kibler.[23] He described the lateral slide test to evaluate the function of the muscles that stabilize, outwardly rotate, and protract the scapula. These muscles include the upper and lower trapezius, serratus anterior, and rhomboid major and minor muscles. A measurement was taken from the inferior angle of the scapula to the nearest thoracic spinous process in three different GH joint positions. Results indicated that baseball pitchers exhibited a difference of 1 cm of lateral slide of the scapula on the injured shoulder. The lateral slide reflected excessive posterior rotation or "winging" of the medial scapular border, indicating weakness of the scapular stabilizers.

Evolution of Diagnosis in Physical Therapy

Musculoskeletal diagnosis in physical therapy was largely influenced by the work of James Cyriax.[24] Cyriax used a clinical assessment system based on selective tissue tension tests (Table 4–4). This approach considered the nature and characteristics of the problem in addition to isolating the tissue at fault. His work introduced the concepts of clinical reactivity and the manner in which different stresses and movements altered the clinical signs and symptoms. Cyriax was concerned with the ability of clinicians to perform ongoing clinical tests that would gauge any subtle changes in the patient's clinical signs and symptoms. The uniqueness of his work added a new body of language to the orthopedic community in detailing and describing musculoskeletal conditions (Table 4–5). By introducing a diagnosis scheme that guided treatment, he provided a foundation for classifications in physical therapy.

One of the first physical therapists to integrate a framework of disablement into evaluation and treatment was McKenzie.[25] His work involved classifying back conditions based on the relationship of impairments, movement, and pain. Although this system is based on the premise that much of spinal dysfunction is attributed to intervertebral disc pathology, patients are classified into one of three groups based on

TABLE 4–4 Selected Tissue Tension Tests

Test Movements	Assessment
Active elevation in abduction	For a painful arc
Active elevation in abduction	For scapulohumeral mechanics
Repeated active elevation in abduction	For pain, overall ROM, quality of movement and muscle endurance
Passive elevation in flexion	For ROM and end feel resistance or pain
Passive elevation in abduction internal rotation, external rotation, adduction, scapular elevation, protraction and retraction.	For ROM and end feel resistance or pain
Resisted abduction, adduction, internal and external rotation, shoulder flexion and extension, and elbow flexion and extension.	For strength, pain and /or weakness due to injury to the contractile elements (muscle-tendon unit)

Adapted from Cyriax,[24] 1978.

TABLE 4–5 Terminology Used to Describe Orthopedic Conditions
As Developed by James Cyriax

Terminology	Definition
End range	The last few degrees of freedom when a tissue or structure is loaded mechanically and passively to the point just before damage occurs.
End feel	The quality of resistance at end range. Examples of end feel include hard or bony, soft tissue, ligamentous, springy, and empty.
Contractile tissue	Tissues, including the muscle belly, musculotendinous junction, tendon, and tenoperiosteal bone, that are directly stressed by the process of isometric contraction during a resisted muscle test.
Noncontractile tissue	Tissues that are not directly mechanically stressed by isometric muscle contraction; includes ligaments, joint capsule, synovial membrane, articular cartilage, and intra-articular menisci.
Capsular pattern	Limitation of pain and movement loss in a joint-specific ratio, usually present with arthritis after prolonged immobilization. The capsular pattern in the glenohumeral joint is greatest limitation in external rotation, followed by abduction, and internal rotation.
Noncapsular pattern	Limitation in a joint in any pattern other than a capsular one reflecting either a derangement that obstructs joint motion, an extra-articular lesion that limits joint motion, or a dysfunction that affects one part of the capsule.

From Cyriax, J: Textbook of Orthopedic Medicine, Vol 1, ed 6. Balliere and Tindall, London, 1975.

presentation of signs and symptoms. The categories of impairments described by McKenzie include dysfunction, derangement, and postural syndrome. Patients with dysfunction syndrome present with limited motion in their lumbar spine with pain at end range. Those with derangement syndrome demonstrate an unstable nucleus pulposus that shifts position and produces pain based on the direction of repetitive active lumbar movement. Patients with postural syndrome present with impaired posture and pain when normal tissues are placed in abnormal positions. Although this treatment-based approach emphasizes impairments, this system is limited to the treatment of patients with spinal pathology.

Maitland[26] also incorporated the work of Cyriax in a more global system of evaluation and treatment based on signs and symptoms. Although tissue pathology influences treatment, the essential elements that guide treatment are clinical signs and symptoms. Use of this system by physical therapists requires that clinicians, when taking a history and performing an evaluation, recognize how clusters of signs and symptoms relate to different movement patterns. The effect of a specific treatment technique or program on reproducible signs and symptoms is reassessed to determine effectiveness.

Recently, an impairment-based diagnostic scheme for the upper extremity was described by Laslett.[27] Using this system, patients with tissue tightness in their shoulders are classified with *dysfunction* and typically present with limited and painful end range motion. These patients may have several pathologies, including myofascial restrictions, adhesive capsulitis, or secondary impingement. Patients with shoulder *derangement* present with full active and passive ROM but with a painful arc or pain or catching in the midrange of humeral elevation. Examples of pathologies in this category include labral tears or osteochondral fractures in the GH joint.

The contributions provided by these professionals have given physical therapists their own unique language and a process of clinical decision making based on the precepts of their professional training as clinical movement experts.

As the profession evolved through the 20th century, the need for a diagnostic classification system that accurately reflected practice patterns in physical therapy became apparent.[1] Today, the use of a disablement paradigm to guide clinical practice has been advocated.[1–5] Reviewing the process of disablement demonstrates how this model conforms to the scope of practice and definition of physical therapy.

PROCESS OF DISABLEMENT

The physical therapy model for musculoskeletal rehabilitation is based on *disablement* and focuses on the evaluation and treatment of impairments.[2] *Disablement* describes how disease or tissue pathology can lead to *impairments* and affect function (Fig. 4–1). For example, patients with severe rotator cuff tendonitis (tissue pathology) can have limited range of motion (impairment) and may not be able to comb their hair with the involved extremity (loss of function). Impairments, as mentioned previously, are the discrete losses or alterations in anatomy, structure, and action in body parts.[2] Specific impairments in the musculoskeletal system include loss of range of motion and muscle strength, abnormal posture, muscle spasms, and pain. Impairments may lead to *functional limitations* if accompanied by a restriction in the ability to perform a physical action, activity, or task in an efficient or expected manner. *Disability* results if an individual is unable to engage in age-specific, gender-specific, or sex-specific roles in a social context. In an effort to provide a framework for understanding and organizing physical therapy practice, the American Physical Therapy Association has incorporated these principals into a comprehensive guide that focuses on optimizing function through evaluation, treatment, prevention, and wellness strategies.[1] The evolution of the disablement model is presented in Chapter 3.

Disease-----Impairment-----Functional Limitations-----Disability

FIGURE 4–1. Nagi's Model of Disablement (Adapted from Nagi, SZ: Some conceptual issues in disability and rehabilitation. In Sussman, MB, (ed): Sociology and Rehabilitation: American Sociological Association, Washington, DC, 1965.)

GUIDE TO PHYSICAL THERAPIST PRACTICE

As stated in the *Guide to Physical Therapist Practice* (the *Guide*),[1] physical therapy seeks to embrace the process of disablement as the foundation for evaluation and treatment. This document includes newly revised descriptions of patient management, as well as preferred practice patterns or categories of diagnoses based on clusters of common impairments (Table 4–6). Preferred practice patterns are diagnostic groups defined by a common set of impairments and functional limitations, rather than pathologies. These practice patterns describe the boundaries within which physical therapists may select a number of clinical paths. Patients with different pathologies but with similar impairments may be classified in the same group. Because many shoulder conditions, regardless of their medical diagnoses, present with a common set of clinical findings, physical therapists should cluster these conditions under a common label of impairments.

Each practice pattern contains five elements, including examination, evaluation, diagnosis, prognosis, and intervention (Fig. 4–2). Through the examination (history, systems review, and tests and measures), the physical therapist identifies impairments, functional limitations, disabilities, or changes in physical function or health. The physical therapist performs an evaluation (makes clinical judgments) for the purpose of establishing the diagnosis and the prognosis. A *diagnosis*, a label encompassing a cluster of signs and symptoms, syndromes, or categories, is a result of the examination process, which includes evaluating, organizing, and interpreting examination data. An example of a musculoskeletal diagnosis for the shoulder is impingement syndrome due to impaired motor control. This diagnosis identifies a specific impairment, which guides treatment.

TABLE 4–6 Musculoskeletal Preferred Practice Patterns

Practice Pattern	Impairments
Pattern A	Primary prevention/risk factor reduction for skeletal demineralization
Pattern B	Impaired posture
Pattern C	Impaired muscle performance
Pattern D	Impaired joint mobility, motor function, muscle performance, and range of motion associated with capsular restriction
Pattern E	Impaired joint mobility, muscle performance, and range of motion associated with ligament or other connective tissue disorders
Pattern F	Impaired joint mobility, motor function, muscle performance, and range of motion associated with localized inflammation
Pattern G	Impaired joint mobility, motor function, muscle performance, range of motion, or reflex integrity secondary to spinal disorders
Pattern H	Impaired joint mobility, muscle performance, and range of motion associated with fracture
Pattern I	Impaired joint mobility, motor function, muscle performance, and range of motion associated with joint arthroplasty
Pattern J	Impaired joint mobility, motor function, muscle performance, and range of motion associated with bony or soft tissue surgical procedures
Pattern K	Impaired gait, locomotion, and balance and impaired motor function secondary to lower extremity amputation

Adapted from the Guide to Physical Therapist Practice, 1998.[1]

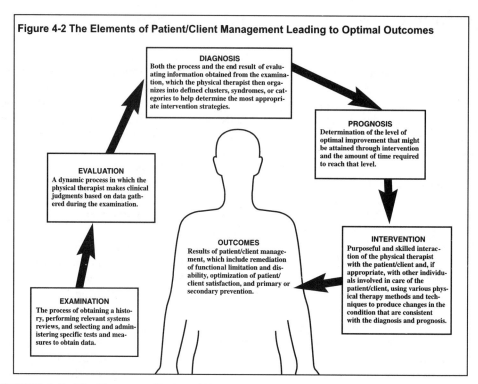

FIGURE 4–2. The Elements of Patient/Client Management Leading to Optimal Outcomes (From Guide to Physical Therapist Practice. Part One: Description of patient/client management and Part Two: Preferred practice patterns. Phys Ther 77:1163, 1997, with permission.)

Diagnosis by physical therapists differs from the medical diagnosis in its overall purpose and scope. Although the medical diagnosis is concerned with identifying the underlying pathology, diagnosis in physical therapy is concerned with determining its characteristics — the cause, nature, and extent of the problem. *Evaluation* in this model focuses on impairments, functional limitations, disabilities, or changes in physical health status resulting from injury, disease, surgical intervention, or other causes.

The *prognosis* is the determination of the optimal level of improvement that might be attained and the amount of time required to reach that level.[1] The prognosis includes establishing short and long-term goals. These goals are affected by degree of tissue pathology or extent of surgical procedure, general health condition of the patient including prior level of activity, and psychological factors. The physical therapist must consider these issues when developing treatment interventions.

Intervention is the purposeful and skilled interaction of the physical therapist with the patient to achieve treatment goals. Examples of musculoskeletal interventions include range of motion exercises, joint and soft tissue mobilization, flexibility exercises, strengthening and endurance training, proprioceptive exercises, and pain control with modalities.

The *Guide* is intended to serve as a changing and evolving document, which parallels the transition from the medical to the physical therapy model. The goal of this transition is to produce a uniform body of knowledge that clearly labels diagnostic categories of *selected* orthopedic conditions based on clusters of similar impairments. The following section presents a classification of shoulder conditions incorporating preferred practice patterns of the APTA.

CLASSIFICATION OF SHOULDER CONDITIONS

The APTA's *Guide to Physical Therapist Practice* classifies *dysfunction* based on clusters of impairments that are commonly attributed to various disorders, procedures, or conditions[1] (Table 4–7). Clustering impairments that occur in repeating patterns and result in functional limitations provide physical therapists with boundaries for effective treatment intervention. As the physical therapist becomes more experienced and proficient in recognizing these patterns in response to specific conditions, the hope is that clinical decision making and treatment pathways will become more refined and consistent. For example, restoring impaired shoulder mobility in a patient with a postoperative anterior stabilization procedure (pattern J) may follow treatment guidelines that are slightly different than restoring impaired mobility in a patient with adhesive capsulitis (pattern D). Protection of the anterior capsule in the early stages of rehabilitation is necessary for the patient who has had an anterior stabilization procedure. Pain and tissue inflammation are the primary limiting factors when restoring impaired mobility in the patient with adhesive capsulitis.

Every musculoskeletal practice pattern may not be appropriate for the shoulder. For example, pattern K refers to lower extremity amputation, which has little relevance for shoulder treatment. Other patterns, such as impaired posture (pattern B) and impaired muscle performance (pattern C), contain impairments that often occur concurrently with other conditions. When applied to the shoulder, impaired posture can be associated with impingement syndrome (pattern F) and impaired muscle performance can exist across multiple patterns (patterns D to J).

The clinician must also rule out all potential causes of shoulder symptoms when examining the shoulder. Chapter 10 integrates two musculoskeletal practice patterns (patterns B and G) and a neuromuscular practice pattern (pattern D) that include common conditions involving referred pain to the shoulder. These conditions include thoracic outlet syndrome, peripheral entrapment neuropathies, reflex sympathetic dystrophy, and adverse neural tension. This chapter integrates the relevant practice patterns to the principles of evaluation and treatment of the shoulder. The purpose of implementing practice patterns is to provide a meaningful classification, which guides treatment for physical therapists.

Pattern D

Practice pattern D involves impaired joint mobility, motor function, muscle performance, and range of motion associated with *capsular restriction.*

CLASSIFICATION

The primary impairment in pattern D is hypomobility due to capsular restriction. The term *adhesive capsulitis* is reserved for conditions where limited ROM is directly attributed to structural changes in periarticular tissues such as capsular contracture and adhesion formation. Because this condition also involves inflammation of the capsule, a patient with adhesive capsulitis could also be classified under musculoskeletal pattern F. Specific causes and pathophysiology of adhesive capsulitis will be discussed in Chapter 7. Secondary impairments in this pattern include decreased motor control and muscle performance. Practice pattern D also includes arthritic conditions of the shoulder girdle, which can also lead to capsular restriction, resulting in limited ROM.

TABLE 4–7 Classifications of Shoulder Conditions

APTA Practice Patterns	Impairments	Procedures/ Tissue Pathology	Clinical Findings
1. Pattern D (Capsular restriction)	a. Motor function b. Muscle performance c. Joint mobility d. ROM	a. Capsulitis b. Bursitis c. Tendinitis	a. Pain b. Limited ROM c. Capsular pattern of restriction d. Altered scapulohumeral rhythm e. Crepitus f. (+) Impingement
2. Pattern E (Connective tissue disorders)	a. Motor function b. Muscle performance c. ROM d. Joint mobility	a. Tendinitis b. Capsulitis c. Bursitis d. Synovitis e. Labral pathology	a. Pain with movements above 90° elevation b. (+) Apprehension c. (+) Sulcus sign d. Altered scapulohumeral rhythm e. (+) Relocation sign
3. Pattern F (Localized inflammation)	a. Motor function b. Muscle performance c. ROM d. Joint mobility	a. Tendinitis b. Bursitis c. Capsulitis	a. (+) Impingement sign b. Pain at end range elevation c. Altered scapulohumeral rhythm d. Weak rotator cuff e. Pain with resisted tests f. Tight posterior capsule
4. Pattern G (Spinal disorders)	a. Motor function b. Muscle performance c. ROM d. Joint mobility	a. Neural tension b. Nerve root	a. (+) Upper limb tension tests b. (+) Thoracic outlet signs c. (+) Nerve root compression signs
5. Pattern H (Fractures)	a. ROM b. Muscle performance c. Joint mobility	a. Scapula b. Humerus c. Clavicle	Same as above
6. Pattern I (Joint arthroplasty)	a. Motor function b. Muscle performance c. Joint mobility d. ROM	a. Glenohumeral AC, SC joint arthritis b. Humeral neck/ head fractures	Same as above
7. Pattern J (Bony/soft tissue surgical procedures)	a. Motor function b. Muscle performance c. Joint mobility d. ROM	a. Stabilization procedures b. Rotator cuff repair c. Capsule/labral repairs d. Debridement	Same as above

PATIENT PRESENTATION

Patients in pattern D present with a chief complaint of limited movement, usually accompanied by pain (Table 4–7). If structural changes are present, passive ROM will be restricted in a capsular pattern, a limitation of movement that occurs in a predictable pattern due to lesions in a joint capsule.[24] The pattern of glenohumeral restriction includes the greatest limitation in external rotation, followed by abduction, flexion, and internal rotation. Capsular limitation usually occurs after a period of immobilization following trauma or surgery (pattern H, I, J). Patients with shoulder hypomobility due to acute inflammation or internal derangement would have limitation in ROM in directions, which stress the inflamed tissue. Other findings include altered scapulohumeral rhythm and pain inhibition of inflamed tissues.

CLINICAL DECISION MAKING

The primary treatment goal in this category is restoring ROM. The concern for clinicians treating patients in this pattern is usually the degree of inflammation and irritability. Irritability is characterized by the following components: (1) pain intensity, (2) rigor of activity needed to elicit the symptoms, and (3) latent response of symptoms or how long it takes for the symptoms to resolve after provocation.[17] A highly irritable condition has a moderate to high intensity that is brought on by light activity and does not resolve within a few minutes. Patients presenting with capsular restriction and low irritability may require aggressive soft tissue and joint mobilization, whereas patients with high irritability may require pain-easing manual therapy techniques. Specific decision making in manual therapy of the shoulder will be discussed in Chapter 13.

Pattern E

Practice pattern E involves impaired joint mobility, muscle performance, and range of motion associated with *ligament* or *other connective tissue disorders.*

CLASSIFICATION

When applied to the shoulder, this pattern is referred to as instability. *Instability of the shoulder* is defined as excessive movement accompanied by specific signs and symptoms that interfere with function.[28] The cause of glenohumeral instability is a combination of ligamentous laxity and lack of neuromuscular control as defined in pattern E (Table 4–7). The ligaments serve as the primary restraints to movement, whereas the muscles around the shoulder provide secondary restraints.[11] The specific pathophysiology of instability will be discussed in Chapter 8. Although the primary impairment is instability, secondary impairments such as poor muscle performance may also exist.

PATIENT PRESENTATION

The chief complaint of patients with pattern E is typically pain with overhead movements, particularly in a position of abduction and external rotation (Table 4–7).

However, patients usually present with full active ROM and passive ROM. A history of the shoulder "slipping" or "popping out" during activities of daily living is often described. Activities usually associated with these symptoms include tennis serves, throwing, swimming backstroke, or playing volleyball. Physical examination may reveal impaired posture (pattern B), including excessive winging of the medial scapular border, downward rotation of the glenoid with excessive thoracic kyphosis.[29] Impaired posture can alter length-tension relationships of the muscles and joint arthrokinematics. Other common impairments include imbalances of the scapular and rotator cuff musculature and altered GH joint proprioception.

A positive apprehension sign, a positive relocation test, and a positive sulcus sign are used to confirm instability.[11] Chapter 8 will discuss special tests for instability.

As pattern E indicates, various tissue pathologies are common with this condition. Increased laxity of the ligaments and capsule require more dynamic control of the rotator cuff to hold the head of the humerus in the glenoid fossa. This increased stress can result in injury to the rotator cuff musculature.[12] Patients with this associated tissue pathology will usually have pain with resisted testing of the rotator cuff musculature. Increased translation can also result in glenoid labrum pathology or encroachment of the subacromial space causing secondary impingement. Patients with these tissue pathologies may test positive using Yergason's test, Speed's test, or impingement sign (see Chap. 8).

CLINICAL DECISION MAKING

Because nothing can be done in physical therapy to change capsular or ligamentous laxity, treatment for patients in this category must address motor control. *Motor control* is defined as the ability to learn or demonstrate the skillful and efficient assumption, maintenance, modification, and control of voluntary postures and movement patterns.[1] Addressing motor control problems involves treatment of impaired posture, abnormal movement patterns, dexterity, coordination, agility, and muscle weakness. Successful treatment results in enough dynamic stability to offset the inherent ligamentous laxity. Specific treatment strategies for neuromuscular control are described in Chapter 14.

Pattern F

Practice pattern F involves impaired joint mobility, motor function, muscle performance, and range of motion associated with *localized inflammation*.

CLASSIFICATION

Pattern F includes impaired ROM, motor function, and muscle performance attributed to inflammation. Conditions causing pain and muscle guarding without the presence of structural changes are included in this pattern (see Chap. 9). In these cases, the primary causes of hypomobility, impaired muscle performance and motor function, are attributed to a protective tissue response.[1] Protective tissue response is limitation in joint mobility due to pain, inflammation, muscle weakness or strain, neurovascular changes, sensory changes, or edema. Examples include the following: (1) sprains and strains of the acromioclavicular, sternoclavicular, and scapulothoracic joints; (2) internal derangements of the GH joint, such as labral pathology and rotator cuff tears; and (3) acute inflammatory conditions due to overuse, such as tendonitis, bursitis, capsulitis, and tenosynovitis. If these conditions are treated with prolonged immobilization or they become chronic, structural changes in the joint may occur (adhesive capsulitis) and patients could also be classified in pattern D.

Primary impingement is a term used to describe many conditions in practice pattern F. Primary impingement is defined as an encroachment of the tendons and/or bursa in the subacromial space between the greater tuberosity of the humerus and the inferior surface of the acromion.[30] Repetitive impingement can occur with overhead activities, leading to tissue microtrauma and inflammation as defined in practice pattern F. Both intrinsic and extrinsic factors can contribute to the development of primary impingement.[30] Intrinsic factors involve structures in the subacromial space and include changes in vascularity of the rotator cuff, degeneration and thickening of the soft tissue structures, and anatomic or bony anomalies. Extrinsic factors include muscle imbalances, motor control problems, tightness of the posterior capsule, and postural changes (pattern B) that can disturb scapulohumeral rhythm. *Scapulohumeral rhythm* is the pattern of concomitant and coordinated movement of the shoulder girdle, which allows the greatest ROM for the upper limb.[31] Normal scapulohumeral rhythm results from synergistic muscle activity between the rotator cuff, scapular stabilizers, and glenohumeral musculature, which allows ideal length-tension relationships and proper arthrokinematics during upper extremity movement. The etiology of this condition will be discussed in greater detail in Chapter 9.

Secondary impingement is caused by glenohumeral instability and is therefore classified in the category of instability (pattern E).

PATIENT PRESENTATION

Patients in practice pattern F typically have pain with movement more than 90° elevation, particularly when combined with forceful internal rotation (Table 4–7). Range of motion may be limited by pain at end range elevation or end range horizontal adduction. Restriction in the acromioclavicular (AC) joint may be noted, as well as weakness of the rotator cuff, and tightness of the posterior capsule. Symptoms are usually reproduced with an impingement test or combined flexion, internal rotation, and horizontal adduction. Pain resulting from impingement usually goes away when humeral distraction is applied, opening up the subacromial space. The most common tissue pathologies associated with this condition include supraspinatus and bicipital tendonitis, subacromial bursitis, and synovitis.

CLINICAL DECISION MAKING

When treating patients in this pattern, a clinician must determine whether inflammation is due to intrinsic or extrinsic factors. Intrinsic factors such as bony anomalies and soft tissue thickening may need to be addressed through surgical intervention. Inflammation is addressed through antiinflammatory modalities and medication. Physical therapy treatment of this pattern usually addresses extrinsic factors. Restoring normal scapulohumeral rhythm requires treatment of impaired motor function, posture, muscle performance, and ROM.

Referred Pain Syndromes: Integration of Musculoskeletal Patterns B and G, and Neuromuscular Pattern D

Referred pain syndromes, integration of musculoskeletal patterns B and G, and neuromuscular pattern D, involve impaired joint mobility, motor function, muscle performance, range of motion, or reflex integrity secondary to *reflex sympathetic dystrophy, spinal disorders, thoracic outlet syndrome,* and *peripheral entrapment neuropathies.*

CLASSIFICATION

This category encompasses practice patterns related to impairments affecting tissues and structures in the upper quarter of the body. The upper quarter of the body includes the occiput and the temporomandibular joint, cervical spine, shoulder girdle and limbs, thoracic spine and contiguous soft tissue, neural, and visceral structures. Chapters 1 and 2 in this text, as well as other authorities, indicate the interrelationship of structure and function in the upper quarter. Several studies have found associated soft tissue and muscle imbalances, and postural changes in the presence of shoulder pain and injury.[23] Referred pain in the shoulder, or symptoms that originate from an area other than the shoulder, is a common finding.[32] Because several tissues in the upper quarter share the same C5 to C6 spinal innervation with the GH joint capsule, physical evaluation requires a thorough upper quarter screening. Referred pain syndromes of the shoulder are discussed in Chapter 10.

Common conditions that can cause altered shoulder movement or pain include cervical/thoracic dysfunction,[33] adverse neural tension,[34] thoracic outlet syndrome,[35] sympathetic pain,[36] and myofascial pain syndromes.[37] This classification addresses the close relationship of signs and symptoms between the cervical/thoracic spine and shoulder girdle. This category may also include postsurgical patients (patterns I and J) who develop reflex sympathetic dystrophy[36] and patients with impaired posture (pattern B).

Impaired posture is commonly associated with referred pain to the shoulder. Posture is the alignment and positioning of the body relative to gravity, center of mass, and base of support.[38] Ideal posture is a state of musculoskeletal balance that protects the supporting structures of the body against injury or progressive deformity.[1] Patients with impaired posture have functional limitation associated with impairments of muscle weakness and imbalance, pain, structural deviations from normal posture, and altered joint mobility.

According to the practice patterns, if impaired posture contributes to radicular symptoms such as pain, paresthesia, analgesia, and motor weakness usually attributed to nerve root or trunk irritation,[36] patients are classified in neuromuscular pattern B. For example, the relationship between impaired posture and referred symptoms includes irritation of the brachial plexus in the presence of forward head posture (thoracic outlet syndrome or adverse neural tension). Forward head posture is typically characterized by rounded shoulders, cervical back bending, and increased thoracic kyphosis.[38] This posture can lead to soft tissue restriction of the anterior shoulder musculature, suboccipital musculature, and shoulder rotators. The relationships among radicular signs, postural impairment, and shoulder symptoms provide a logical basis for clustering these patterns into one category.

PATIENT PRESENTATION

Physical examination may reproduce symptoms during cervical/thoracic spine provocation tests, upper limb tension tests, and thoracic outlet syndrome tests (Table 4–7). Patients in this classification may have full, pain-free ROM, and special tests of the shoulder may fail to yield any positive results. Additional findings can include impaired posture (as described previously), altered sensation, changes in deep tendon reflexes, and muscle weakness. If sympathetic involvement exists, findings may include trophic changes in the skin, hypersensitivity throughout the upper extremity, and circulatory disturbances.

CLINICAL DECISION MAKING

Determining treatment for patients in this category should involve consideration of the source of the symptoms and may involve mobilization of the cervical/thoracic spine, soft tissue structures, and nerves as they relate to shoulder dysfunction. If impaired posture is contributing to the dysfunction, clinicians may consider patient education for proper stretching, strengthening, and ergonomic postures.

Pattern H

Pattern H involves impaired joint mobility, muscle performance, and range of motion associated with *fracture.*

CLASSIFICATION

Patients in this category will have an upper extremity fracture that affects function of the shoulder complex. Primary impairments in this category are restricted range of motion and decreased muscle performance attributed to disuse.

PATIENT PRESENTATION

Patients usually present following a period of immobilization ranging from 3 to 6 weeks. Hypomobility of the GH joint, with possible involvement of the AC or sternoclavicular (SC) joints, is usually noted. Atrophy of the deltoid and rotator cuff musculature may be observed. As a result of this atrophy, a "squaring" of the acromion may be noted. Resisted muscle testing may yield generalized muscle weakness of the shoulder girdle musculature.

CLINICAL DECISION MAKING

Treatment of patients in this category will focus on addressing impaired joint mobility and impaired muscle performance. Clinicians treating patients following a fracture are faced with many considerations. Patient age, presence of osteoporosis, location of the fracture, type of fracture, and type of reduction can all affect rehabilitation. Although most fractures heal within 5 to 8 weeks, clinicians must understand the individual healing constraints that guide treatment.

Patterns I and J

Patterns I and J involve impaired joint mobility, motor function, muscle performance, and range of motion associated with *joint arthroplasty* or *surgical procedures.*

CLASSIFICATION

Clinicians treating patients following soft tissue surgical procedures or total joint arthroplasty must consider healing constraints when addressing impaired ROM, motor function, and muscle performance. The type of surgical approach used will affect the rehabilitation program. Some procedures require the surgeon to perform an arthrotomy to create a larger field of vision or to have more room for surgical repair. However, arthrotomy involves opening the joint capsule, resulting in more tissue damage than arthroscopy. Additional tissue damage may occur when a surgeon uses muscle resection instead of muscle splitting. Muscle splitting is the process of entering a joint capsule through intervals in the muscle belly, rather than cutting through muscle fibers and resecting the tissue. More pain, swelling, and muscle inhibition occur with more tissue damage. Surgical fixation and, in the case of joint arthroplasty, the type of prosthesis used and use of cement should also be considered in rehabilitation.

PATIENT PRESENTATION

Similar to practice pattern H (fractures), patients in practice patterns I and J usually present following a period of immobilization ranging from 3 to 6 weeks. Hypomobility of the shoulder girdle is usually noted resulting from the period of immobilization and soft tissue scarring. Atrophy of the deltoid and rotator cuff musculature may be observed, resulting in a "squared" appearance of the acromion. Resisted muscle testing may yield generalized muscle weakness of the shoulder girdle musculature.

CLINICAL DECISION MAKING

When treating impairments in a patient who has had a soft tissue surgical procedure or a total shoulder arthroplasty, several considerations must be addressed. The extent of the tissue pathology, location of tissue pathology, and type of surgical fixation will affect treatment progression. By knowing the location, extent of tissue damage, and type of fixation, a clinician will know which exercises and motions are safe and which to avoid. In addition, clinicians must understand soft tissue healing constraints to ensure that patients are progressed quickly enough to avoid complications, but not at a rate that can compromise the surgical procedure.

CHAPTER SUMMARY

The medical model of diagnosing pathology to determine treatment strategies is not consistent with the practice of physical therapy for identifying and correcting impairments to optimize function. Subsequently, the impairment-based diagnosis of shoulder conditions was developed to provide a framework for developing clinical guidelines for rehabilitation.

Differential diagnosis of selected shoulder conditions formally introduced and popularized by Codman,[7] recognized the importance of clinical diagnosis by clustering signs and symptoms to pathology. His system of differential diagnosis served as a template for the evolution of the medical model. Neer[10] further refined the process of differential diagnosis by offering a comprehensive description of mechanical impingement with specific correlated impairments. The identification and correction of the underlying impairment became as important to treatment as identifying the tissue pathology. Patients with rotator cuff tendonitis were differentiated with either glenohumeral hypermobility or hypomobility. Restoration of normal shoulder mobility to prevent recurrent problems was a primary goal of treatment.

The role and scope of physical therapy practice based on the theoretical framework of movement science became increasingly focused on the identification and correction of patients with impairments and functional limitations. Therapists such as McKenzie and Maitland, spurred by Cyriax, formulated systems of physical therapy diagnosis based on impairments. These systems provided the framework for treatment consistent with the scope and goals of physical therapy practice. The process of disablement recently outlined by the APTA into "preferred practice patterns," provided boundaries within which physical therapists can choose different clinical paths. Impairment-based categories of shoulder injuries are designed to help physical therapists practice in a framework consistent with the process of disablement; that is, the impact of conditions on function. For physical therapists to remain accountable to the public they serve, like other health-care professionals, they must practice in a manner consistent with the scope of their practice.

REFERENCES

1. Guide to Physical Therapist Practice. Part One: Description of patient/client management; and Part Two: Preferred practice patterns. Phys Ther 77:1163, 1998.
2. Dekker, J, et al: Diagnosis and treatment in physical therapy: An investigation of their relationship. Phys Ther 73:568, 1993.
3. Guccione, AA: Physical therapy diagnosis and the relationship between impairment and function. Phys Ther 71:499, 1991.
4. Sahrman, SA: Diagnosis by the physical therapist—A prerequisite for treatment: A special communication. Phys Ther 68:1703, 1988.
5. Rose, SJ: Physical therapy diagnosis: Role and function. Phys Ther 69:535, 1989.
6. Jette, AM: Diagnosis and classification by physical therapists: A special communication. Phys Ther 69:967, 1989.
7. Codman, EA: The Shoulder, ed 2. Thomas Todd, Boston, 1934.
8. International Classification of Impairments, Disabilities, and Handicaps. World Health Organization, Geneva, Switzerland, 1980.
9. Nagi, SZ: Some conceptual issues in disability and rehabilitation. In Sussman, MB, (ed): Sociology and Rehabilitation. American Sociological Association, Washington, DC, 1965, p100.
10. Neer, CS: Impingement lesions. Clin Orthop 173:70, 1973.
11. Jobe, FW, and Pink, M: Classification and treatment of shoulder dysfunction in the overhead athlete. J Orthop Sports Phys Ther 18:427, 1993.
12. Meister, MD, and Andrews, JR: Classification and treatment of rotator cuff injuries in the overhand athlete. J Orthop Sports Phys Ther 18:413, 1993.
13. Litchfield, R, et al: Rehabilitation for the overhead athlete. J Orthop Sports Phys Ther 18:433, 1993.
14. Wilk, KE, and Arrigo, C: Current concepts in the rehabilitation of the athletic shoulder. J Orthop Sports Phys Ther 18: 365, 1993.
15. Gowan, ID, et al: Electromyographic analysis of the shoulder during pitching. Am J Sports Med 15:586, 1987.

16. Glousman, R, et al: Dynamic electromyographic analysis of the throwing shoulder with glenohumeral instability. J Bone Joint Surg 70A: 2220, 1988.
17. McMaster, WC, et al: Shoulder torque changes in the swimming athlete. Am J Sports Med 20:323, 1992.
18. Alderink, GL, and Kuck, DJ: Isokinetic strength of high school and college-aged pitchers. J Orthop Sport Phys Ther 7:163, 1986.
19. Chandler, TJ, et al: Shoulder strength, power, and endurance in college tennis players. Am J Sports Med 20:455, 1992.
20. Brown, LP, et al: Upper extremity range of motion and isokinetic strength of the internal and external shoulder rotators in major league baseball players. Am J Sports Med 16:577, 1988.
21. Albert, MS, and Wooden, MJ: Isokinetic evaluation and treatment. In Donatelli, R (ed): Physical Therapy of the Shoulder. Churchill Livingstone, New York, 1997, p 401.
22. Falkel, JE, and Murphy, TC. Case principles: Swimmers shoulder, In Malone, TR (ed): Shoulder Injuries. Williams and Wilkins, Baltimore, 1988.
23. Kibler, WB: Role of the scapula in the overhead throwing motion. Contemp Orthop 22:525, 1991.
24. Cyriax, J: Textbook of Orthopedic Medicine, Vol 1, Diagnosis of soft tissue lesions, ed 7. Sailiere and Tindall, London, 1978.
25. McKenzie, RA: The Lumbar Spine: Mechanical Diagnosis and Therapy. Spinal Publications, Waikanae, New Zealand, 1989.
26. Maitland, GD: Vertebral Manipulation, ed 5. London: Butterworth, London, 1987.
27. Laslett, M: Mechanical Diagnosis and Therapy: The Upper Limb. Mark Laslett, New Zealand, 1996.
28. Matsen III, FA, et al: Mechanics of glenohumeral instability. Clinics Sports Med 10: 783, 1991.
29. Kvitne, RS, and Jobe, FW: The diagnosis and treatment of anterior instability in the throwing athlete. Clin Orthop 291:107, 1993.
30. Greenfield, SH, and Thein, LA: Impingement syndrome and impingement related instability. In Donatelli, RA (ed): Physical Therapy of the Shoulder, ed 3. Churchill Livingstone, New York, 1997, p 229.
31. Norkin, C, and Levangie, P: Joint Structure and Function: A Comprehensive Analysis, FA Davis, Philadelphia, 1985.
32. Overton, LM: Causes of pain in the upper extremities: A differential diagnosis study. Clin Orthop 51:27, 1967.
33. Dillon, W, et al: Cervical radiculopathy: A review. Spine 11 (suppl)10:988, 1986.
34. Markey, KL, et al: Upper trunk brachial plexopathy: The stinger syndrome. Am J Sports Med 21:650, 1993.
35. Strukel, RJ, and Garrick, JG: Thoracic outlet compression in athletes. Am J Sports Med 6:3, 1978.
36. Caillet, R: Sympathetic referred pain. In Caillet, R: Shoulder Pain. FA Davis, Philadelphia, 1981.
37. Travell, JG, and Simons, DG: Myofascial Pain and Dysfunction: The Trigger Point Manual. Williams and Wilkins, Baltimore, 1983.
38. Kendall, HO, et al: Muscles: Testing and Function, ed 2. Williams and Wilkins, Baltimore, 1971.

CHAPTER 5

Clinical Examination of the Shoulder

Kevin Cappel, MS, PT, SCS, ATC, CSCS
Michael A. Clark, MS, PT, CSCS
George J. Davies, Med, PT, SCS, ATC, CSCS
Todd S. Ellenbecker, MS, PT, SCS, CSCS

INTRODUCTION

According to the *Guide to Physical Therapist Practice*, physical assessment of a patient involves the following four components: examination, evaluation, diagnosis, and prognosis.[1] The *examination* refers to the process of obtaining a history, performing relevant systems review, and selecting and administering specific tests and measures to obtain data. *Evaluation* is a dynamic process involving clinical decision making by the physical therapist based on data gathered during the examination. The information and data obtained in the examination and evaluation are organized to define clusters of signs and symptoms that are unique to a specific condition or syndrome. This categorization process, *diagnosis*, helps determine the most appropriate intervention strategies. Based on the information from these three components, clinicians formulate a *prognosis*, the level of optimal improvement that might be obtained through intervention delivered for a specified time period.

The interrelationship of the multiple joints composing the shoulder girdle makes evaluation and treatment difficult.[2] Impairment at one joint can affect function of the entire shoulder complex, making a comprehensive examination even more challenging. The mobility of the shoulder joint, in conjunction with the demands placed on the shoulder complex during activities of daily living, work, and recreational and competitive sports, result in a high incidence of injuries. Therefore, an understanding of shoulder activity and mechanics (see Chapters 1 and 2) with patterns of impairments allows the clinician to perform more efficient examination procedures and treatment interventions. This chapter describes the elements of examination and evaluation, including specific tests and measures used to assess shoulder impairments and dysfunction.

EXAMINATION AND EVALUATION PROCEDURES

The examination process in physical therapy is quite different from the assessment process in medicine. The goal of the physical therapy examination is to obtain a thorough history and use an adequate number of tests for accurate diagnosis of a patient within appropriate practice patterns. As stated in Chapter 5, the goals of a physical therapy examination are to:

1. Determine whether the findings from the examination and evaluation suggest that a referral to a medical specialist is indicated. The clinician must decide if there is a physical therapy problem.
2. Determine the impairments:
   a. Does the patient require increased mobility?
   b. Does the patient require improved muscle performance?
   c. Does the patient require improved motor control?
   d. Does the patient require symptomatic management or treatment of inflammation?
   (Regardless of the practice pattern, treatment will address one or more of these questions.)
3. Determine the functional limitations and the relationship between the impairments and functional limitations.
4. Determine the reason(s) for specific impairments, based on Preferred Practice Patterns.

The number of special tests described for shoulder examination often presents a dilemma for the clinician. Some textbooks list more than 60 special tests for the shoulder,[3] but it is unlikely that a clinician will perform all of these tests. The senior author has developed a testing sequence that has been used for several years, which provides an efficient mechanism for examining the shoulder.[4] This testing sequence is presented in the Special Tests section of this chapter. The integration of the Preferred Practice Patterns also provides a framework for an efficient examination process.

Ensuring that the patient's condition is appropriate for physical therapy and identifying specific impairments according to practice patterns facilitates treatment intervention. The practice patterns provide the parameters of a treatment based on soft tissue healing, inflammation, and irritability. For example, the goal of addressing hypomobility might be similar for all patients with restricted range of motion, but the techniques used to restore motion might be different. Using the practice patterns helps to guide how fast or how slow this goal might be accomplished based on soft tissue healing and inflammation.

The nature and extent of shoulder impairments might not always be evident. As part of the physical therapy assessment process, the clinician should determine the tissue pathology that is involved. Ultimately, the examination and evaluation process should result in a diagnosis.

History

A thorough subjective assessment of patients with shoulder dysfunction is an important element of the evaluation process.[5] The components described below should be included as part of a history.

CHIEF COMPLAINT AND DESCRIPTION OF SYMPTOMS

The patient's chief complaint or complaints typically involve pain, limited motion, weakness, instability, sensory changes, and crepitus (grinding and/or grating between the articular surfaces). The examiner attempts to quantify the degree, severity, and exact location of these factors based on the patient's subjective responses through a sequential, organized dialogue with the patient. During the subjective evaluation of the shoulder, the examiner attempts to delineate and localize the symptoms to the injured segment or segments. If a patient reports radicular symptoms into the distal upper extremity, constant pain without change or relief, referred pain to the head or neck, spinal pain, or psychological issues, further objective evaluation outside the upper extremity kinetic chain or referral to a specialist might be indicated.[6]

ONSET

Whereas many variations exist in the types of questions to be asked, the following four questions are essential when determining the onset:

1. What is the problematic area?
2. How did the problem occur?
3. When did the problem develop?
4. Where did the problem occur?

Whereas these might seem overly simplistic, these questions provide succinct, basic information[5] that can help distinguish between microtrauma and macrotrauma or help identify intrinsic and extrinsic predisposing factors to guide treatment.

LOCATION OF SYMPTOMS

Determining the location of the symptoms will guide the objective portion of the evaluation process. Isolating the area of discomfort is often difficult for the patient with an overuse injury to the rotator cuff because of the close proximity of the tendons at their humeral insertion.[7] The rotator cuff muscles conjoin at their insertion along the humerus. In addition, the biceps tendon is ensheathed by the subscapularis and supraspinatus tendon. These anatomical configurations complicate the isolation of a direct point of injury in these structures.[7]

Embryologically, the shoulder is derived from C4, C5, and C6. Tissues sharing these same spinal dermatomes, sclerotomes, and myotomes can refer pain to the shoulder. A patient presenting with referred symptoms to the lateral aspect of the shoulder or upper extremity requires objective testing to rule out other joints and soft tissue structures, including the cervical spine, which might be causing the pain. Confirmation of the location of patient symptoms is often achieved through the use of a body chart.[6]

IRRITABILITY AND BEHAVIOR OF SYMPTOMS

Irritability is classified by assessing the severity of the symptoms, aggregating and easing factors, and a latent response.[5,8] Typically, analog scales are used and recommended for quantifying a patient's pain level or severity. A patient rates the resting pain and pain during activity on a 10 point scale. The patient's ratings are used for comparison between visits and following treatment or activity trials.

Using the analog scale involves asking the patient to rate the pain from 0 to 10, with "0" being no pain, and "10" being the worst pain they have ever encountered. By assessing aggravating and easing factors, the clinician gains information on the level of activity needed to provoke the symptoms. A highly irritable condition might be aggravated by low levels of activity, followed by a long latent response (the amount of time required for the symptoms to resolve). For example, patients who experience a pain level of 8 to 10 brought on by reaching above their head with symptoms not resolving for 2 to 3 hours would be classified as highly irritable. Conversely, patients who experience a pain level of 8 to 10 for a few seconds when serving a tennis ball would not be classified as highly irritable. In the first instance, care is necessary to avoid provoking symptoms during the assessment process because the symptoms will not resolve for a few hours. As a result, completing the assessment on the first day will be unlikely.

Additional attempts at quantifying the patient's pain and functional limitations are commonly achieved using rating scales.[9–11] These scales are generally used to evaluate the outcome of a specific surgical procedure, or to determine the effectiveness of a treatment process. The use of specific scales for assessing outcomes of shoulder function are discussed in Chapter 6.

The severity of symptoms is not the only factor that determines the level of irritability. Because certain positions can exacerbate shoulder symptoms, a clinician should also assess sleeping positions when assessing the behavior of symptoms. Inquiring whether the patient can sleep on the involved side is one question to be used to evaluate the presence of night pain and sleeping position. In an MRI study, Salem-Bertof et al.[12] demonstrated that subacromial space was narrower in a position of scapular protraction compared to scapular retraction. In a side lying position, the scapula is protracted, possibly resulting in narrowing of the subacromial space. A patient who presents with primary glenohumeral (GH) joint impingement should be discouraged from resting in a side lying position.

Assessing the level of activity during the history will help guide treatment. For example, when questioning an athlete involved in overhead activities who has pain with throwing or serving, confirming the presence of pain when throwing or serving does not provide enough information to properly diagnose and formulate a treatment plan. The examiner needs to determine the stage of the throwing or serving motion in which the pain occurs and the number of repetitions needed to produce the symptoms. This information provides insight into what structure or structures are involved. Each stage of the throwing motion or tennis serve involves specific muscular recruitment patterns and joint kinematics, which can assist in identifying whether the source of the symptoms is compressive forces or tensile forces.[5] Subtle instability of the GH joint during the cocking phase of overhead activities can produce impingement or compressive symptoms.[13–15] Conversely, a feeling of instability or loss of control at the GH joint during the follow-through phase with predominantly an eccentric contraction of the rotator cuff can indicate a tensile rotator cuff injury.[15] Additional questions regarding a change in sports equipment, ergonomic environment, and training history and habits provide information that is imperative in understanding the stresses leading to the injury.

SYSTEMS REVIEW

Some systemic diseases such as gout, syphilis, gonorrhea, sickle cell anemia, hemophilia, rheumatic disease, and metastatic cancer (breast, prostrate, kidney, lung, thyroid) might also present as shoulder pain.[16] Other conditions affecting the structures in the chest and abdomen can also refer pain to the shoulder girdle. These conditions include: disease processes involving the cervical spine (bone tumors, metastasis, tuberculosis, cervical cord tumors, nodes in the neck, mastodynia), axilla, thorax, thoracic spine, chest wall (angina, pericarditis, aortic aneurysm, pulmonary tuberculosis, Pancoast's tumor, lung cancer, spontaneous pneumothorax, breast cancer, hiatal hernia), and abdomen (liver disease, ruptured spleen, peptic ulcer, gallbladder disease, hiatal hernia, upper urinary tract infection). In addition, pain of cardiac and diaphragmatic origin is often experienced in the shoulder.[16]

PAST HISTORY

An understanding of the patient's past history of shoulder injury helps guide treatment and determine the prognosis. For example, a clinician treating a patient with instability must determine whether the patient is experiencing a "one time" anterior dislocator from a traumatic event (TUBS classification of Matsen), or if the patient has chronic instability of the GH joint from repetitive stresses and an atraumatic onset of injury (AMBRI classification of Matsen).[17] Although two patients might have similar physical findings, a patient with multiple episodes of atraumatic instability is a more likely candidate for surgery. Another example of the importance of obtaining a thorough history relating to shoulder pathology is demonstrated during the examination of a mature athlete with a rotator cuff injury from overhead activity. Complete questioning of the patient might reveal a fall onto the lateral aspect of the shoulder, possibly 20 to 30 years ago, or a shoulder separation during high school football. This type of information can aid in understanding the patient's impingement-type symptoms. Encroachment of the subacromial space because of degenerative changes in the acromioclavicular (AC) joint from previous injury has been reported as an etiological factor in impingement lesions.[18]

The clinician should also ask about any treatment intervention used previously and its level of effectiveness. Additionally, information about previous surgical procedures, steroid injections, therapeutic modalities, and exercise programs can help formulate an evaluation-based treatment program for a patient.

ACTIVITIES OF DAILY LIVING: VOCATIONAL AND AVOCATIONAL GOALS

Knowledge of the patient's goals assists the clinician in developing an assessment and treatment plan that addresses the functional demands of a specific vocational or avocational activity. Testing the shoulder in positions that reproduce functional movement patterns of each patient will lead to a more accurate diagnosis and will help to formulate a more individualized treatment program.

At the completion of the history and the subjective examination, the clinician should have formulated an idea regarding primary impairments, what structures might be involved, and what tests and measures will be needed during the physical examination to confirm a diagnosis.

Physical Tests and Measures

The physical examination establishes a database that is used for patient reassessment during the course of rehabilitation.[6,8,19] The components of the objective physical examination are described in Box 5–1. The physical examination accomplishes two major objectives. One objective of the physical examination is to provide a series of provocative tests to either implicate or rule out the involvement of specific tissue structures. Knowing the tissue structure and the degree of pathology helps determine whether the patient is a candidate for rehabilitation. If the patient is suitable, the diagnosis of tissue pathology helps guide the treatment plan. Clinicians use this information to determine how much or how little can be done in treatment.

The other objective of the physical examination is to identify the impairments

---

BOX 5–1 Components of the Objective Physical Examination

Observation and posture
Posture
Gait evaluation
Anthropometric measurements
Referral/related joint clearing tests
Palpation
Neurological examination
- Sensation
- Reflexes
- Manual muscle testing
- Proprioception/kinesthetic testing
Active range of motion testing
- Codman's scapulohumeral rhythm
- Painful arc syndrome
- Shoulder shrug sign
- Apley's scratch tests
- Capsular pattern limitations
PROM testing
- End-feels
- Pain resistance sequence
- Accessory joint motion
Flexibility Testing
Special Tests
- Thoracic outlet syndrome tests
- Biceps brachii tests
- Transverse humeral ligament tests
- Impingement syndrome tests
- Rotator cuff partial or full thickness tear tests
- Acromioclavicular joint tests
- Glenoid labrum tests
- Instability tests
- Shoulder functional testing algorithm
Isokinetic testing
- Bilateral comparisons
- Unilateral strength ratios
- Peak torque/body weight ratios
- Descriptive normative data
- Total arm strength
Functional testing
- Functional Throwing Performance Index
- Closed kinetic chain upper extremity stability test
Biomechanical analysis
Medical tests

associated with the tissue pathology. In some cases, tissue pathology leads to impairments, although in other cases, impairments can cause tissue pathology.

The physical examination should always start with the uninvolved side for the following reasons:

1. Provides a database for a bilateral comparison.
2. Allows the patient to "experience the tests" to be performed on the involved side, and therefore decreases apprehension or anxiety about the testing procedures.
3. Provides a starting reference point to be used for reassessment during rehabilitation.
4. Provides information that can be used for clinical research.
5. Allows the clinician to learn what is "normal" for that patient, that is, how much passive anterior translation occurs on the load and shift test on the uninvolved side, so that an appropriate comparison can be made.

INITIAL OBSERVATION

The physical examination begins when the patient is first seen by the clinician. This initial observation can reveal a great deal of information. General observations of upper extremity positioning and active movement patterns during shaking hands and taking off a shirt, for example, offer the clinician a general idea of upper extremity function. A patient with shoulder pain typically protects the upper extremity by using compensatory movements when performing functional activities.[3,6,19-24]

Throughout the examination process, the clinician also needs to assess the patient's willingness to move the involved extremity,[6,19,21] noting consistency of motion. A patient who can easily move an arm overhead while disrobing, but can only minimally elevate the extremity while active range of motion is being assessed, demonstrates an inconsistency. The clinician must then determine if the inconsistency is attributed to physiological or psychosocial impairments.[23]

Proper exposure is necessary to allow visual inspection of the shoulder complex during the examination process. Males should disrobe from the waist up; females should wear a gown that allows adequate exposure of the shoulder girdle.[3,6,19-24] A methodical inspection is performed to assess soft-tissue and structures. Bony prominences and joint geometry for all joints in the shoulder girdle are viewed for asymmetry or deformity. Enlargement of the sternoclavicular (SC) or AC joints should be noted. Elevation of the distal end of the clavicle suggests a previous AC joint sprain or dislocation.[3,21,24] Depression of the clavicle and shoulder girdle might be because of loss of shoulder elevation, possibly associated with chronic spinal nerve injury or fascioscapulohumeral muscular dystrophy.[23]

Observation of muscle symmetry and contours should be noted because specific muscle atrophy might suggest certain diagnoses.[24] Atrophy of the deltoid from axillary nerve neuropathy results in a squared appearance of the lateral shoulder, exposing the lateral acromion.[21,24] Excessive prominence of the scapular spine is an indication of supraspinatus and infraspinatus wasting, which can be attributed to pathology of the musculotendinous unit, cervical nerve root, suprascapular nerve, or upper brachial plexus.[23,24] Atrophy of the posterior deltoid is often observed in patients with multidirectional instability.[24] Tendon rupture produces noticeable muscle contour changes, as in the "Popeye" muscle that results from a long head of the biceps tendon rupture. Detection of muscle bulk changes in patients who are deconditioned or obese requires astute visualization enhanced by active contraction and or palpation.[23]

The girth and lengths of both arms, upper extremity alignment, and relationships to the trunk as they hang by the sides are noted. Shoulder heights should be examined. Caution is necessary when interpreting differences, which might be caused by upper extremity dominance.[6,19,24]

POSTURE

Posture, the optimal alignment of the patient's body that allows the neuromuscular system to perform actions requiring the least amount of energy to achieve the desired effect,[25] is evaluated to determine scapular and spinal alignment. The shoulder girdle should be evaluated from anterior, lateral, and posterior views in both sitting and standing. Assessment also should include the cervical and thoracic spine because muscular attachments connect the shoulder girdle to the spine.[19,25]

Although posture varies among individuals, an optimal posture does exist.[6,19] Optimal posture in a relaxed standing position can be defined in relation to the hypothetical line of gravity acting vertically downward. Using a plumbline to represent gravity, normal alignment can be described in both the sagittal and frontal planes. In an ideal sagittal alignment, a plumb line traverses through the patient's ear, lateral midacromion, scapula, greater trochanter, midlateral knee between the popliteal fossa and the patella, and anterior to the lateral malleolus.[6]

Clinicians must also assess static and dynamic scapular orientation. Although the exact height might differ from side to side because of unilateral dominance, the spines of the scapulae typically begin medially at the level of the third thoracic vertebra (T3). The scapula should extend from the T2 spinous process, with the inferior scapular angle at the level of the T7 spinous process and the medial border of the scapula positioned 5 to 9 cm from the spinous process.[3,22,23]

Because extremity dominance can affect scapular orientation,[26] bilateral comparisons should always be noted when performing a postural assessment for the purpose of normalization. Greater unilateral activity usually results in greater asymmetry, particularly in pitchers and tennis players.[26] Static scapular winging should be noted because this postural deviation might be associated with long thoracic nerve neuropathy or weakness of the serratus anterior and lower trapezius.[23] Scapular winging, which often becomes more noticeable during dynamic functional activities, might be associated with glenohumeral dysfunction. Observing the patient performing a wall push-up might demonstrate more pronounced scapular winging.[3,6,19,21–24]

Changes in normal postural alignment during relaxed standing or sitting can potentially activate a long-term postural impairment with associated muscle imbalances and impaired joint mobility and motor function. A sedentary individual who sits or stands with posterior pelvic tilt, lumbar flexion, increased thoracic flexion (kyphosis), and a forward head position usually has rounded shoulders. Prolonged positioning in this posture significantly alters the normal arthrokinematics of the shoulder girdle, resulting in abnormal scapulohumeral rhythm. This position can also result in adaptive shortening of the anterior chest and shoulder musculature with lengthening and weakness of the posterior musculature.[6,19,25] Additionally, decreased range of motion might result from limited scapular rotation during arm elevation and decreased trunk and rib expansion.[23] Repetitive functional overhead activities in this position could potentially predispose the shoulder to microtraumatic soft-tissue injury, including impingement.

GAIT EVALUATION

As part of the initial observation, gait is examined to observe freedom of arm swing, reciprocal upper extremity movement, position of the arms and scapulae, and motion of the trunk and lower extremities.[6,19] Any noticeable breakdown along the kinetic chain in terms of inflexibility, improper motion, muscle imbalances, or weakness can cause disruption and breakdown in the kinetic chain.[25]

ANTHROPOMETRIC MEASUREMENTS

Anthropometric measurements have limited value in shoulder evaluation. Girth measurements taken at the midupper arm, elbow, midforearm, and wrist might show differences from the opposite extremity, possibly suggesting effusion or distal dependent edema.[6,19]

REFERRAL AND RELATED JOINT CLEARING

All structures capable of causing referred symptoms to the shoulder complex must be evaluated for possible involvement. The cervical spine, the shoulder girdle and upper extremity, and the thorax are collectively referred to as a kinetic chain. The kinetic chain principle recognizes the interrelationships of each joint segment to adjoining segments (see Chap. 10). Involvement of one structure can significantly affect other structures in the kinetic chain and result in dynamic compensatory changes.[3,6,19,25] The structures and syndromes described below can refer pain or cause dysfunction in the shoulder girdle.

Cervical Spine

Problems in the cervical spine can be ruled out through an accurate history and by a series of provocative tests. The patient performs active cervical spine range of motion in the six directions (flexion, extension, right/left lateral flexion, and right/left rotation). Overpressure is applied to the end range of motion to determine if noncontractile structures are responsible for the referring symptoms. Isometric resisted tests performed at midrange of each direction are used to stress the contractile units. Passive spring testing is performed on each cervical segment to assess accessory motion. If these tests do not reproduce symptoms, the cervical spine can be ruled out as a source of pain.

The cervical quadrant test is a nonspecific yet excellent test to determine cervical involvement. The head is extended, laterally flexed, and rotated to the ipsilateral side. Overpressure is then applied, which further compresses the posterolateral disc, facet joint, and foraminal space on the side of motion. Although this test does not always isolate a particular cervical level or structure, a reproduction of the patient's symptoms suggests involvement of the cervical spine.[3,6,19,22,23]

Temporomandibular Joint

To check for local swelling or tenderness resulting from the temporomandibular joint, the patient opens and closes his or her mouth to demonstrate changes in range of motion, presence of clicks, or pain with movement.[6,19] In extreme cases, pain can be referred to the shoulder region. Shoulder symptoms originating from this area are usually detected while obtaining the patient's history.

Thoracic Outlet Syndrome

Thoracic outlet syndrome (TOS) usually includes symptoms of pain, numbness, or tingling in the shoulder girdle and upper extremity.[27-33] Various conditions can cause or contribute to this condition, including poor posture, fascial fusions of muscles, malunion of old clavicular fractures, pseudoarthrosis of the clavicle, exostosis of the first rib, adverse neural tension, and a cervical rib. Many tests are used to diagnose this condition, but these tests have low reliability and specificity.[27-33]

Costosternal Joint

Swelling in the area of the costosternal joint might indicate inflammation or subluxation of the joint (Tietze's Syndrome). Both conditions will be tender to palpation. However, if costosternal subluxation is the primary problem, the symptoms usually decrease when the subluxation is manually reduced by finger pressure. Additionally, elevating and lowering the arms or breathing deeply might elicit symptoms if a costosternal subluxation exists.

The application of manual compression of the ribs followed by sudden release is one method of evaluating these conditions. If pain occurs with testing, the joint or joints are palpated to assess for abnormal motion and to identify which joint might be referring pain into the shoulder girdle.[6,19]

Costovertebral and Costotransverse Joints

Inspection of these joints rarely shows swelling unless a complete dislocation is present. If subluxation is present, mild tenderness on palpation might be demonstrated. Deep diaphragmatic breathing might reproduce pain and refer symptoms to the shoulder.[6,19]

Thoracic Spine

Visual inspection might reveal a postural deviation at the location of an injured vertebra. Injured vertebrae will usually be tender on compression of the spinous process during spring testing. Normal physiological range of motion might also be limited because of a spinal injury.[3,6,19,23] Limitation in thoracic extension results in a reduction of shoulder elevation range of motion. Scoliosis, which can cause asymmetrical movement of the upper extremity, also might be a source of shoulder pain.

Lumbar Spine

Symptoms originating from the lumbar spine can alter posture and affect shoulder motion, particularly in an athletic patient involved in overhead sports.[25,34]

Carpal Tunnel Syndrome

Examination for carpal tunnel syndrome can be performed by tapping over the volar carpal ligament (Tinel's Sign), which would reproduce pain in the distribution of the median nerve. Phalen's Test might reproduce the symptoms by maximally flexing the patient's wrist and maintaining that position for a prolonged period of time.[3,22]

Neural Tissue Provocation Testing

The upper limb tension tests are sometimes referred to as the upper limb equivalent of the straight leg raise test of the lower limb. The patient is placed to stress various positions of the brachial plexus. The primary test stresses the median nerve and C5 to C7 nerve roots. Other tests are designed to assess neural tension of various major nerves of the upper extremity. The patient lies supine while the examiner holds

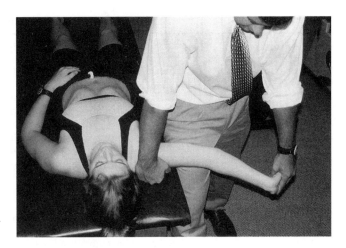

FIGURE 5–1. Upper limb tension test.

the shoulder girdle fixed in depression. The upper extremity is then moved into abduction, followed by external rotation of the shoulder, elbow extension, forearm supination, and wrist extension (Fig. 5–1). If the patient experiences pain or a burning sensation in the area of the cubital fossa or tingling in the thumb and the first three fingers, the test might be classified as positive. To confirm the diagnosis of adverse neural tension of the median nerve, the examiner can reproduce the symptoms with passive wrist extension or side bending of the cervical spine to the contralateral side. The available range of elbow passive extension when compared with the normal side can also give some indication of the degree of restriction.[3,35] When assessing neural tension, clinicians must first determine the level of irritability to prevent an exacerbation. Additionally, patients with glenohumeral instability might not be appropriate candidates for some of the upper limb tension tests because those tests place excessive stress on the anterior capsule.

Elbow and Forearm

Elbow pathology can be associated with symptoms in the shoulder complex. A thorough assessment of range of motion includes flexion, extension, supination, pronation, ulnar deviation, and radial deviation.[22,36] Decreased range of motion in the elbow can significantly affect the osteokinematics and arthrokinematics of the shoulder girdle. For example, decreased supination at the elbow can result in excessive external rotation at the shoulder as a compensatory movement. Clinicians must also rule out peripheral nerve entrapments when assessing the elbow.[6,35]

PALPATION

Various structures are palpated when examining the shoulder girdle (Table 5–1). Palpation is performed for the following reasons:

- To check for any changes in skin temperature suggestive of an inflammatory process or a chronic condition.
- To determine whether the patient has any sensory deficits.
- To localize specific sites of swelling.
- To determine circulatory status by checking distal pulses.

TABLE 5–1 Shoulder Girdle Palpation

Compartment	Common Palpation Points
Anterior compartment	a. Sternoclavicular joint (sprain, subluxation, dislocation)
	b. Clavicle (fracture)
	c. Coracoid process (fracture, strain short head of biceps)
	d. Anterior acromion (strain anterior deltoid, coracoid ligament fibrosis)
	e. Lesser tuberosity (strain pectoralis major, strain subscapularis)
	f. Greater tuberosity (tendonitis supraspinatus, fracture)
	g. Bicipital groove (strain long head of biceps, subluxation)
	h. Scalene (strain, spasm, pain)
	i. Biceps tendon (strain, tendonitis)
	j. Biceps (strain, rupture)
Superior compartment	a. Acromioclavicular joint (sprain, subluxation, dislocation)
	b. Supraspinatus tendon (tendonitis)
	c. Subacromial/subdeltoid bursa (bursitis)
	d. Upper trapezius (strain, spasm, myogeloses)
	e. Levator scapula (strain, spasm)
Lateral compartment	a. Deltoid (strain, wasting)
	b. Supraspinatus (tendonitis, strain)
	c. Acromion (fracture)
	d. Deltoid insertion (insertional strain, rotator cuff referral site, myositis ossificans)
Posterior compartment	a. Trapezius (strain, spasm)
	b. Scapula (fracture)
	c. Thoracic spine (vertebral alignment, joint sprains)
	d. Infraspinatus (strain)
	e. Teres minor (strain)
	f. Triceps (strain)
	g. Rhomboids (strain)
	h. Posterior capsule pain secondary to posterior or anterior subluxation
	i. Scapulothoracic bursitis at the inferior medial angle of the scapula
Inferior compartment	a. Axilla (deformities, enlarged nodes, dislocated humeral head)
	b. Pectoralis major (strain)
	c. Latissimus dorsi (strain)
	d. Lymph nodes (swelling)
	e. Brachial artery (pulses)

- To identify point tenderness.
- To identify bony or soft tissue deformities.

Typically, the shoulder complex can be divided into compartments to perform specific palpation. Symptoms reproduced with palpation in these compartments are frequently associated with specific underlying pathologies.[3,6,19,21–23] Clinicians might choose to perform palpation early in the physical examination, at the end, or in certain cases, throughout. Regardless, palpation should always be performed in a systematic manner to aid in organizing information. Additionally, palpation usually proceeds from general areas to specific structures and from superficial to deep tissues.

NEUROLOGICAL EXAMINATION

Components of the neurological examination to be performed include manual muscle testing and evaluation of sensation and reflexes.[3,6,19,21–24]

Sensation

Sensation should be assessed for each dermatome of the involved upper extremity to detect abnormalities or differences between sides. A Semmes Weinstein sensation kit can be used to quantify the level of sensation in a particular dermatome by applying monofilaments of different diameters.

Reflexes

The biceps (C5), brachioradialis (C6), and triceps (C7) reflexes should be assessed to determine the presence of hypo- or hyperreflexia. If a response is difficult to obtain, subjects can be asked to clench their teeth, look in the opposite direction, or clasp their hands. This Jendrassik's maneuver facilitates the reflex response.[6,19]

Manual Muscle Testing

Manual muscle testing provides a clinical assessment of muscle strength and innervation of myotomes. Manual muscle testing of the hand, wrist, elbow, and shoulder girdle musculature allows the examiner to estimate a patient's strength by providing manual resistance to specific movements. The strength of muscle groups can be compared bilaterally to determine weakness.[22,36]

Manual muscle testing of the shoulder complex should include an accurate assessment of the following motions: flexion, extension, abduction, adduction, horizontal abduction, horizontal adduction, external rotation, internal rotation, elevation, depression, retraction, and protraction. Specific manual muscle testing protocols might be obtained from books such as Kendall and McCreary[37] and Daniels and Worthingham.[38] Clinical myotome assessment should include the following[6,19]:

- C1 = Cervical Rotation
- C2, C3, C4 = Scapular Elevation
- C4 = Diaphragm
- C5 = Shoulder Abduction
- C6 = Wrist Extension
- C7 = Wrist Flexion
- C8 = Thumb Extension
- T1 = Abductor Digiti Minimi

Proprioceptive and Kinesthetic Testing

Testing proprioceptive and kinesthetic awareness is important when planning a treatment program. Most clinicians will incorporate this testing and rehabilitation for patients with ankle or knee problems, but fail to test proprioception in the shoulder. Recently, the importance of testing proprioception has been stressed, particularly in patients with instability. Smith and Brunolli[39] were some of the first researchers to document methods of evaluating proprioception and kinesthesia in the shoulder complex. Numerous other authors have established the importance of adequate proprioception training in patients with shoulder injuries who receive different treatment interventions.[40–45] However, several of these studies have used equipment that is more suited to a laboratory environment than a clinical setting, therefore limiting the generalizability of the results. Furthermore, the use of equipment such as a motorized wheel does not simulate functional movement patterns. Davies and Hoffman[43] have described a clinically useful method to assess shoulder kinesthesia by using a goniometer or inclinometer. Proprioceptive and kinesthetic deficits are present in many patients with shoulder dysfunctions, but if proprioception and kinesthesia are not measured objectively, a clinician might not know whether there is an actual deficit present.

ACTIVE RANGE OF MOTION TESTING

Active range of motion (AROM) testing assesses the patient's willingness to move, the quantity of movement, and the quality of movement. Active movements of the shoulder complex are evaluated prior to passive movements, allowing the objective portion of the examination to be conducted from general to specific. Active range of motion uses both the contractile and noncontractile tissues of the joint, whereas passive range of motion (PROM) emphasizes the noncontractile structures.[46] Therefore, pain or limitation found in a specific AROM will be followed by PROM of the same movement to distinguish the tissue(s) involved.

AROM should be assessed in all physiological planes, including the plane of the scapula, and in all joints of the shoulder complex. The scapular plane, or scaption, is defined as 30° anterior to the frontal plane. Benefits inherent in scapular plane movement include optimal osseous congruency between the humeral head and glenoid fossa, length tension relationship of glenohumeral and scapulothoracic muscles, and minimal tension on the anterior joint capsule compared with movement in the coronal or frontal plane. Normal values for full ROM of these movements are available from several sources.

While measuring the quantity of shoulder AROM, the examiner should be observing the quality of movement, willingness to move the arm, any aberrant movements, and sequence of symptoms that occur. This information is helpful in determining the structures involved. It also lets the examiner know how intensive or nonintensive the remaining examination should be.[46]

Shoulder Shrug Sign

As compensation for a pathology, patients will use surrounding muscles to aid in elevation of the upper extremity. The upper trapezius is often recruited for shoulder elevation, resulting in the entire complex initially moving as one unit. Often the patient leans to the opposite side in an attempt to move the upper extremity through a greater range of motion. For example, as patients attempt to abduct their right upper extremity by recruiting their right upper trapezius, they will laterally flex to their left at the trunk to achieve a greater range. The shrug sign is often a result of pain, weakness, rotator cuff tear, or selective capsular hypomobility.[24]

Lateral Scapular Slide Test

Clinical documentation of scapulothoracic dysfunction using the lateral scapular slide test has been described by Kibler[47] and modified for the overhead position by Davies and Dickhoff-Hoffman.[43] This procedure involves measuring the relationship of the scapula relative to the thoracic spinous processes at different positions of the GH and ST joints. Kibler[47] stated that more than 1 cm asymmetry between the two sides correlates with pathologies such as GH joint instability and impingement.

Painful Arc Syndrome

Pain that occurs only during the mid-range of upper extremity elevation has been termed the painful arc syndrome.[46,48] This painful arc, only in the range of 60° to

120° elevation, can be attributed to bursitis, rotator cuff tendonitis, capsular laxity, selective hypomobility, or a combination of these conditions. The pain results from compression of structures between the acromion and coracoacromial ligament and the head of the humerus. The pain disappears when the structure has passed beneath the acromion. If the pain does not subside or if it increases, the examiner must consider the possible involvement of the AC joint. The painful arc might also be present to a lesser extent during forward flexion or passive abduction.

Apley's Scratch Tests[3]

A gross examination of the patient's AROM can be accomplished by using combinations of the physiological movements. Apley's Scratch Tests are a series of three movements that involve placing the hand of the involved side (1) on the opposite shoulder, (2) behind the head, and (3) in the lumbar spine area. The first movement is a combination of shoulder flexion, horizontal adduction, and internal rotation. The second movement involves shoulder abduction and external rotation. The final movement combines shoulder extension, adduction, and internal rotation. These composite movements can be used as objective measures by identifying the distance of the thumb relative to a specific landmark. For example, a clinician can measure the distance of the thumb to the spinous process of C7 when performing the behind-the-head position. This measurement can be used for comparison with the contralateral side or used for reassessment from one treatment to the next. Although using these movements might save time, if a restriction is detected the examiner should also assess individual movements to determine the source of the limitation.

Capsular Pattern Limitations

A lesion of the joint capsule or synovial membrane might result in a characteristic loss of motion, referred to as a *capsular pattern*.[46] The capsular pattern for the GH joint is external rotation limited more than abduction, abduction limited more than flexion, and flexion limited more than internal rotation. Joints that are not controlled by muscles, such as the AC and SC joints, lack specific capsular patterns. The limitations of these joints are described as pain occurring at the extreme ranges of movement.

Cyriax[46] believes that the presence of a capsular pattern indicated an arthritic condition in the joint, that is, osteoarthritis, rheumatoid arthritis, or traumatic arthritis (inflammation) following a sprain. He also believes that the examiner cannot discern the type of arthritis present by the capsular pattern, because each type presents with the same pattern. Other components of the evaluation will allow the examiner to isolate the cause.

Davies and DeCarlo[6] state that a glenohumeral capsular pattern exists only in a shoulder with complete capsular involvement, such as adhesive capsulitis. They feel that conditions involving selected hypomobility are more common and display the greatest limitation in internal rotation, not external rotation or abduction.

Research on other peripheral joints has concluded that a consistent capsular pattern might not exist. Hayes et al.[49] conducted a study quantifying joint limitations in 79 subjects with osteoarthritis of the knee. They concluded that few subjects demonstrated a capsular pattern as defined by Cyriax. They felt that the idea of a patterned ROM loss would be useful, but a proportional definition should be abandoned. Given the lack of research evidence favoring capsular patterns, continued use of this term is primarily based on empirical findings and tradition.[50]

PASSIVE RANGE OF MOTION TESTING

Assessing passive range of motion (PROM) determines the integrity of the noncontractile tissues such as ligaments, joint capsules, fascia, connective tissue, bursae, or neurovascular structures. Pain felt in the same direction with both active and passive motion usually involves the noncontractile structures, whereas pain felt in opposite directions is more likely to indicate muscle-tendon unit or contractile tissue involvement. Findings from the resisted motion portion of the exam used in conjunction with the AROM/PROM data will help to isolate the involved tissue(s).

End-Feels

As with active movements, the examiner must assess more than the amount of motion. The resistance felt by the examiner at the extreme of passive motion is an essential diagnostic tool. Cyriax[46] refers to the resistance encountered at the end ranges of movement as "end-feels." The summary in Box 5-2 describes end-feels according to Cyriax.

Sequence of Pain with Resistance

The sequence of pain with resistance can offer additional information about musculoskeletal dysfunction. This pain-resistance sequence as described by Cyriax[46]

BOX 5-2 End-Feels According to Cyriax

The first three end-feels—bone-to-bone, capsular, and tissue approximation—are normal for specific joints of the body. However, a bony end-feel that is detected in a joint that normally has a capsular end-feel would be classified as abnormal. The remaining three end-feels are classified as abnormal because they are often caused by some type of lesion. The reliability of end-feel classification has been questioned,[65] but the system continues to be used by clinicians when assessing PROM.

a. **Bone-to-bone:** An abrupt halt to movement from two bony surfaces coming into contact with one another without the presence of pain. Movement beyond this end-feel would be contraindicated. Passive abduction of the shoulder to 180° will produce this end-feel when the humeral head/shaft comes into contact with the acromion.

b. **Capsular:** An end-feel described as stretching leather, normally occurring in the shoulder and hip at the extremes of rotation. The presence of this end-feel encountered prior to reaching full range of motion can be indicative of chronic lesion.

c. **Tissue Approximation:** An end-feel produced from the approximation of soft tissue structures, normally felt at the end range of shoulder horizontal adduction. This end-feel will be limited by soft-tissue approximation of the pectorals and anterior deltoid.

d. **Empty:** An end-feel resulting from voluntary cessation of movement by the patient, usually because of pain. The patient interrupts the movement before the examiner is able to determine the resistance at full ROM.

e. **Spasm:** An end-feel experienced with involuntary muscle guarding that might be caused by an acute or subacute lesion.

f. **Springy:** An end-feel resulting from an internal joint derangement that causes a rebound from the full ROM. This type of end-feel is typically felt at end range knee extension when movement is limited by a torn meniscus. At the shoulder, lesions of the glenoid labrum could produce a springy end-feel. Examples of glenoid pathologies include Bankart lesions and types III and IV SLAP lesions. Types III and IV SLAP lesions both involve bucket handle displacements of the superior labrum that could result in a springy block end-feel.

can be used by clinicians when planning treatment programs. Findings from these tests are summarized in Box 5–3. Although the validity and reliability of the pain-resistance sequence have been questioned,[49] this system is frequently utilized to determine the chronicity of a lesion.

Accessory Joint Motion

After assessing the physiological motions through active and passive movements, the accessory motions within the various joints of the shoulder complex need to be assessed. Full physiological movement (osteokinematics) of a joint is dependent on normal accessory motion (arthrokinematics) within the joint. Passive accessory motion has been defined as movement occurring between joint surfaces produced by forces exerted by the examiner.[51] Patients are unable to produce these movements in isolation of physiological motion.

Accessory motion testing is used to gain insight about joint function based on the amount of motion occurring. Although quantification of accessory motions is not well documented, some literature estimates that these movements are less than 4 mm in most joints.[3] Accessory motion at the GH joint is greater than most joints because the humeral head is four times as large as the glenoid fossa. A study conducted on eight subjects determined that the normal shoulder has 8 mm of anterior translation, 9 mm of posterior translation, and 11 mm of inferior translation.[52] The investigators found little difference in laxity between normal shoulders and unstable shoulders requiring surgical intervention. Papilion and Shall[53] measured anterior and posterior translation of the GH joint using spot radiographs, in which translation was expressed as a percentage of displacement of the humeral head relative to the glenoid. The findings showed that normal translation is up to 14% anteriorly and 37% posteriorly. However, results of this study cannot be generalized to a normal population as subjects were examined under general anesthesia, which might have caused a greater degree of translation.

BOX 5–3 Pain Resistance Sequence According to Cyriax

a. **Pain before resistance** (acute lesion): The onset of pain prior to reaching the end ROM indicates an acute condition. Any additional resistance felt is usually attributed to muscle guarding. Initial treatment focuses on control of pain and inflammation through the use of various modalities. Progressive stretching or ROM exercises to a painful range might be contraindicated during this stage.

b. **Pain with resistance** (subacute lesion): Pain and resistance occurring simultaneously indicates a subacute condition. The treatment can be more aggressive than an acute condition, but the examiner must remain cautious to avoid exacerbating the inflammatory process. The clinician may choose to continue controlling pain and inflammation. Gentle stretching and mobilizations to restore lost motion also are initiated.

c. **Pain after resistance** (chronic lesion): Little pain, if any, is experienced after the examiner encounters resistance. Any overpressure that is added to the extreme of the range might produce an increase in patient discomfort, but the pain stops when the overpressure is released. Aggressive stretching and mobilizations without restrictions can be implemented in the treatment plan.

Accessory motion testing helps the examiner assess specific end-feel[46] and determine the presence of an inflammatory process.[54] Symptom reproduction might indicate an inflamed joint structure. Ligamentous integrity can also be assessed through accessory motion testing. Specific testing of the shoulder complex ligaments will be described further in this chapter.

Testing accessory motions of the shoulder complex involves analyzing several joints in several directions. All testing should be performed with each joint in a loosely packed or resting position to minimize articular surface congruence and to maximize ligamentous laxity.[3] Bilateral comparisons are frequently used by examiners to determine whether the affected joint is hypomobile, normal, or hypermobile. Although intratester reliability has been shown to be reliable, particularly when looking at side-to-side differences, the intertester reliability and validity of accessory testing has not been consistently documented.

FLEXIBILITY TESTING

Muscular flexibility is assessed to determine whether muscle imbalances are contributing to a patient's symptoms. A shortened musculotendinous unit can result in abnormal osteokinematic and arthrokinematic movements. Tightness of the anterior musculature can result in rounding of the shoulders, often associated with impingement and thoracic outlet syndrome. This tightness is usually attributed to the pectoralis major and minor. Flexibility of the pectoralis is assessed by positioning the patient supine with hands behind the head and retracting the patient's elbows toward the plinth. If the lateral epicondyles touch the plinth, the muscles have normal flexibility. The patient should remain in the supine position to test the pectoralis minor, and the clinician must stabilize the thorax to prevent substitution patterns. The arms are elevated above the patient's head while maintaining the lumbar spine on the plinth. Normal flexibility is found if the thumbs touch the plinth. These tests should be performed with controlled force because excessive overpressure can exacerbate impingement and thoracic outlet symptoms. A lack of consistency and normative data exists in the literature regarding appropriate techniques for performing flexibility tests of the shoulder girdle. More research is needed in this area to correlate flexibility deficits with specific dysfunctions.

SPECIAL TESTS

Special tests are assessment procedures used to implicate particular structures during the examination. These tests are used to (1) confirm the specific structure(s) involved, (2) help determine the degree of tissue damage, and (3) determine whether the patient is a suitable candidate for physical therapy. After completion of the previously described components of the examination, the clinician should have a good idea about which underlying structures are causing the patient's symptoms and the severity of the injury. These special tests serve to corroborate the previous subjective and objective findings and to further rule out or implicate structures that might be involved. Although these tests might not have high reliability and validity, they represent the best noninvasive examination procedures available. *A comprehensive examination does not require that all these tests be performed on every patient. The clinician must determine which special tests are appropriate based on patient presentation and preferred practice pattern.* An efficient sequence of special tests for the shoulder is described in Figure 5–2.

Thoracic Outlet Syndrome Tests

When performing thoracic outlet syndrome tests, decreased or disappearing pulse or reproduction of neurological symptoms indicates a positive test.[3,27–33,55–57] Numerous tests are presented in the literature[27–33] and used clinically to make a diagnosis despite the high incidence of false positives. Ironically, a thorough history and assessment of impairments in patients with thoracic outlet syndrome might be more helpful in treatment planning than performing numerous special tests. Patients with this condition often present with impaired posture, such as scapular protraction and internal rotation of the GH joints, and muscle imbalances, such as tightness of the anterior chest and scalene musculature and weakness of the posterior shoulder musculature. Regardless of which special tests are positive or negative, treatment usually will address these impairments. Specific examination and treatment of thoracic outlet syndrome will be discussed in Chapter 10.

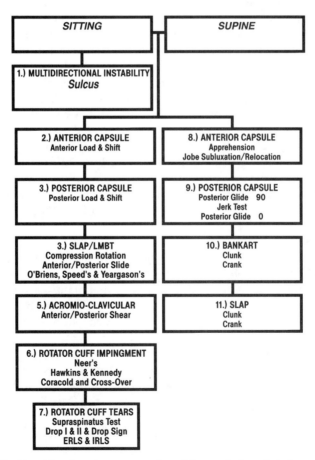

FIGURE 5–2. Algorithm-based sequence of special tests during clinical examination.

Allen Maneuver (Scaleni Traction)

With the patient in a sitting position, the clinician flexes the patient's elbow to 90° and abducts the shoulder to 90°. The shoulder is then extended horizontally, rotated laterally, and retracted while the patient then rotates his/her head away from the test side. A positive test is indicated by a diminution or loss of the radial pulse.[3,55]

Adson Maneuver (Scaleni Compression)

Probably the most common method of testing for thoracic outlet syndrome, this test is designed to selectively evaluate whether the anterior and middle scalene muscles are the primary source of pain resulting from occlusion of arterial blood flow. The patient's head is rotated to the ipsilateral test side. The patient then extends the head while the examiner laterally rotates and extends the patient's shoulder. At the same time the patient is asked to take a deep breath and hold it. A disappearance of pulse indicates a positive test.[3,5,27]

Halstead Maneuver (Scaleni Traction)

With this test, the examiner finds the radial pulse and applies a downward traction on the test extremity while the patient's neck is hyperextended and rotated to the contralateral side. Absence or disappearance of a pulse indicates a positive test for thoracic outlet syndrome.[3]

Costoclavicular Syndrome Test (1st Rib/Clavicle Compression)

The examiner palpates the patient's radial pulse and then draws the patient's shoulder down and back into a retracted position. This maneuver narrows the costoclavicular space by approximating the clavicle to the first rib and compressing the neurovascular structures. A positive test, demonstrated by an absence of a pulse, indicates thoracic outlet syndrome. This test is particularly effective in evaluating patients who complain of symptoms while wearing a backpack or heavy coat.[3,27]

Pectoralis Minor Syndrome Test (Wright's Maneuver)

Wright advocates moving the arm so that the hand is brought over the head with the elbow and arm in the coronal plane. If the pectoralis minor is tight, this movement can compress the middle portion of the axillary artery and compromise neurovascular function. This test is best performed in a supine position to eliminate the effects of gravity. With the patient supine, the clinician hyperabducts the patient's arm overhead while palpating the radial pulse. A positive test is indicated by absence of the patient's pulse.[3,27,57]

Roos Tests

For this test, the patient stands and abducts the arms to 90°, externally rotates the shoulders, and flexes the elbows to 90°. The patient then opens and closes the hands slowly for 3 minutes. If the patient is unable to maintain the position for 3 minutes or suffers ischemic pain, heaviness of the arm, or numbness and tingling of the hand during the 3 minutes, the test is positive for thoracic outlet syndrome on the affected side.[3,6,19,33]

Provocative Elevation Test

For this test, the patient is asked to elevate both arms above the transverse plane of the shoulder and then rapidly open and close the hands 15 times. If fatigue, cramping, or tingling occurs during the test, the test is positive for vascular insufficiency and thoracic outlet syndrome.[3,21]

Readers are encouraged to read Calliet[2] and Lephart et al.[42] for a critical analysis of these tests. Rayan and Jensen[27] evaluated the accuracy of these tests on normal subjects and found a high number of false positive tests. When these tests were used by the authors of this chapter, over 50% false positive tests were detected on normal subjects. Yet clinicians often base their treatments on the results of these tests. Rayan[33] provides a critical review of the literature regarding what many of these thoracic outlet syndrome tests really mean, as well as some recommendations on ways to make the tests more reliable and clinically meaningful.

Biceps Brachii Tests

Yergason's Test

With the patient's elbow flexed to 90° and stabilized against the thorax with the forearm pronated, the examiner resists supination while the patient also externally rotates the arm against resistance. The examiner can concomitantly palpate the long head of the biceps tendon. Tenderness in the bicipital groove indicates a positive result. The tendon might sublux out of the groove, indicating bicipital tendonitis or involvement of the transverse humeral ligament.[3,58]

Speed's Test

The patient positions the involved extremity at 90° of shoulder flexion with external rotation, elbow extension, and forearm supination. The examiner resists shoulder forward flexion. Because the long head of the biceps is a secondary shoulder flexor and forearm supinator, resistance during shoulder flexion with the forearm supination places maximal force on the long head of the biceps. A positive test is indicated by increased tenderness in the bicipital groove, indicating bicipital tendonitis.[3]

Ludington's Test

The patient clasps both hands on top of the head, interlocking the fingers to support the weight of the upper limbs. This action allows maximum relaxation of the biceps tendon in its resting position. The patient then alternately contracts and relaxes the biceps muscles, while the clinician palpates the biceps tendon. If the test is positive, no contraction can be palpated on the affected side. A positive result indicates a rupture of the long head of the biceps tendon.[59]

Gilchrest's Sign

While standing, the patient lifts a 5-pound weight overhead. The arm is externally rotated and lowered eccentrically in the frontal plane. Any discomfort or pain located within the bicipital groove is a positive test and indicates bicipital tendonitis. In some cases, an audible snap might be felt between 100° and 90° of abduction.[3,6,19]

Heuter's Sign

During normal muscle recruitment, some accessory supination will occur during resisted elbow flexion with the forearm pronated. This recruitment strategy occurs because the biceps attempts to assist the brachialis muscle to flex the elbow; which is referred to as a Heuter's Sign. If this movement is absent, the biceps mechanism has been disrupted.[60]

Transverse Humeral Ligament Tests

Lippman Test

The patient sits or stands while the clinician holds the arm in a neutral position with the elbow flexed to 90°. Using the other hand, the clinician palpates the biceps tendon within the bicipital groove and moves the biceps tendon from side to side within the bicipital groove. A positive test is confirmed if sharp pain is elicited within the bicipital groove, indicating bicipital tendonitis.[3,6,19]

Long Head of Biceps Subluxation Test

This test is used to assess the integrity of the transverse humeral ligament. The subject's arm is passively abducted and externally rotated while the examiner places pressure on the bicipital groove. The arm is internally and externally rotated, while the examiner palpates the biceps tendon to determine stability within the bicipital groove. A positive test produces an audible or palpable snap accompanied by pain.[3,6,19]

Rotator Cuff Impingement Syndrome Tests

Clinical signs of impingement might include pain over the anterior aspect of the shoulder in the area of the acromion and greater tuberosity, pain referred to the lateral aspect of the shoulder at the site of the deltoid insertion, a painful arc of movement with abduction, and positive impingement signs.[61] Several tests have been described for GH joint impingement. See Chapters 8 and 9 for discussions of both primary and secondary GH joint impingement and the role of these tests in clinical decision making.

Neer's Impingement Sign

Clinical application of Neer's impingement sign involves forcibly elevating the upper extremity while holding the shoulder in forward flexion and internal rotation (Fig. 5–3). This motion produces an impingement of the supraspinatus between the greater tuberosity and the anterior inferior surface of the acromion. Variations of this test include both neutral and externally rotated humeral positions with the full forward flexion.[62,63]

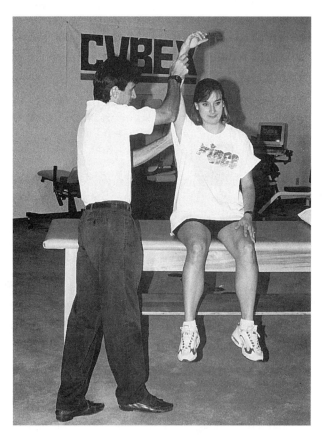

FIGURE 5–3. Neer impingement sign.

Hawkins' Impingement Sign

Hawkins' impingement sign is performed by elevating the shoulder to 90° in the scapular plane. The humerus is then forcibly internally rotated, impaling the supraspinatus tendon against the anterior-inferior acromion and coracoacromial ligament[21,64–66] (Fig. 5–4).

Coracoid Impingement Sign

A variation of Hawkins' impingement sign has been called the coracoid impingement sign. This procedure is performed with the shoulder flexed to 90° in the sagittal plane rather than in the scapular plane as demonstrated by Hawkins. The coracoid impingement test can indicate impingement of the subscapularis, long head of the biceps, and supraspinatus.[6,67]

Cross-Over Impingement Test

The cross-over, or cross-arm, impingement test involves horizontal adduction of the shoulder with overpressure at end range of motion. The shoulder is placed in approximately 90° of flexion and then horizontally adducted across the body. Interpretation of this test varies based on the location of pain described by the patient.[6] An anterior pain distribution denotes impingement of the long head biceps, and/or subscapularis. Lateral pain is primarily indicative of a supraspinatus impingement syndrome. Pain described over the superior aspect of the shoulder is generally indicative of pathology of the AC joint, resulting from the compression of the distal clavicle against the acromion.[47,68] Pain reported in the posterior aspect of the shoulder

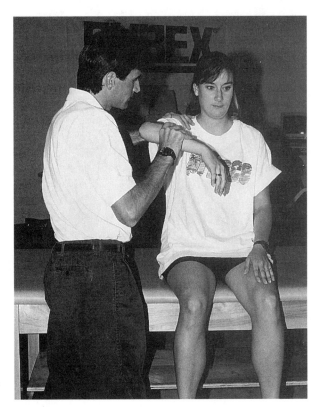

FIGURE 5–4. Hawkin's impingement sign.

implicates the infraspinatus, teres minor, or posterior capsule, as this position places the posterior structures in an elongated position (Fig. 5–5).

Rotator Cuff Rupture Tests

Clinical tests to determine a complete tear or rupture of the rotator cuff, specifically the supraspinatus, have been reported in the literature.[6,61,69–71] The supraspinatus muscle is important in assisting GH joint abduction and stabilizing the humeral head into the glenoid fossa. These functions form the basis for these clinical tests.[72,73]

Drop Arm Test

The drop arm test for evaluation of a complete rotator cuff tear involves passive abduction of the shoulder in the coronal plane to 90°. The patient is then asked to sustain this position while the clinician taps the patient's arm near the elbow. If the patient's arm drops, it indicates a full thickness tear of the rotator cuff.[70] Placement of one of the clinician's hands or arms just below the patient's arm during the tapping procedure is recommended because of pain elicited with the sudden adduction of the arm in the presence of a full thickness rotator cuff tear.

A variation of the drop arm test involves passively raising the patient's arm into full abduction. The patient then eccentrically lowers the arm with the arm in a "palm-down" position. A positive test is present when the patient eccentrically lowers the arm to approximately 90° and then drops the arm into adduction without control. Placement of the clinician's hand or arm under the patient's arm during the

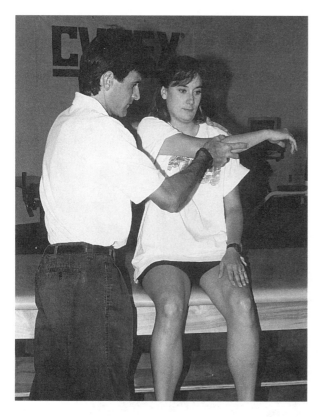

FIGURE 5–5. Cross-over impingement sign.

eccentric adduction is also recommended during this test to support the extremity if the patient does not have adequate control. Upper extremity substitution patterns should be noted with this test. Many patients with rotator cuff weakness often "cheat" by using lateral trunk flexion to the contralateral side. Patients might also compensate with excessive scapular elevation and upward rotation because of activation of the upper trapezius muscle during the eccentric lowering phase of this test.

Lag Sign Tests

Hertel et al.[69] have described a new series of physical examination tests designed to differentiate partial from full thickness rotator cuff tears. Details regarding the tests and the sensitivity and specificity are described in the study.

Supraspinatus Isolation Test

The supraspinatus isolation test is used to assess strength of the supraspinatus muscle[74,75] and is reported to isolate the supraspinatus based on the GH joint position used.[73] The shoulder is placed at 70° to 90° of elevation in the scapular plane with full internal rotation of the humerus (Fig. 5–6). Internal rotation of the humerus decreases the mechanical efficiency of the deltoid and increases the activity of the supraspinatus as compared to abduction of the shoulder in the coronal plane with other positions of humeral rotation.[73] Internal rotation of the humerus also causes a prestretch to the supraspinatus and increases the mechanical advantage. Therefore more EMG activity and muscle force is produced. Substitution patterns encountered during this test include contralateral lateral flexion of the trunk and scapular elevation.

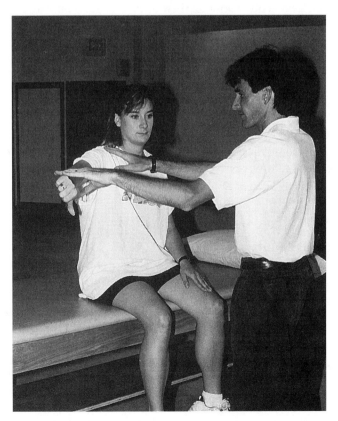

FIGURE 5–6. Supraspinatus test.

Acromioclavicular Joint Tests

Testing of the AC joint can be accomplished through observation and palpation. A first-degree injury to the AC joint will usually result in observable swelling. Second- and third-degree sprains will also have elevation of the distal end of the clavicle relative to the acromion. This "step deformity" of the shoulder is often tender on palpation, but can frequently be reduced with a caudal force applied to the distal end of the clavicle.[68,76,77]

Acromioclavicular Shear Test

During this test, the examiner stands to the patient's side with both hands cupped around the deltoid. The anterior hand is placed on the clavicle and the posterior hand is placed along the scapular spine. Compressing the hands produces a shearing force at the AC joint. A positive test reproduces the patient's symptoms. An increase in translation is expected with an acromioclavicular sprain, indicating a hypermobile joint.[6,34]

Cross-Over Impingement Test

As previously stated, the cross-over impingement test can be used to identify pathology of the AC joint. Forced horizontal adduction of the shoulder with internal rotation will cause compression at the AC joint, and the patient will usually experience pain at that joint.[64]

Active Compression Test

Recently, O'Brien et al.[34] described the active compression test. The patient elevates the arm to approximately 90°, adducts past the midline, and internally rotates the arm. The examiner then applies a manual muscle test. This position "locks and loads" (compresses) the AC joint and might replicate or increase the patient's pain. In the second part of the test, the patient externally rotates the arm to decrease compression at the AC joint. In this position, the pain should decrease or go away. The type of acromioclavicular sprain is dependent on the number of ligaments torn and the direction and magnitude of the displaced clavicle.[78,79] These findings have been divided into different grades by O'Brien et al.[78,79]

Painful conditions resulting from pathology other than a sprain can involve the AC joint.[80] A frequent cause of pain and dysfunction in the AC joint is osteoarthritic degenerative changes. Another source of symptoms can result from long thoracic nerve neuropraxia. This condition causes scapular winging, which might increase stress at the AC joint and result in secondary inflammation. Systemic disorders, such as rheumatoid arthritis or hematogenous osteomyelitis, can also result in a painful AC joint.

Glenoid Labrum Tests

The active compression test also implicates involvement of the superior labrum anterior-posterior lesion.[34] Clinical tests have been reported in the literature to test the integrity of the glenoid labrum. In a recent study[81] comparing clinically applied labral tests and MRI, the clinical tests were found to be more accurate in properly diagnosing labral tears as confirmed via arthroscopy.

Clunk Test

The clunk test is performed with the patient in a supine position, with the arm in varying degrees of elevation from 120° to 180°.[20,82] The hands of the examiner are placed just distal to the humeral head with a compressive force applied along the axis of the humeral shaft into the glenoid cavity.[22] A circumduction movement pattern around the perimeter of the glenoid is performed while the GH joint surfaces are

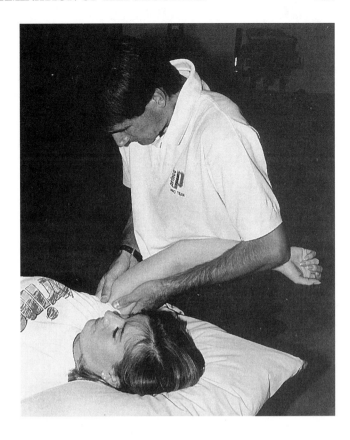

FIGURE 5–7. Clunk test.

compressed (Fig. 5–7). A positive test is identified by a "clunk" produced with the circumduction motion. Reproduction of the patient's pain, as well as a locking sensation, are also described as characteristic findings of a positive test.

Alterations of the clunk test include the combination of humeral rotation with a circumduction movement pattern while compression is applied to the joint surfaces. A similar patient position is used with the examiner grasping the elbow flexed to 90° and exerting a long axis compression while the shoulder is rotated and circumducted. Attempts to "catch" a portion of the torn labrum during rotation and compression of the humeral head are the main factors of this test.

Compression-Rotation Test

The compression-rotation test has been described by Matsen[83] for testing the glenoid labrum. The patient is placed in a supine position with the GH joint abducted to 90° in the coronal plane.[6] The humeral head is compressed into the glenoid fossa while the extremity is moved into internal and external rotation (Fig. 5–8). Similar to the clunk test described previously, a positive test includes a "clunk" as well as a painful locking sensation.

Anterior Slide Test

Whereas advances in arthroscopic surgery have assisted in the identification of labral lesions in the superior aspect of the glenoid, termed a SLAP lesion (superior labrum anterior and posterior), clinical diagnosis of this lesion has been difficult. Kibler[84] has developed the Anterior Slide test as a means of testing the superior labrum of the shoulder in a clinical setting. The patient is examined in either the

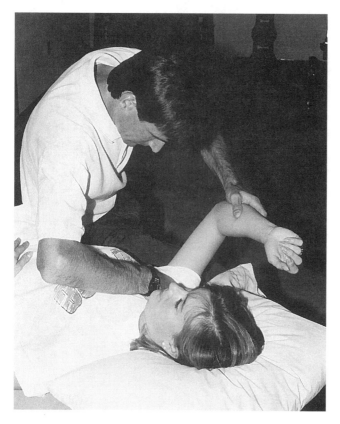

FIGURE 5–8. Circumduction labral test.

seated or standing position, with hands on the hips, and thumbs pointing posteriorly.[84] One of the examiner's hands is positioned with the end of the index finger extending over the anterior aspect of the acromion. The examiner's other hand is placed behind the elbow and upper arm, and the patient is asked to push against this force. Pain localized to the anterior aspect of the shoulder under the examiner's hand and a pop or click in the anterior-superior aspect of the shoulder are considered signs of a positive test.

Internal Impingement Syndrome

An impingement syndrome was identified by Walch et al.[85] and subsequently described by others.[86–89] This condition involves impingement of the posterior portion of the supraspinatus and the anterior portion of the infraspinatus on the posterior aspect of the superior labrum. This type of impingement has been diagnosed using the Jobe subluxation/relocation test when the patient has posterior pain. The pain increases with the subluxation part of the test but decreases or goes away during the relocation phase of the test.

Instability Tests

The understanding of pathomechanics leading to shoulder instabilities has advanced in the last several years. Knowledge of the primary and secondary restraints in controlling motion has led to a better understanding of subtle instabilities in the shoulder. Many publications have contributed to an increased understanding of the "circle concept" of the shoulder.[90–105] The *circle concept* states that increased translation

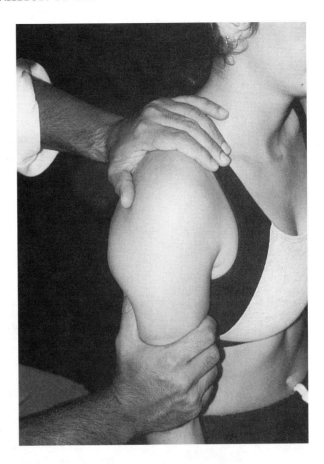

FIGURE 5–9. Start position of sulcus sign.

of the humeral head occurs in one direction when one side of the joint capsule is injured. Complete dislocation of the shoulder causes injury on both sides of the joint.

As the shoulder is assessed for instabilities, clinicians must examine for straight plane instability, multiplane instability, degree of instability, direction of instability, cause of the instability, force required to cause the instability, chronology of the instability, recurrence rate, and whether the instability is volitional or involuntary. Although many clinicians advocate attempting to grade or quantify the degree of instability, the literature reports no consistency in grading instabilities.[90,92,94–97,101,102,104,105]

An increased understanding of the concept of multidirectional instability (MDI) has developed over the last several years.[97] Multidirectional instability is defined as shoulder dislocation or subluxation that occurs in more than one direction. MDI can be a combination of anterior, posterior, and inferior excursion of the humeral head relative to the glenoid fossa. Clinical findings associated with MDI include a sulcus sign (Fig. 5–9 and Fig. 5–10). A *sulcus sign* is a "steplike" appearance between the acromion and the superior aspect of the humeral head that occurs when a light traction force is applied to the upper extremity in an inferior direction. In some cases, a sulcus sign is apparent when the patient has the arm resting in a neutral position. In the presence of an MDI, determining the primary and secondary components of the instability is also important.[97]

Load and Shift Test

The load and shift test (drawer test, glide test)[104,105] has become the "gold standard" test for the assessment of anterior and posterior instability of the shoulder

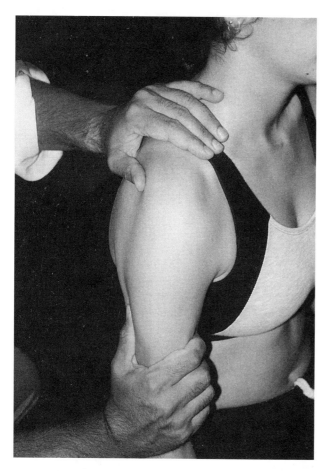

FIGURE 5–10. Sulcus sign with distraction applied.

(Fig. 5–11). With this test, the examiner creates a loading force to reduce the humeral head centrally in the glenoid fossa. To perform this maneuver, the examination initially involves assessment of the patient sitting while the examiner is located beside and behind the side to be examined. Once the humeral head is loaded, directional stresses are applied. The examiner places one hand over the shoulder and scapula to stabilize the shoulder girdle and uses the other hand to grasp the humeral head. As the humeral head is loaded, anterior and posterior forces are applied and translation is noted. Next, the elbow is held and inferior traction is applied to assess inferior translation. The area adjacent to the skin is observed for a sulcus sign. Until the development of better clinical methods, such as shoulder arthrometers, to assess the laxity or translation in the shoulder, much of the testing and clinical findings will remain empirically based.

Apprehension Sign

A patient with anterior instability will usually exhibit an apprehension sign to protect the anterior capsule.[3] When testing for apprehension, the shoulder is passively moved into external rotation while the arm is held at 90° of abduction and the elbow flexed to 90°. As the examiner moves the arm farther into external rotation, the patient will guard to prevent further movement.

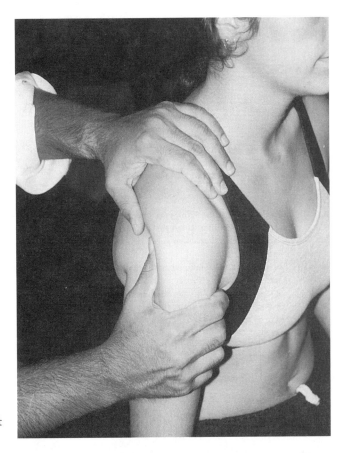

FIGURE 5–11. Load and shift test.

Relocation Test

The relocation test has been used to distinguish between primary impingement and primary instability.[21] During this test, the examiner places the upper extremity in 90° of abduction with 90° of elbow flexion while the patient lies supine. The examiner then externally rotates the shoulder to approximately 90° or until the patient experiences pain. In this position, a posteriorly directed force is applied to the anterior aspect of the head of the humerus (Fig. 5–12). Patients with anterior instability and secondary impingement will experience a decrease in pain as the head of the humerus

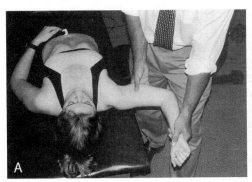
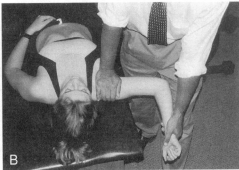

FIGURE 5–12. Relocation test. *(A)* Start position. *(B)* Finish position.

Functional Throwing Performance Index

Patient Name:_____ GC#_____ DOB_____

Dominant Arm:_____ Diagnosis:_____

(Davies) Functional Throwing Performance Index (FTPI)
Materials and Protocol

Materials

Distance:	15 feet
Height:	4 feet
Target Size:	1 foot x 1 foot square
Ball:	20 inch circumference rubber playground ball

Testing Protocol

1. Normal throwing mechanics are encouraged. Patient should use the "crow-hop" technique when throwing and not just standing still at the 15 foot line.
2. Patient performs 4 gradient submaximal to maximal warmups (25, 50, 75, 100 percent of controlled volutional effort).
3. Patient performs 5 maximal controlled volutional throws and must also catch the ball on the rebound. (Consequently, the effort is not really 100% effort because the ball would bounce too hard and the patient would not be able to throw, catch, and control the motion).
4. The patient throws as many times as he/she can in 30 seconds with control and accuacry.
5. Three 30 second tests are performed.
6. Data analysis:
    1. The number of throws in 30 seconds are counted.
    2. The number of throws that land within the target are counted.

FUNCTIONAL THROWING PERFORMANCE INDEX

FTPI=$\dfrac{\text{Accuracy in Target Square}}{\text{Total Number of Throws}}$ X 100   FTPI= _____ %

Status/Post (Weeks):_____

Trial	1	2	3	4	x̄
Throws					
Accuracy					
FTPI					

In:_____ Out:_____

Status/Post (Weeks):_____

Trial	1	2	3	4	x̄
Throws					
Accuracy					
FTPI					

In:_____ Out:_____

Status/Post (Weeks):_____

Trial	1	2	3	4	x̄
Throws					
Accuracy					
FTPI					

In:_____ Out:_____

Status/Post (Weeks):_____

Trial	1	2	3	4	x̄
Throws					
Accuracy					
FTPI					

In:_____ Out:_____

Norms	Males	Females
Throws	15	13
Accuracy	7	4
FTPI	47%	29%
Range	33%-60%	17%-41%

FIGURE 5–13. Functional throwing performance index. (Courtesy of Gundersen Lutheran Sports Medicine, Lacrosse, Wisconsin.)

is reduced posteriorly. The posterior reduction relieves the impingement occurring between the undersurface of the rotator cuff and the posterosuperior glenoid.

FUNCTIONAL TESTING

Functional Throwing Performance Index

Few functional tests of the shoulder are described in the literature. Davies and Hoffman[43] described the Functional Throwing Performance Index (FTPI) as a way to assess an overhead motion within the confines of most clinical settings (Fig. 5–13). Hoffman also cites an unpublished reliability test performed by Quincy et al.[43] that demonstrates a 0.91 reliability using ICCs. Additionally, Rankin et al.[106] performed a test-retest reliability analysis of Davies' clinically oriented Functional Throwing Performance Index (FTPI) over extended time intervals. The reliability of the FTPI was 0.83 and the individual reliability results fell within the expected normal values established by Davies for males and females in 100% of the cases.

Unilateral Upper Extremity Stance Stability

Because many clinicians are using closed kinetic chain exercises as part of rehabilitation programs,[8,43,107] a few clinicians have tried to identify closed kinetic chain tests to evaluate this activity in the shoulder[43,108–110] (Fig. 5–14). Ellenbecker and Roetert[111] used a Cybex Fastex to assess upper extremity unilateral stance in a closed chain. The shoulder was placed in 80° of flexion in a simulated "one arm push-up" position. A 20-second stance stability test was performed using only unilateral upper extremity support without visual input. Postural sway was calculated and used to determine the ability of an individual to balance and remain stationary during the test duration. The results of this research showed that despite large differences between upper extremity muscles in open chain isokinetic testing, placing the extremity in a closed chain position did not produce significant differences between extremities in these unilaterally dominant populations. This finding is in contrast to previous research using primarily open kinetic chain upper extremity testing. Further research is necessary to validate and provide rationale for using upper extremity closed chain testing and training methods in rehabilitation of the shoulder.

Closed Kinetic Chain Upper Extremity Stability Test

Goldbeck and Davies[109] performed test-retest reliability of the closed kinetic chain upper extremity stability test developed by Davies. A paired sample t-test was performed on the data, which revealed a correlation coefficient of 0.927. Therefore, this test has become a mainstay to assess closed kinetic chain function in the upper extremity in the clinical setting.

BIOMECHANICAL ANALYSIS

The clinician might require more diagnostic information than is obtainable from an office examination. If an injury is the result of repetitive microtrauma, the patient should be observed performing the particular activity (e.g., throwing, tennis, swimming). Quantification of the kinetic data of the shoulder complex can be accomplished using various biomechanical techniques. This type of assessment will

CKC UE Stability Test

Patient Name:_____ GC#:_____ D.O.B._____
MD:_____ PT:_____ D.O.S./D.O.I._____
Diagnosis:_____ Ht:_____in   Wt:_____ lbs

Procedure:

1.   Subject assumes push-up (male) or modified push-up (female) position.
2.   Subject has to move both hands back and forth from each line as many times as possible in 15 sec. Lines are three feet apart.
3.   Count the number of lines touched by both hands.
4.   Begin with one submaximal warm-up. Repeat 3 times and average.
5.   Normalize score by following formula:

$$\text{Score} = \frac{\text{avg.\# of lines touched}}{\text{height (in)}}$$

6.   Determine Power by following formula: (68%= Trunk, head, arms)

$$\text{Power} = \frac{68\% \text{ weight} \times \text{avg.\# of lines touched}}{15}$$

Data:

Date_____

	1	2	3	$\bar{x}$
Touches				

Score_____
Power_____

Date_____

	1	2	3	$\bar{x}$
Touches				

Score_____
Power_____

Date_____

	1	2	3	$\bar{x}$
Touches				

Score_____
Power_____

Date_____

	1	2	3	$\bar{x}$
Touches				

Score_____
Power_____

Norms	MALES	FEMALES
AVERAGE TOUCHES	18.5	28.5
AVERAGE POWER	150	135
AVERAGE SCORE	.26	.31

FIGURE 5–14. CKC UE stability test. (Courtesy of Gunderson Lutheran Sports Medicine, Lacrosse, Wisconsin.)

enable the clinician to evaluate and treat any pathomechanics that might be involved. This approach addresses the cause of the problem rather than the symptoms.

Tools and studies used in a biomechanical analysis commonly include force platforms, motion analysis, electromyography, accelerometry, and pressure systems. Force platforms and pressure systems are seldom used for shoulder examinations because the upper extremity primarily functions as an open kinetic chain. Forces imparted to the shoulder from various ground reaction forces can be determined with force platforms, but the level of introduced error is significant.

The majority of biomechanical studies conducted on the upper extremity involves motion analysis or electromyography, with the focus on either a throwing or a swing motion. Whereas two-dimensional (2D) kinematic analyses are frequently used, three-dimensional (3D) analyses provide greater detail of the joint.[112] Two-dimensional analysis limits the data collection to three degrees of freedom: two translational and one rotational. The addition of the third dimension provides information about all three axes, thereby supplying six degrees of freedom. The use of 3D analysis gives greater detail to the position of the various shoulder structures during movement. Laboratory research uses specialized equipment such as high-speed video cameras, synchronized lighting, and motion analyzers aided with various computer programs to accomplish greater accuracy and increased information regarding the shoulder's position in space.

Standard video recording equipment, frequently used for 2D kinematic analysis, might be more practical clinically because of expense and spatial constraints. While 2D analysis does not provide the examiner with a scientific analysis of a patient's kinematics, it does allow patients to view their own pathomechanics and can serve as comparative data for posttreatment mechanics.

Electromyography (EMG) provides the examiner with insight into the magnitude and rate of muscle firing. When multiple muscles are analyzed, the sequence of firing can be determined. These data can be sequenced with a video analysis to determine muscle function. Normal shoulder movement requires specific patterns of muscle recruitment to maintain the proper arthrokinematics and osteokinematics. Several studies have determined the muscle patterning for various movements in sports such as baseball, tennis, and swimming.[110,113–117]

FUNCTIONAL QUESTIONNAIRES

Many types of self-reports are used to assess function. Although this method of assessment relies on subjective information, the data generated by self-reports can provide objective information. The use of functional questionnaires for the shoulder is discussed in Chapter 6.

MEDICAL TESTS

Additional medical tests may be used to corroborate an examination and confirm the diagnosis.[3] Some of the tests that may be performed to confirm the diagnosis include: *radiographs* (fracture, dislocation, arthritis, acromioclavicular problems, impingement), *arthrograms* (adhesive capsulitis, supraspinatus tear), *CT scans* (labral pathologies), *MRI* (rotator cuff pathology, bursitis, tendonitis, muscle strains), *angiograms* (thoracic outlet syndrome), and EMGs (peripheral neuropathy).[3,6]

INTEGRATION OF EVALUATIVE FINDINGS WITH PREFERRED PRACTICE PATTERNS

By performing a detailed physical examination, a clinician can determine whether the patient is a suitable candidate for rehabilitation. The examination process will also help detect the presence of tissue pathology or inflammation, which might influence treatment. However, the main goal of the physical examination is to identify the primary impairments limiting a patient's function. In some cases the impairments might lead to tissue pathology or inflammation, while in others the impairment might be the result of a specific tissue pathology or procedure. Many of the physical findings found in each practice pattern are outlined in Chapter 4. The following section reviews the primary examination findings and tissue pathology applicable to each practice pattern related to the shoulder.

Pattern D: Impaired Joint Mobility, Motor Function, Muscle Performance, and Range of Motion Associated With Capsular Restriction

SUBJECTIVE EXAMINATION

History
- Period of muscle guarding or disuse following injury
- Period of immobilization following injury or procedure
- History of diabetes

Onset
- Usually insidious, occurring over several weeks or months

Area of Pain
- Can affect the entire glenohumeral area
- Might have referred pain to deltoid area

Aggravating Factors
- Usually excessive active movement of the shoulder, particularly external rotation or elevation of the upper extremity

Easing Factors
- Rest
- Anti-inflammatory medication
- Possibly passive motion

PRIMARY PHYSICAL FINDINGS

Observation
- Apprehensive or guarded movements of the involved extremity when removing clothing

Posture
- Possibly a forward head posture
- Internally-rotated, rounded shoulders and increased kyphosis

Active Range of Motion
- Capsular pattern of limitation
- Pain with movement of the shoulder
- Shoulder shrug sign indicating poor scapulohumeral rhythm

Passive Range of Motion
- Decreased accessory motion at the GH joint
- Possible hypomobility of the AC and SC joints

Neurological Assessment
- Motor testing (MMT) revealing weakness of the shoulder girdle musculature

Special Tests
- Positive impingement tests

POSSIBLE TISSUE PATHOLOGY
- Capsulitis
- Tendonitis: supraspinatus, long head of the biceps
- Bursitis

PROGNOSIS
- Dependent on the length of time between onset and treatment
- Other dependent factors including the degree of irritability and the amount of limitation in range of motion

INTERVENTION
- Anti-inflammatory modalities
- Manual therapy techniques
- Motor control techniques
- Muscle performance and strengthening

Pattern E: Impaired Joint Mobility, Muscle Performance, and Range of Motion Associated With Ligament of Other Connective Tissue Disorders

SUBJECTIVE EXAMINATION

History
- Reports of subluxation
- Reports of dislocation
- Pain and sensation of shoulder "giving way" with overhead activities

Onset
- Possible history of physical trauma resulting in subluxation/dislocation
- Insidious onset with overhead activities

Area of Pain
- Usually around the GH joint
- Possible referred pain to the deltoid area

Aggravating Factors
- Overhead activities
- Laxity involving only the anterior capsule aggravated by excessive external rotation or extension
- Laxity involving the posterior capsule aggravated by excessive horizontal adduction

Easing Factors
- Rest
- Avoidance of end range of shoulder movements or overhead activities

PHYSICAL EXAMINATION

Observation
- Might have arm immobilized in a sling
- Might have arm guarded at the side

Posture
- Possible scapular protraction and/or downward rotation of the glenoid fossa
- Possible scapular winging (excessive posterior rotation of the medial scapular border)

Active Range of Motion
- Hypermobility
- Possible altered scapulohumeral rhythm
- Possible pain at the end range of shoulder motion

Passive Range of Motion
- Hypermobility
- Increased GH joint play (excessive translation)
- Possible hypomobility of posterior capsule (restricted posterior glide of the humeral head)

Neurological Assessment
- Weak rotator cuff and scapular stabilizers
- Normal sensation

Special Tests
- Possible positive instability tests
- Possible positive impingement test
- Possible positive labral tests
- Possible positive biceps tendon tests

POSSIBLE TISSUE PATHOLOGY
- Capsulitis
- Tendonitis: supraspinatus, long head of the biceps
- Glenoid labrum
- Transverse humeral ligament

PROGNOSIS
- Dependent on the number of episodes of instability and the amount of activity needed to cause instability

INTERVENTION
- Address weak rotator cuff and scapular stabilizers
- Address posterior capsule tightness
- Address motor control

Pattern F: Impaired Joint Mobility, Motor Function, Muscle Performance, and Range of Motion Associated With Localized Inflammation

SUBJECTIVE EXAMINATION

History
- Reports of insidious or sudden onset with trauma

Onset
- Usually because of trauma or overuse

Area of Pain
- With GH joint involvement, area of pain usually confined to the subacromial space
- Possibly localized to AC joint or SC joint

Aggravating Factors
- Overhead activities
- Horizontal adduction

Easing Factors
- Rest
- Avoidance of overhead activities

PHYSICAL EXAMINATION

Observation
- Possible arm guarding at side

Posture
- Internally rotated shoulders
- Possible scapular protraction
- Possible scapular winging

Active Range of Motion
- Painful arc from 60° to 120° of elevation
- Pain only at the end range of elevation
- Altered scapulohumeral rhythm

Passive Range of Motion
- Possible restricted posterior capsule
- Possible hypomobility of AC or SC joints

Neurological Testing
- Weak rotator cuff
- Weak scapular musculature

Special Tests
- Positive impingement tests
- Painful empty can test
- Possible positive biceps tendon tests

POSSIBLE TISSUE PATHOLOGY
- Long head of the biceps
- Supraspinatus
- Subacromial bursa

PROGNOSIS
- Prognosis depends on the underlying impairments and length of history.
- Inflammation resulting from instability or primary mechanical impingement might have a worse prognosis than inflammation resulting from overuse or muscle weakness.

INTERVENTION
- Anti-inflammatory modalities
- Possible joint and soft tissue mobilization
- Possible postural correction
- Possible strengthening of the rotator cuff and scapular musculature
- Possible neuromuscular control to enhance scapulohumeral rhythm

Pattern G: Impaired Joint Mobility, Motor Function, Muscle Performance, Range of Motion, or Reflex Integrity Secondary to Spinal Disorders

SUBJECTIVE EXAMINATION

History
- Reports of insidious or sudden onset with trauma

Onset
- Usually because of trauma or overuse

Area of Pain
- Usually diffuse area of symptoms
- Involvement of shoulder girdle and possibly the cervical spine and upper extremity

Aggravating Factors
- Usually related to specific movement patterns of the shoulder girdle and cervical spine

Easing Factors
- Rest
- Avoidance of specific movement patterns

PHYSICAL EXAMINATION

Observation
- Arm guarding at side

POSTURE
- Internally rotated shoulders
- Possible scapular protraction and scapular winging

Active Range of Motion
- Pain depending on position of the shoulder girdle and cervical spine
- Possible altered scapulohumeral rhythm
- Usually no restriction in ROM

Passive Range of Motion
- Usually no restriction

Neurological Testing
- Possible weakness
- Possible changes in deep tendon reflexes
- Possible sympathetic responses

Special Tests
- Positive cervical spine tests
- Positive thoracic outlet tests
- Positive neural tension tests
- Positive tests for reflex sympathetic dystrophy

POSSIBLE TISSUE PATHOLOGY
- Peripheral nerve
- Nerve root
- Cervical facet joints
- Cervical disc

Prognosis
- Dependent on the underlying impairments, length of history, and degree of tissue pathology

INTERVENTION
- Anti-inflammatory modalities
- Possible soft tissue or neural mobilization
- Possible postural correction
- Possible strengthening of the rotator cuff and scapular musculature
- Possible neuromuscular control to enhance scapulohumeral rhythm

Patterns H, I, and J: Impaired Joint Mobility, Motor Function, Muscle Performance, and Range of Motion Associated With Fractures, Joint Arthroplasty, and Soft-Tissue Surgical Procedures

Patients in these three practice patterns will have similar findings related to postinjury or postsurgical immobilization. These findings include decreased ROM, muscle weakness, disuse atrophy, and impaired motor control. The tissue pathology will vary according to the site of the lesion.

SUBJECTIVE EXAMINATION

History
- Involvement of bony fracture or surgery

Onset
- Sudden

Area of Pain
- Variable according to site of fracture or type of surgical procedure

Aggravating Factors
- Movements that stress the injured or healing tissues

Easing Factors
- Rest
- Avoiding excessive motion

PHYSICAL EXAMINATION

Observation
- Usually immobilized in a sling

Posture
- No remarkable findings

Active Range of Motion
- Limited based on site of fracture and type of surgical procedure
- Altered scapulohumeral rhythm

Passive Range of Motion
- Capsular restriction because of immobilization

Neurological Testing
- Weak rotator cuff and scapular musculature from disuse
- Possible decreased sensation around the incision

Special Tests
- Not applicable

POSSIBLE TISSUE PATHOLOGY
- Bony tissues: scapula, humerus, clavicle
- Soft tissues: Rotator cuff; glenoid labrum, joint capsule, ligamentous structures

PROGNOSIS
- Dependent on the age and activity level of the patient and degree of tissue pathology

INTERVENTION
- Modalities for pain control
- Joint and soft tissue mobilization when healing allows
- Possible postural correction
- Strengthening of the rotator cuff and scapular musculature when healing allows
- Neuromuscular control when healing allows

CHAPTER SUMMARY

This chapter provides an overview of examination for the shoulder complex, including a review of many commonly used evaluation procedures. New concepts for shoulder examination are introduced, along with scientific and clinical rationale for their use. Understanding and implementing this system of examination involves experience and practice. By implementing a system that identifies the relationship between tissue pathologies, impairments, and functional limitations, clinicians will use an examination that guides treatment.

The need for a standardized format for examining the shoulder complex has been suggested by the Research Committee for the American Shoulder and Elbow Surgeons.[117] Developing a standardized consensus to determine the best examination approach for the shoulder complex is difficult because the system must be comprehensive, reliable, and valid. Additionally, an examination approach should promote uniformity within a profession, enhance communication between professions, and facilitate the measurement of outcome studies. Although these practice patterns might need further development as they are adapted to the clinical setting, this system can serve as a blueprint from which consistent examination and treatment are established.

REFERENCES

1. Guide to Physical Therapist Practice. Part One: Description of patient/client management and Part Two: Preferred practice patterns. Phys Ther 77:1163, 1998.
2. Calliet, R: Shoulder Pain, ed 2. FA Davis, Philadelphia, 1981.

3. Magee, DJ: Orthopedic Physical Assessment, ed 3. WB Saunders, Philadelphia, 1997.
4. Davies, GJ, et al: An algorithm based examination for special tests of the shoulder complex. Manuscript submitted for publication, 1998.
5. Maughon, TS, and Andrews, JR: The subjective evaluation of the shoulder in the athlete. In Andrews, JR, and Wilk, KE (eds): The Athlete's Shoulder. Churchill Livingstone, New York, 1994.
6. Davies, GJ, and DeCarlo, MS: Examining the shoulder complex. In Bandy, W (ed): Current Concepts in Rehabilitation of the Shoulder. Sports Physical Therapy Section Home Study Course, 1995.
7. Clark, JM, and Harryman, DT: Tendons, ligaments and capsule of the rotator cuff. J Bone Joint Surg 74(Am):713, 1992.
8. Gould, JA, and Davies, GJ: Orthopaedic and sports rehabilitation concepts. In Gould, JA, and Davies, GJ (eds): Orthopaedic and Sports Physical Therapy. CV Mosby, St Louis, 1985.
9. Ellman, H: Arthroscopic subacromial decompression. Analysis of one to three year results. Arthroscopy 3:173, 1987.
10. Rowe, CR, et al: The Bankart procedure: a long-term end-result study. J Bone Joint Surg 60(Am):1, 1978.
11. Altchek, DW, et al: Arthoscopic acromioplasty. J Bone Joint Surg 72(Am)1198, 1990.
12. Salem-Bertoft, E, et al: The influence of scapular retraction and protraction on the width of the subacromial space: an MRI study. Clin Orthop 296:99, 1993.
13. Jobe, FW, and Pink, M: The athlete's shoulder. J Hand Ther 2:107, 1994.
14. Walch, G, et al: Impingement of the deep surface of the supraspinatus tendon on the posterosuperior glenoid rim: an arthroscopic study. J Shoulder Elbow Surg 1:238, 1992.
15. Andrews, JR, and Alexander, EJ: Rotator cuff injury in throwing and racquet sports. Sports Med Arthroscopy Rev 3:30, 1995.
16. Goodman, CC, and Snyder, TEK: Systemic origins of musculoskeletal pain: associated signs and symptoms. In Goodman, CC, and Snyder, TEK (eds): Differential Diagnosis in Physical Therapy. WB Saunders, Philadelphia, 1990.
17. Matsen, FA, et al: Mechanics of glenohumeral instability. Clin Sports Med 10:783, 1991.
18. Neer, CS: Impingement lesions. Clin Orthop 173:70, 1983.
19. Davies, GJ, et al: Functional examination of the shoulder complex. Phys Sports Med 9:82, 1981.
20. Andrews, A, and Gillogy, S: Physical examination of the shoulder in throwing athletes. In Zatins, B, et al (eds): Injuries to the Throwing Arm. WB Saunders, Philadelphia, 1985.
21. Hawkins, RJ, and Bokor, DJ: Clinical evaluation of shoulder problems. In Rockwood, CA, and Matsen, FA (eds): The Shoulder. WB Saunders, Philadelphia, 1990.
22. Hoppenfeld, S: Physical Examination of the Spine and Extremities. Appleton-Century-Crofts, New York, 1976.
23. Kelley, MJ, and Clark, WA: Orthopedic Therapy of the Shoulder. JB Lippincott, Philadelphia, 1995.
24. Silliman, JF, and Hawkins, RJ: Clinical examination of the shoulder complex. In Andrews, JR, and Wilk, KE (eds): The Athlete's Shoulder, Churchill Livingstone, New York, 1994.
25. Ayub, E: Posture and the upper quarter. In Donatelli, R (ed): Physical Therapy of the Shoulder. Churchill Livingstone, New York, 1987.
26. Davies, GJ, and Ellenbecker, TS: Total arm strength rehabilitation for shoulder and elbow overuse injuries. Orthopaedic Physical Therapy Home Study Course, LaCrosse, WI, 1993.
27. Rayan, GK, and Jensen, C: Thoracic outlet syndrome: Provocative examination maneuvers in a typical population. J Shoulder Elbow Surg 4:113, 1995.
28. Bateman, JE: Neurologic painful conditions affecting the shoulder. Clin Orthop 173:44, 1983.
29. Bennet, RM: The painful shoulder. Postgrad Med 73:153, 1983.
30. CIBA Publication. Thoracic Outlet Syndrome. CIBA, Summit, NJ, 1971.
31. Lord, JW: Thoracic Outlet Syndromes. Ann Surg 173:700, 1971.
32. Smith, KF: The thoracic outlet syndrome: a protocol of treatment. J Orthop Sports Phys Ther 1:89, 1979.
33. Rayan, GM: Thoracic outlet syndrome. J Shoulder Elbow Surg 7:440, 1998.
34. O'Brien, SJ, et al: The active compression test: A new and effective test for diagnosing labral tears and acromioclavicular joint abnormality. Am J Sports Med 26:610, 1998.
35. Elvey, RL: The investigation of arm pain. In Grieve, GP (ed): Modern Manual Therapy of the Vertebral Column. Churchill Livingstone, Edinburgh, 1986.
36. Hislop, HJ, and Montgomery, J: Muscle Testing, ed 6. WB Saunders, Philadelphia, 1995.
37. Kendall, FP, et al: Muscles: Testing and Function ed 4. Williams & Wilkins, Baltimore, 1993.
38. Daniels, L, and Worthingham, C: Muscle Testing. Techniques of Manual Examination, ed 5. WB Saunders, Philadelphia, 1986.
39. Smith, R, and Brunolli, J: Shoulder kinesthesia after anterior glenohumeral joint dislocation. Phys Ther 69:106, 1989.
40. Davies, GJ: The acute effects of fatigue on shoulder rotator cuff internal/external rotator isokinetic power and kinesthesia (abstract). Phys Ther 73: 1993.
41. Borsa, PA, et al: Functional assessment and rehabilitation of shoulder proprioception for glenohumeral instability. J Sport Rehab 3:84, 1994.
42. Lephart, SM, et al: Proprioception of the shoulder joint in healthy, unstable and surgically repaired shoulders. J Shoulder Elbow Surg 3:371, 1994.

43. Davies, GJ, and Dickhoff-Hoffman, S: Neuromuscular testing and rehabilitation of the shoulder complex. J Orthop Sports Phys Ther 18:449, 1993.
44. Voight, ML, et al: The effects of muscle fatigue and the relationship of arm dominance to shoulder proprioception. J Orthop Sports Phys Ther 23:348, 1996.
45. Lephart, SK, et al: The role of proprioception in the management and rehabilitation of athletic injuries. Am J Sports Med 25:130, 1997.
46. Cyriax, J: Textbook of Orthopaedic Medicine, Vol I: Diagnosis of Soft Tissue Lesions. Bailliere Tindall, London, 1982.
47. Kibler, WB: Role of the scapular in the overhead throwing motion. Contemp Orthop 22:525, 1991.
48. Kessel, L, and Watson, M: The painful arc syndrome. J Bone Joint Surg 59(B):166, 1977.
49. Hayes, KW, et al: An examination of Cyriax's passive motion tests with patients having osteoarthritis of the knee. Phys Ther 74:697, 1994.
50. Rothstein, JM: Cyriax reexamined. Phys Ther 74:1073, 1994.
51. Riddle, DL: Measurement of accessory motion: Critical issues and related concepts. Phys Ther 72:865, 1992.
52. Matsen, FA, et al: Mechanics of glenohumeral instability. Clin Sports Med 10:783, 1991.
53. Papilion, JA, and Shall, LM: Fluoroscopic evaluation for subtle shoulder instability. Am J Sports Med 20:548, 1992.
54. Grieve, GP: Common Vertebral Joint Problems. Churchill Livingstone, New York, 1981.
55. Allen, EV: Thromboangiitis obliterans: Methods of diagnosis of chronic occlusive arterial lesions distal to the wrist with illustrative cases. Am J Med Sci 178:237, 1929.
56. Adson, AW, and Coffey, JR: Cervical rib: A method of anterior approach for relief of symptoms by division of the scalenus anticus. Ann Surg 85:839, 1927.
57. Wright, IS: The neurovascular syndrome produced by hyperabduction of the arm. Am Heart Assn 29:1, 1945.
58. Yergason, RM: Supination sign. J Bone Joint Surg 13(Am):160, 1931.
59. Ludington, NA: Rupture of the long head of the biceps flexor: Cubiti muscle. Ann Surg 77:358, 1923.
60. Post, M: Physical Examination of the Musculoskeletal System. Year Book Medical Publishers, Chicago, 1987.
61. Jobe, FW, and Bradley, JP: The diagnosis and nonoperative treatment of shoulder injuries in athletes. Clin Sports Med 8:419, 1989.
62. Neer, CS: Impingement lesions. Clin Orthop 173:70, 1983.
63. Neer, CS, and Welsh, RP: The shoulder in sports. Orthop Clin North Am 8:583, 1977.
64. Hawkins, RJ, and Kennedy, JC: Impingement syndrome in athletes. Am J Sports Med 8: 151, 1980.
65. Hawkins, RJ: Basic science and clinical application in the athlete's shoulder. Clin Sports Med 10:963, 1992.
66. Hawkins, RJ, and Hobeika, P: Physical examination of the shoulder. Orthop 6:1270, 1983.
67. Ianotti, JP (ed): Rotator Cuff Disorders. American Academy of Orthopaedic Surgeons, Chicago, 1991.
68. Bergfeld, JA, et al: Evaluation of the acromioclavicular joint following first and second degree sprains. Am J Sports Med 6:153, 1978.
69. Hertel, R, et al: Lag signs in the diagnosis of rotator cuff rupture. J Shoulder Elbow Surg 5:307, 1996.
70. Moseley, HF: Disorders of the shoulder. Clin Symp 12:1, 1960.
71. Walch, G, et al: The "drooping" and "hornblower's" signs in evaluation of rotator-cuff tears. J Bone Joint Surg 80(B):624, 1998.
72. Kronberg, NL, et al: Muscle activity and coordination in the normal shoulder. An electromyographic study. Clin Orthop 257:76, 1990.
73. Townsend, H, et al: Electromyographic analysis of the glenohumeral muscles during a baseball rehabilitation program. Am J Sports Med 19:264, 1991.
74. Jobe, FW, et al: An EMG analysis of the shoulder in throwing and pitching. Am J Sports Med 11:3, 1983.
75. Jobe, FW, and Bradley, JP: The diagnosis and nonoperative treatment of shoulder injuries in athletes. Clin Sports Med 3:419, 1989.
76. Petmon, SA: Arthritis and arthroplasty. In Hawkins, RJ, and Misamore GW (eds): Shoulder Injuries in the Athlete. Churchill Livingstone, New York, 1996.
77. Ellman, et al: Eady degenerative joint disease simulating impingement syndrome: Arthroscopic findings. Arthroscopy 8:482, 1992.
78. Allman, FL: Fractures and ligamentous injuries of the clavicle and its articulation. J Bone Joint Surg 49(A):774, 1967.
79. Rockwood, CA, and Young, DC: Disorders of the acromioclavicular joint. In Rockwood, CA, and Matsen, FA (eds): The Shoulder. WB Saunders, Philadelphia, 1990.
80. Bach, BR, and Novak, PJ: Chronic acromioclavicular joint pain. Phys Sports Med 21:63, 1993.
81. Liu, SH, et al: Diagnosis of glenoid labrum tears: a comparison between magnetic resonance imaging and clinical examinations. Am J Sports Med 24:149, 1996.
82. Walsh, DA: Shoulder evaluation of the throwing athlete. Sports Med Update 4:24, 1989.
83. Matsen FA, et al: Glenohumeral joint instability. In Rockwood, CA, and Matsen, FA (eds): The Shoulder. WB Saunders, Philadelphia, 1990.

84. Kibler, WB: Specificity and sensitivity of the anterior slide test in throwing athletes with superior glenoid labrum tears. Arthroscopy 11:296, 1995.
85. Walch, G, et al: Impingement of the surface of the supraspinatus tendon of the posterosuperior glenoid rim: An arthroscopic study. J Shoulder Elbow Surg 1:238, 1992.
86. Jobe, CM, et al: Evidence for a superior glenoid impingement upon the rotator cuff (abstract). J Shoulder Elbow Surg (suppl) S19, 1993.
87. Jobe, CM: Posterior superior glenoid impingement. J Shoulder Elbow Surg 11:530, 1995.
88. Davidson, PA, et al: Rotator cuff and posterior-superior glenoid labrum injury associated with increased glenohumeral motion. J Shoulder Elbow Surg 4:384, 1995.
89. Jobe, CM: Superior glenoid impingement. Clin Orthop 330:9 8, 1996.
90. Bigliani, LU (ed): The Unstable Shoulder. American Academy Orthopaedic Surgeons, Rosemont, IL, 1995.
91. Jobe, FW, et al: Shoulder pain in the overhand or throwing athlete: The relationship of anterior instability and rotator cuff impingement. Orthop Rev 18:963, 1989.
92. Gerber, C, and Ganz, R: Clinical assessment of instability of the shoulder. J Bone Joint Surg 66(B):551, 1984.
93. Glousman, R, et al: Dynamic electromyographic analysis of the throwing shoulder with glenohumeral instability. J Bone Joint Surg 70(A):220, 1988.
94. Haayman, DT, et al: Translation of the humeral head on the glenoid with passive glenohumeral motion. J Bone Joint Surg 72(A):1134, 1990.
95. Hawkins, RJ, et al: Translation of the glenohumeral joint with the patient under anesthesia. J Shoulder Elbow Surg 5:286, 1996.
96. Lippitt, SB, et al: In vivo quantification of the laxity of normal and unstable glenohumeral joints. J Shoulder Elbow Surg 3:215, 1994.
97. Mallon, VU, and Speer, KP: Multidirectional instability: Current concepts. J Shoulder Elbow Surg 4:54, 1995.
98. Matsen, FA, et al: The Shoulder- a Balance of Mobility and Stability. American Academy Orthopaedic Surg, Rosemont, IL, 1993.
99. Matsen, FA, et al: Practical Evaluation and Management of the Shoulder. WB Saunders, Philadelphia, 1994.
100. Norwood, LA, and Terry, GC: Shoulder posterior subluxations. Am J Sports Med 12:25, 1984.
101. Protzman, RR: Anterior instability of the shoulder. J Bone Joint Surg 62(A):909, 1980.
102. Richards, RR, et al: A standardized method for the assessment of shoulder function. J Shoulder Elbow Surg 3:347, 1994.
103. Iannotti, JP, et al: Magnetic resonance imaging of the shoulder: Sensitivity, specificity, and predictive value. J Bone Joint Surg 73(A):17, 1991.
104. Cofield, RH, and Irning, JF: Evaluation and classification if shoulder instability: With special reference to examination under anesthesia. Clin Orthop 223:32, 1987.
105. Baker, CL, et al: Arthroscopic evaluation of acute initial shoulder dislocations. Am J Sports Med 18:25, 1990.
106. Rankin, SA, et al: Test-retest reliability analysis of Davies' clinically oriented Functional Throwing Performance Index (FTPI) over extended time intervals. Unpublished Master Science Degree, University of Kentucky, 1996.
107. Ellenbecker, TS: Rehabilitation of shoulder and elbow injuries in tennis players. Clin Sports Med 14:87, 1995.
108. Inman, VT, et al: Observations on the function of the shoulder joint. J Bone Joint Surg 26 (A):1, 1944.
109. Goldbeck, TG, and Davies, GJ: Test-retest reliability of the closed kinetic chain upper extremity stability test: A clinical field test. Manuscript submitted for publication, 1998.
110. Pappas, AM, et al: Biomechanics of baseball pitching. Am J Sports Med 13:216, 1985.
111. Ellenbecker, TS, and Roetert, EP: A bilateral comparison of upper extremity unilateral closed chain stance stability in elite tennis players and professional baseball pitchers (abstract). Med Sci Sports Exerc 28:SlG5, 1996.
112. Feltner, NL, and Dapena, J: Dynamics of the shoulder and elbow joints of the throwing arm during a baseball pitch. Int J Sports Biomech 2:235, 1986.
113. Perry, J: Anatomy and biomechanics of the shoulder in throwing, swimming, gymnastics and tennis. Clin Sports Med 2:247, 1983.
114. Ryu, RK, et al: An EMG analysis of shoulder function in tennis players. Am J Sports Med 16:481, 1988.
115. Kibler, BW: Biomechanical analysis of the shoulder during tennis activities. Clin Sports Med 14:79, 1995.
116. Moynes, DR, et al: Electromyography and motion analysis of the upper extremity in sports. Phys Ther 66:1905, 1986.
117. Nuber, G, et al: Fine wire EMG analysis of the shoulder during swimming. Am J Sports Med 14:7, 1986.

APPENDIX 5A: ISOKINETIC ASSESSMENT

INTRODUCTION

The use of isokinetics in the clinical evaluation of the GH joint is indicated because of the fast contractile velocities of upper extremity activities of daily living and sport-specific movement patterns, as well as the open kinetic chain atmosphere in which the upper extremity functions.[1,2] Whereas several reliability studies have been published regarding isokinetics in the lower extremity using the knee extension-flexion movement pattern,[2,3] several recent investigations have demonstrated high test-retest reliability for isokinetic measurement of the shoulder.[4–7]

Dynamic strength assessment using isokinetics is important for identifying the relative strength and balance of the musculature surrounding the GH joint. Initial isokinetic testing and training in rehabilitation of the shoulder typically utilizes the pattern of internal and external rotation.[1,2,8–19] The external-internal rotation movement pattern is most commonly used and is recommended as the preferable testing pattern in patients with rotator cuff tendonitis.[20]

The modified base position (30/30/30 position) has been recommended by Davies[2] for testing and training the internal and external rotators of the GH joint. The modified base position is obtained by tilting the dynamometer approximately 30° from the horizontal base position (Fig. 5A–1). Tilting the dynamometer into this

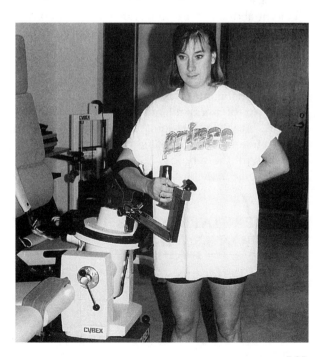

FIGURE 5A–1. Modified base isokinetic testing position.

121

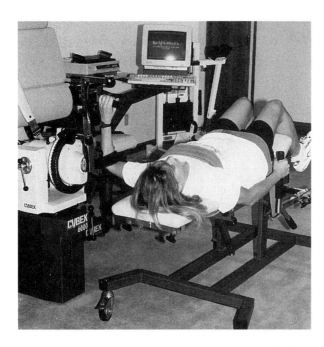

FIGURE 5A–2. Cybrex isokinetic test position for internal/external rotation with 90 degrees of glenohumeral joint abduction.

position places the GH joint in 30° of abduction and slight forward flexion in the scapular plane,[2] which is characterized by enhanced bony congruity and a neutral GH joint position. This alignment results in a midrange position for the capsular ligaments and scapulohumeral musculature.[21] Isokinetic testing requires consistent application of the patient to the dynamometer, because research has indicated that significant differences in internal and external rotation strength occur with varying positions of GH joint abduction, flexion, and horizontal abduction-adduction.[22–24]

Five maximal repetitions are recommended for peak torque and work performance data collection. In a sample of upper extremity athletes, maximum peak torque and single repetition work performance occurred in repetitions two to four.[25] Varying the testing speed through a velocity spectrum from 60° to 300° per second has been used in rehabilitation of the shoulder and in research investigations.[1,2] Isokinetic assessment of internal and external rotation strength is also performed with the shoulder in 90° of GH joint abduction (Fig. 5A–2). This test position allows greater stabilization in either a seated or supine test position on most dynamometer systems. Placement of the shoulder in abduction also simulates an overhead throwing position used in sport activities.[26]

INTERPRETATION OF SHOULDER INTERNAL-EXTERNAL ROTATION TESTING

Bilateral Differences

Assessment of an extremity's strength relative to the contralateral side forms the basis for standard data interpretation,[2] which is similar to isokinetic testing of the lower extremity. This practice is more complicated in the upper extremity because of limb dominance, particularly in the unilaterally dominant sport athlete.[1,2] In normal, untrained individuals, isokinetic testing of the upper extremities has not identified a significant strength dominance in males or females for peak torque and single repetition work values.[27,28]

Unilateral Strength Ratios

Using isokinetic strength data to evaluate the degree of balance of muscle groups surrounding a joint is assessed by a unilateral strength ratio.[2] The strength ratio of external-internal rotation has been reported as a 2:3 ratio or 66% in normal, uninjured subjects through the velocity spectrum.[2,27] Alteration of this ratio has been reported in unilaterally dominant upper extremity athletes such as baseball and tennis players.[21,22,29,30] A ratio below 66% might be detected in overhead athletes (athletes involved in overhead sports such as baseball, volleyball, and tennis), who selectively strengthen the internal rotators relative to the external rotators on the dominant arm, as well as in patients with GH joint instability and impingement.[23,31]

Unilateral strength ratios for shoulder extension-flexion are 5:4, and adduction-abduction are 2:1.[2,27] Biasing of these ratios toward greater extension and adduction strength has been reported in unilaterally dominant upper extremity athletes.[32,33] Additional isokinetic testing has been reported utilizing the movement pattern of protraction-retraction.[34] A 1:1 ratio (92%–116%) of muscular performance between the scapular retractors and protractors was reported by Davies[34] from a sample of 250 shoulders tested with approximately 60° of shoulder elevation.

Peak Torque/Body Weight, Work/Body Weight Ratios (Normalized Relative Data)

The use of normalized data allows for comparison between patients or groups of patients, regardless of the subject's body weight.[2] These ratios play an important part in the utilization of normative data research in clinical application.[1,2,30,33] However, the practice of normalizing data using body weight does not consider specific body composition and might skew the results.

Descriptive Normative Data

Using population and apparatus-specific normative data assists the clinician in the interpretation of isokinetic test results.[2] The importance of using this type of normalized data has been reported by Gross et al.[35] and Francis and Hoobler.[36] Isokinetic profiles for specific populations of upper extremity athletes have been established. These profiles offer additional information regarding other bilateral comparison (dominance), and unilateral strength ratios (muscle balance). Comparing normative data relative to body weights allows for comparison within a population.

Total Arm Strength

Some clinicians advocate evaluating the strength of the entire upper extremity.[36,37,38] This assessment might identify weaknesses associated with particular pathologies and might help isolate a specific shoulder injury or pathology. Knowing this information facilitates the development of a rehabilitation program because it considers all the muscular impairments for the upper extremity and any resulting dysfunction or disability.

SUMMARY

Prior to using isokinetics for rehabilitation or testing, patients should be screened to ensure they are appropriate candidates for this type of exercise. Patients should have the proper amount of ROM and motor control needed to perform the task. Clinicians should be careful to avoid using speeds or placing the patient in positions that exacerbate the condition. Using mechanical stops help prevent overstressing the joint capsule. Although an isokinetic score might not be the sole indicator of function, a correlation exists between this measure of muscle performance and shoulder dysfunction, particularly in the overhead athlete. Therefore, isokinetic ratios can be used in conjunction with other functional tests, to gauge progress and to determine when a patient might be ready to return to overhead activities.

REFERENCES

1. Ellenbecker, TS: Rehabilitation of shoulder and elbow injuries in tennis players. Clin Sports Med 14:87, 1995.
2. Davies, GJ: A Compendium of Isokinetics in Clinical Usage, ed 4. S & S Publishers, LaCrosse, WI, 1992.
3. Timm, K: The physiological and mechanical reliability of selected isokinetic dynamometers. Isok Exerc Sci 2:182, 1992.
4. Perrin, DH: Reliability of isokinetic measures. Athl Train 21:319, 1986.
5. Frisiello, S, et al: Test-retest reliability of eccentric peak torque values for shoulder medial and lateral rotation using the Biodex isokinetic dynamometer. J Orthop Phys Ther 19: 341, 1994.
6. Malerba, JL, et al: Reliability of dynamic and isometric testing of shoulder external and internal rotators. J Orthop Sports Phys Ther 18:543, 1993.
7. Hageman, PA, et al: Effects of position and speed on eccentric and concentric isokinetic testing of the shoulder rotators. J Orthop Sports Phys Ther 11:64, 1989.
8. Davies, GJ, Ellenbecker, TS: Eccentric isokinetics. Orthop Phys Ther Clin North Am 1:297, 1992.
9. Scoville, CR, et al: End range eccentric antagonistic/concentric agonists strength rations: A new perspective in shoulder strength assessment. J Orthop Sports Phys Ther 25:203, 1997.
10. Davies, GJ: The need for critical thinking in rehabilitation. J Sport Rehab 4:1, 1995.
11. Davies, GJ, et al: Open kinetic chain assessment and rehabilitation. Athl Train: Sports Health Care Perspective 1:347, 1995.
12. Davies, GJ, et al: Assessment of strength. In Malone, TR, et al (eds): Orthopaedic and Sports Physical Therapy, ed 3. CV Mosby, St. Louis, 1997, p 225.
13. Davies, et al: Computerized isokinetic testing of patients with rotator cuff (RTC) impingements demonstrates specific external rotators power deficits. (Abst). Phys Ther 77: S105, 1997.
14. Davies, GJ, and Ellenbecker, TS: Application of isokinetic testing and rehabilitation. In Andrews, JR, et al (eds): Physical Rehabilitation of the Injured Athlete. WB Saunders, 1998, p 219.
15. Davies, GJ, and Manske, R: The evaluation of torque acceleration energy (TAE) in 110 patients with shoulder conditions. Unpublished Data, LaCrosse, WI, 1998.
16. Ellenbecker, TS, et al: Concentric vs eccentric isokinetic strengthening of the rotator cuff: Objective data vs functional test. Am J Sports Med 16:64, 1988.
17. Heiderscheit, B, et al: The effects of isokinetic versus plyometric training of the shoulder internal rotators. J Orthop Sport Phys Ther 23:125, 1996.
18. Fortun, C, et al: The effects of plyometric training on the shoulder internal rotators (abstract). Phys Ther 78:58, 1998.
19. Manske, R, and Davies, GJ: The effects of rehabilitation on torque acceleration energy (TAE) in 60 patients with TAE deficits of the index test. Unpublished Data, LaCrosse, WI, 1998.
20. Holm, I, et al: External rotation-best isokinetic movement pattern for evaluation of muscle function in rotator cuff tendonosis: A prospective study with a 2-year follow-up. Isok Exerc Sci 5:121, 1996.

21. Saha, AK: Dynamic stability of the glenohumeral joint. Acta Orthop Scand 42:491, 1971.
22. Greenfield, B, et al: Isokinetic evaluation of shoulder rotational strength between the plane of the scapula and the frontal plane. Am J Sport Med 18:124, 1990.
23. Soderberg, GJ, and Blaschak, MJ: Shoulder internal and external rotator peak torque production through a velocity spectrum in differing positions. J Orthop Sports Phys Ther 8:518, 1987.
24. Walmsley, RP, and Szybbo, C: A comparative study of the torque generated by the shoulder internal and external rotator muscles in different positions and at varying speeds. J Orthop Sports Phys Ther 9:217, 1987.
25. Arrigo, CA, et al: Peak torque and maximum work repetition during isokinetic testing of the shoulder internal and external rotators. Isok Exer Sci 4:171, 1994.
26. Dillman, CJ, et al: Biomechanics of pitching with emphasis upon shoulder kinematics. J Orthop Sports Phys Ther 18:402, 1993.
27. Uvey, FM, et al: Normal values for isokinetic testing of shoulder strength. Med Sci Sports Exerc 16:127, 1984.
28. Gallagher, MA, et al: The effect of age, speed and arm dominance on shoulder function in untrained men. J Shoulder Elbow Surg 5:25, 1996.
29. Ellenbecker, TS, and Mattalino, AJ: Concentric isokinetic internal and external rotation strength in professional baseball pitchers. J Orthop Sports Phys Ther 5:275, 1997.
30. Wilk, KE, et al: The strength characteristics of internal and external rotator muscles in professional baseball pitchers. Am J Sports Med 21:61, 1993.
31. Warner, JP, et al: Patterns of flexibility, laxity, and strength in normal and shoulders with instability and impingement. Am J Sports Med 18:366, 1990.
32. Ellenbecker, TS: A total arm strength isokinetic profile of highly skilled tennis players. Isok Exerc Sci 1:9, 1991.
33. Wilk, KE, et al: The abductor and adductor strength characteristics of professional baseball pitchers. Am J Sports Med 23:307, 1995.
34. Davies, GJ, and Dickhoff-Hoffman, S: Neuromuscular testing and rehabilitation of the shoulder complex. J Orthop Sports Phys Ther 18:449, 1993.
35. Gross, MT, et al: Intramachine and intermachine reliability of the Biodex and Cybex II for knee flexion and extension peak torque and angular work. J Orthop Sports Phys Ther 13:329, 1991.
36. Francis, K, and Hoobler, T: Comparison of peak torque values of the knee flexor and extensor muscle groups using the Cybex II and Lido 2.0 isokinetic dynamometers. J Orthop Sports Phys Ther 8:480, 1987.
37. Davies, GJ, and Ellenbecker, TS: Total arm strength rehabilitation for shoulder and elbow overuse injuries. Orthopaedic Physical Therapy Home Study Course, LaCrosse, WI, 1993.
38. Schexneider, MA, et al: An isokinetic estimation of total arm strength. Isok Exerc Sci 1:117, 1991.

APPENDIX 5B: CLINICAL BIOMECHANICAL ASSESSMENT

Determining the cause of the initial injury is an important aspect of any evaluation. Among pitchers, the initial injury might result from overuse of the arm or from abnormal or faulty mechanics. In either case, tissues around the shoulder girdle might experience unusually high stresses during each pitch. To determine if faulty mechanics were responsible for the injury, an assessment of throwing mechanics must be performed. Prior to performing a biomechanical evaluation, the examiner must understand the mechanics of throwing and pitching and have a very good understanding of baseball.

NORMAL PITCHING MECHANICS

The overhead pitching motion has been analyzed by several researchers.[1–13] Pitching a baseball involves repeated, coordinated movements of the entire body. Because the pitcher always starts from the same position on the field and throws to the same target, pitching a baseball is an easy motion to analyze. Other overhead movements that are not as controlled, such as throwing from the outfield or throwing a football, are not as easy to study. Repetitive movements of overhead pitching, combined with motion analysis technology in the area of biomechanical research, allow the medical community to have better comprehension of its normal biomechanics. Through understanding normal pitching mechanics, a clinician can better identify abnormal mechanics that can cause injury or predispose a pitcher to future injury.

The classic pitching motion can be broken into five different phases: windup, early cocking phase, late cocking phase, acceleration, and follow through, which some experts have subdivided into the deceleration and follow-through phases.[2–4]

Windup

The windup begins when the pitcher initiates motion and concludes when the lead knee (left knee for a right-hander) reaches its peak height.[4] A windup allows the pitcher to position himself properly, develop rhythm, and possibly provide a distraction or deception for the hitter. The windup also allows the pitcher to develop a "personality" to the motion. However, a faulty windup can establish a poor position for the remainder of the pitching motion, possibly leading to inaccuracy, inefficiency, inconsistency, and injury. The pitcher should maintain good balance and be in a position to transfer weight toward the target. If adequate balance and transfer of weight do not occur during the windup, the pitcher might compromise in a later phase.

126

Early Cocking

The early cocking phase immediately follows the windup and concludes when the lead foot is on the ground.[4] In this author's opinion, this phase requires the most detailed assessment. The early cocking phase is the sequence of motion that occurs before the dynamic and explosive phases, creating the propulsion of the ball. Therefore, it is performed at a much slower and more controlled rate compared to that of the late cocking and acceleration phases. This phase has four essential elements that need to be assessed: stride offset, stride angle, the amount of horizontal extension to the throwing arm, and trunk involvement.

STRIDE OFFSET

Stride offset refers to *where* the lead foot lands. An imaginary line is drawn between the midfoot of the pitcher's back leg (immediately in front of the rubber) and the target. The perfect stride offset would have the lead foot landing directly on the imaginary line. However, an acceptable range would include 3 inches to either side of that line.[5] This variable is best observed from the anterior camera view angle, during the frame where the lead foot becomes flat on the mound. If a right-handed pitcher lands with his lead foot to the pitcher's right of the line, he has a closed stride offset. If a right-handed pitcher lands with his lead foot to the pitcher's left of the line, he has an open stride offset.

Pitchers with closed stride offsets will usually demonstrate an inability to complete the follow-through motion. The lead foot becomes the axis of rotation for the late cocking, acceleration, and follow-through phases. If this axis is placed too far to the right (closed offset) of the intended motion (imaginary line), completing the follow-through motion would be difficult because a great deal of rotation to the pitcher's left would be required.

A greater problem exists when a pitcher lands with an open stride offset. When the foot lands in a position of open stride offset, the hips must follow the motion of the foot and open prematurely. In most cases, premature opening of the hips also causes the lead shoulder (nonthrowing shoulder) to open slightly. When the lead shoulder opens too early, the throwing shoulder moves into a position of greater horizontal extension that increases anterior translation of the GH joint.[4,6,7] This premature opening might increase the valgus stress to the medial aspect of the elbow.[7,8]

STRIDE ANGLE

Stride angle refers to the angle at which the lead foot (left foot for a right-handed pitcher) lands, or in other words, *how* the foot lands. This movement is observed best from the anterior camera angle during the frame where the lead foot becomes flat on the mound. Studies have shown that the optimal stride angle should be between 6° to 27° closed.[4] This measurement means that a right-handed pitcher should land with the lead foot adducted 6° to 27° relative to the imaginary reference line. Any deviation left of this ideal range for a right-hander is considered an open stride angle.

The results of an abnormal stride angle are very similar to those of an abnormal stride offset. A closed stride angle might prevent adequate hip rotation needed to complete the follow-through phase. Conversely, an open stride angle forces the lead hip to open prematurely. Based upon the descriptive data about injured pitchers, collected by these authors over 5 years, an open stride angle led to premature opening of the lead hip more frequently than an open stride offset.

HORIZONTAL EXTENSION

Horizontal upper extremity extension is defined as the movement of an abducted arm posterior to the frontal plane. This movement is also observed best from the anterior camera angle. However, instead of assessing a particular frame, the clinician should observe the entire early cocking phase for assessment of horizontal extension. Ideally, the throwing arm should not extend beyond the frontal plane for two reasons. First, the head of the humerus loses joint congruency with the glenoid labrum when the humerus moves beyond the frontal plane. Greater horizontal extension will result in a greater amount of anterior translation of the humerus, which might result in anterior instability.[4] Second, the pitcher can conceal the ball longer from the hitter, theoretically allowing less time for the hitter to react to the pitch.

TRUNK INVOLVEMENT

The trunk plays a critical role in transferring forces generated from the lower extremities to the upper extremities and recruits large muscles of the trunk to help create additional forces. The trunk is best evaluated from the side camera angle throughout the entire motion of the early cocking phase with special emphasis at the point at which the lead foot makes contact with the mound.

At the beginning of the early cocking phase, the lead leg and hip should initiate movement toward the target. Shoulders that move forward before the hips indicate that the pitcher might have been off balance during the windup phase. This abnormal movement might also indicate that the pitcher is rushing the motion and not allowing the legs and trunk to maximally generate force for the pitch.

Evaluating the efficiency of trunk involvement can best be observed when the lead foot makes contact with the mound. When viewing this frame, it is useful to drop a plumb line from each shoulder joint and compare the line to the respective hip joint (right shoulder to right hip, and left shoulder to left hip). The observer should see that the shoulder plumb line is posterior to the respective hip joint. If the plumb line is anterior to the hip, the shoulders have preceded the hips and the trunk is not generating optimal muscle force. The pitcher might compensate by recruiting the scapulothoracic and rotator cuff musculature to generate the force to propel the ball.

Late Cocking

The late cocking phase follows the early cocking phase and concludes when the throwing arm reaches maximal external rotation. A sequential rotation of the trunk toward the target should begin with the hips and end with the shoulders.[6] The extreme amount of external rotation ROM results from GH motion, scapulothoracic motion, and trunk extension. Mechanical errors usually do not occur in this phase.

Acceleration

The acceleration phase begins at the point of maximal external rotation and ends at the point of ball release, which lasts approximately 50 milliseconds.[4] Because of this short duration, very little information can be gathered from this phase without highly sophisticated motion analysis equipment.

Follow-Through

The follow-through phase includes all motion from the point of ball release until motion ceases. The purpose of the follow-through is to allow the body to decelerate the large forces generated during the late cocking and acceleration phases. The ideal finishing position involves 180° of body rotation from the windup position (left rotation for a right-handed pitcher) with the pitching shoulder facing the batter.[6] This position allows the large posterior muscles of the trunk and lower extremities to decelerate the motion.

DESCRIPTIVE STUDY OF PATHOMECHANICS AND CORRELATION TO INJURIES OF THE UPPER EXTREMITY

Introduction

Over the past 6 years, the authors have been performing biomechanical analysis of overhand throwers. Emphasis has been placed on patients who have been referred by physicians with a throwing injury. The largest number of patients examined has been baseball pitchers, totaling 124 subjects. Retrospective chart and video reviews have been performed to collect data for this study.

Subjects

This study included 124 pitchers with different areas of pain. The average age of the subjects was 17.2 years with a range of 11 to 37 years. Categories by injured body segment include shoulder (n=57), elbow (n=46), humerus (n=5), and other (n=16).

Patients with shoulder pathology were subdivided into five different primary diagnoses: anterior instability (n=27), rotator cuff impingement (n=14), rotator cuff tendonitis (n=12), posterior instability (n=3), and rotator cuff repair (n=1). The average age of those patients seen with a shoulder injury was 18.0 years.

Patients with elbow pathology were subdivided into five different primary diagnoses: valgus overload syndrome (n=30), distal bicipital tendonitis (n=5), lateral compression syndrome (n=6), extension overload syndrome (n=2), and general elbow pain (n=4). The average age of those patients with an elbow injury was 16.6 years.

Patients with pathology of the humerus (n=5) included four patients diagnosed with proximal humeral apophysitis and one patient sustaining a traumatic distal humeral fracture while throwing a pitch. The average age of all humeral patients was 14.7 years, but the average age of the four patients sustaining the apophysitis injuries was 12.7 years.

The "other" group included patients with lower extremity and trunk injuries.

Materials and Methods

Patients were evaluated by a physical therapist or one of the authors who performed the biomechanical analysis. Patients would warm up on an upper body ergometer and perform their own flexibility routines. Each patient would then begin playing catch from approximately 30 feet and gradually increase the distance and intensity of throws until ready to pitch from the mound. This progression was done at the pace of the patient in an attempt to simulate a normal routine.

An indoor pitching mound with an elevation of 10 inches was positioned so the front edge of the rubber was 60.5 feet from the target. A Panasonic PV–810 video camera was positioned 3 feet forward of the rubber and 15 feet to the side of the patients' throwing arm. The videograph was collected at a shutter speed of 1/4000 second with a 2000-watt spotlight to eliminate as many shadows as possible. After removing their shirts to allow better visibility of joint angles and limb placements, patients threw fastballs into a 9 × 9 foot netted cage; a minimum of three pitches were recorded. Occasionally, other pitches were recorded if symptoms were present with a specific pitch.

An anterior view was the second position used for data collection. The video camera was placed just inside the netted cage on the throwing arm side of the patient. A Plexiglas barrier was placed in front of the camera for protection. Again, at least three pitches were recorded on the videotape for future qualitative analysis. Upon completion of the data collection, the patient would ice the injured area.

The videograph was viewed and analyzed on a Panasonic AG 7300 VCR and Sony PVM–1341 monitor. The analysis performed was qualitative because digitization equipment was not available. Therefore, measurements were made with a goniometer on the monitor, or an estimate of the actual position was made.

Results

The pathomechanics identified included an open stride angle, excessive horizontal extension, open stride offset, and trunk involvement. Seventy-eight (63%) of the pitchers demonstrated lower extremity pathomechanics (stride angle or stride offset), 55 (44%) demonstrated upper extremity pathomechanics (horizontal extension), and 33 (27%) demonstrated trunk pathomechanics.

Of the 57 pitchers with a shoulder diagnosis, 27 (47%) had an open stride angle, 20 (35%) demonstrated excessive horizontal extension, 11 (19%) had pathomechanics of the trunk, and eight (14%) had an open stride offset.

Of the 46 pitchers with an elbow diagnosis, 24 (52%) had an open stride angle, 17 (37%) demonstrated excessive horizontal extension, 12 (26%) had trunk involvement pathomechanics, and nine (20%) had an open stride offset.

The 103 pitchers with both elbow and shoulder diagnoses were combined with the following pathomechanics: 51 (49.5%) with an open stride angle, 37 (35.9%) with excessive horizontal extension, 24 (23.3%) with trunk involvement, and 17 (16.5%) with an open stride offset.

Conclusion

Based on this descriptive study, it could be theorized that abnormal pitching mechanics that include an open stride angle, an excessive amount of horizontal extension, an open stride offset, or an inefficient trunk involvement could lead to injury of the shoulder or elbow. Further study in this area using quantitative measures is certainly needed.

REFERENCES

1. Pappas, et al: Biomechanics of baseball pitching: A preliminary report. Am J Sports Med 13:216, 1983.
2. Atwater, AE: Biomechanics of overarm throwing movements and of throwing injuries. Exerc Sport Sci Rev 7:43, 1979.
3. Fleisig, GS, et al: Kinetics of baseball pitching with implications about injury mechanisms. Am J Sports Med 23:233, 1995.
4. Feltner, M, and Dapena, J: Dynamics of the shoulder and elbow joints of the throwing arm during a baseball pitch. Int J Sports Biomech 2:235, 1986.
5. Elliot, B, et al: Timing of the lower limb drive and throwing limb movement in baseball pitching. Int J Sports Biomech 4:59, 1988.
6. Dillman, et al: Biomechanics of the Shoulder in Sports: Throwing Activities. Post Graduate Studies in Physical Therapy. Pennington, NJ, Forum Medical, 1990.
7. Leisig, GS, and Barrentine, SW: Biomechanical aspects of the elbow in sports. Sports Med Arthroscop Rev 3:149, 1995.
8. Schwab, GH, et al: Biomechanics of elbow instability: The role of the medial collateral ligament. Clin Orthop 146:42, 1980.
9. Werner, SL, et al: Biomechanics of the elbow during baseball pitching. J Orthop Sports Phys Ther 17:274, 1993.
10. Moynes, DR, et al: Electromyography and motion analysis of the upper extremity in sports. Phys Ther 66:1905, 1986.
11. Barrentine, SW, et al: Kinematic analysis of the wrist and forearm during baseball pitching. J Appl Biomech 14:24, 1998.
12. Perry, J: Anatomy and biomechanics of the shoulder in throwing, swimming, gymnastics and tennis. Clin Sports Med 2:247, 1983.
13. Dillman CJ, et al: Biomechanics of pitching with emphasis upon shoulder kinematics. J Orthop Sports Ther 18:402, 1993.

CHAPTER 6

Functional Outcome Measures for the Shoulder

Jill Binkley, PT, MClSc, FCAMT, FAAOMPT

INTRODUCTION

Physical therapists routinely need to document the status of their patients and determine if changes have occurred following one or more treatments. Improvement might be detected as a decrease in pain on a pain scale, increased range of motion, or an ability to do something that could not be performed previously. This information is used to make decisions about continuing, discontinuing, or changing an intervention. Information regarding the outcomes of an intervention is used to guide clinical decision making. It is also used for systematic data collection, such as for a quality assurance program or for research. In addition, outcome measurement is a critical component of formal clinical studies when comparing interventions. The selection of appropriate measures of patient progress and outcome is critical. The literature is deficient, however, in assisting clinicians to evaluate and interpret the variety of self-report functional outcome measurement scales available.

In clinical practice, physical therapists assess patients' status through informal inquiry, such as, "How are you doing today, are you able to do more with your shoulder?" and through measures of impairment such as pain, range of motion, and strength. Impairment measures alone are not adequate measures of outcome. Consider an athlete with tendonitis resulting in an inability to pitch in baseball. For this patient, measures of impairment such as pain intensity, shoulder range of motion, and strength might not adequately reflect the nature of the disability and the changes that occur with physical therapy intervention. An appropriate measure of function might be the only outcome measure with which to document change in such a patient.

Patients' goals for physical therapy intervention are typically related to function, such as improved ability to throw, comb hair, or go to work. The inclusion of outcome measurements of functional ability is important to match therapists' goals and approach the goals of patients. In summary, whereas measures of impairment remain important in planning intervention, measures of function are a critical component of measuring outcomes.

132

USING FUNCTIONAL OUTCOME MEASURES IN CLINICAL PRACTICE

Incorporating standardized functional outcome measurements into clinical practice provides many benefits. Primarily, patient care is enhanced because the focus is on functional goals that are critical to the patient. Patient-clinician communication is improved when patients feel that the clinician comprehends their functional limitations. Clinical decision making regarding continuation, change, or discontinuation of treatment is improved. Finally, communication with referral sources and payers regarding patients' functional level and the goals and outcomes of physical therapy needs to be clear, providing evidence about the quality of physical therapy intervention. Payers are beginning to demand regular documentation of patients' functional levels and updates on functional goals and outcomes.

METHODS OF MEASURING FUNCTION FOR PATIENTS WITH SHOULDER CONDITIONS

Two principal categories of measures are used to evaluate function in patients with orthopaedic dysfunction: self-report functional scales and observed functional performance tests. Self-report functional scales, which vary in length from one page to many pages, are completed by patients in the clinic or through phone surveys. Examples of these scales include the SF-36 health status scale and the Shoulder Pain and Disability Index.[1-7] In some cases, the term *health status measure* is applied to more global scales that include physical, psychological, and social function. The term *functional status scale* is sometimes reserved for those scales that primarily include physical function. In this chapter, the terms *functional status scale* or *functional status measure* will refer to any self-report scale used for assessing any combination of physical, psychological, or social function.

Functional performance tests require a patient to complete a single task or battery of functional tasks while being observed by a physical therapist. In general, the measurement properties of functional performance measures available for patients with orthopaedic dysfunction are only beginning to be documented. In addition, functional performance measures can be time-consuming to implement into clinical practice. While performance measures have a role in clinical practice, self-report functional scales are recommended as fundamental measures of functional status and outcome. Many functional scales are available, consisting of documented measurement properties that are efficient and economical to incorporate into orthopaedic physical therapy practice. Self-report functional scales will, therefore, be the focus of this chapter.

Types of Self-Report Functional Status Outcome Measures

Self-report functional status outcome measures, in which patients respond verbally or with pen and paper to questions regarding their functional status, are the easiest measures of functional outcome to incorporate into clinical practice. Functional status measures are classified as *generic, condition-specific,* and *patient-specific.* The appendix at the end of this chapter provides an overview of the various functional scales used for the shoulder.

Generic measures are designed to be applicable across a broad spectrum of diseases, conditions, and demographic and cultural subgroups.[8] Examples of generic scales include the Sickness Impact Profile (SIP)[9] and the SF–36.[5–7] Condition-specific measures are intended to assess disability and clinically important changes in disability within a specific group (e.g., patients with shoulder dysfunction). Examples of condition-specific scales relevant to the shoulder include the Shoulder Pain and Disability Index (SPADI)[1–4] and the Disabilities of the Arm, Shoulder, and Hand (DASH) measure.[10–12] Health care policy makers and clinical researchers are interested in acquiring data on groups, whereas clinicians are interested in obtaining information and making decisions concerning individual patients. Both generic and condition specific measures have been conceived with the former interest in mind. More recently, a growing interest is being seen in using functional status outcome measures that are applicable to individual patients. In response to this need, a third type of outcome measure has emerged, the patient-specific measure.[13–18] The goal of patient specific outcome measures is to aid clinicians in making decisions about the functional status of individual patients. Several patient-specific measures exist.[13,14,17–19] When comparing existing patient specific outcome measures, the measurement properties of the Patient Specific Functional Scale (PSFS)[17–19] are more fully documented in diverse patient populations.

Criteria for Selecting a Functional Status Outcome Measure

Several criteria are required for selecting a functional status outcome measure for use in clinical practice. These include the following:

1. The scale has been developed using a systematic approach to item-generation and scoring.
2. The scale is reliable and valid, and includes sensitivity to change.
3. There is no ceiling or floor effect.
4. The measurement properties of the scale are reported in clinically meaningful terms to assist in decision making.
5. The scale is efficient to implement into clinical practice.

SCALE DEVELOPMENT

Development of a functional status outcome measure that is scientifically sound and clinically useful is a complex process.[20] The initial step is to develop the questions for the scale. Item generation is usually carried out by interviews with expert clinicians, questions to patients, and reviews of existing scales, if applicable. The nature of the items included in the scale is critical to its measurement properties. For example, some scales include questions that are impairment items, such as pain, range of motion, or instability.[21–24] For example, with the Subjective Shoulder Rating Scale, fear of dislocation and shoulder range of motion are included in the score.[4,21] Range of motion is estimated on a 5-point scale. Thus, the inclusion of impairment data might impact the measurement properties of the scale when the reliability of the impairment measure is lower than that of the functional scale. In addition, functional change might be obscured in cases in which range of motion or fear of dislocation is not changing, but function is improving. Finally, information is lost when continuous data (e.g., range of motion in degrees) are converted to ordinal data (e.g., 5-point scale). Several functional scales that are designed to evaluate shoulder disability include separate pain and function domains. This approach allows isolated clinical interpretation of these issues.[2,21,24]

Once items are determined, the initial version of the scale is pilot-tested by administering the scale to a group of appropriate patients. Items are then systematically reviewed for inclusion or exclusion in the final scale. A critical aspect in scale development is item scaling. Scaling addresses the issue of how the items will be rated. For example, responses might be dichotomous (e.g., yes or no) or rated using an interval scale (e.g., a 7-point scale from "unable to perform the task" to "no difficulty"). The type of scale selected, number of scale points, and labels for scale points are examples of factors that impact the reliability, validity, and sensitivity to change of a measure.

RELIABILITY AND VALIDITY OF FUNCTIONAL STATUS OUTCOME MEASURES

Reliability and validity, including sensitivity to change, are termed the *measurement properties* of a test or measure. *Reliability* refers to the repeatability of the measure and reflects the measurement error associated with a measure. For a test or measure to be reliable, it must remain stable when a patient has not changed.[25] Reliability is often assessed by administering a scale or test at two points in time when a change in a patient's condition is not expected. *Validity* addresses the extent to which a test or measure truly measures what is intended. In the case of a functional scale, its validity is the extent to which the scale captures patients' true functional capacity.[25]

The capacity of a measure or tool to detect change in an individual patient or groups of patients has been termed *responsiveness*.[20,26,27] Responsiveness, however, does not address the validity of a change, or whether the change measured truly reflects a clinically important change. The term *sensitivity to change* will be used in this chapter to encompass both concepts of the capacity of a measure to detect change and the validity or meaningfulness of the change.[26] Examining the validity of a change requires the use of an external measure, such as a patient-clinician rating of change, or the use of a construct in which there is evidence that one group will change at a different rate than another (e.g., comparison of patients with acute versus chronic conditions).

Important clinical implications arise when selecting a tool that does not have established or acceptable measurement properties for the patient population in which it will be used clinically. For example, if a scale has poor reliability, a clinician will be unable to distinguish true change in a patient's status from measurement error. Additionally, when a measure shown to be sensitive to valid change in a particular population (e.g., postsurgical patients) is used for patients with other conditions (e.g., degenerative joint disease) the scale might not be as sensitive to change in the second group. The risk of incorporating into practice a functional status outcome measure without documented measurement properties is significant. If a scale is incorrectly designed, patients might be improving, but the functional improvement might not be detected.

CEILING AND FLOOR EFFECT

A *ceiling effect* occurs when patients "top out" on the scale, achieving normal function when in fact some disability remains. A *floor effect* occurs when the patients "bottom out," being rated as completely disabled when in fact they are not. Ideally, few patients will "bottom out" or "top out" on a given scale, so that functional change will not be obscured by lack of a place to move on the scale. For example, an athlete given a scale with relatively easy activities, such as eating, might reach the maximum functional ability on the scale, but be unable to pitch a baseball. The difficulty of scale items, as well as the patient population for administration, affects whether a scale demonstrates ceiling and floor effects. If the scale is designed for use in a wide range of patients and conditions, care must be given during scale development to have a wide range of easy and hard activities to prevent ceiling and floor effects.

MEASUREMENT PROPERTIES AND CLINICAL DECISION MAKING

The physical therapist must be able to interpret functional status scale scores to provide information that is germane to clinical decision making. In order to interpret scale scores, the error associated with a single measure and a measure of change on the scale must be available to the physical therapist. In addition, the amount of change on a given scale that is clinically meaningful is critical to clinical decision making. These properties must be documented for any scale that is to provide information on the level and progress of functional status.

CLINICAL EFFICIENCY

Ease of administration and scoring are critical, particularly for cases in which complex calculations or a computer is required to compute a score. Functional scores might not be available to clinicians for day-to-day decision making. For situations in which a scale is scored outside the clinic, such as through the use of a database, clinicians should be aware that the application of functional measures for establishing initial functional level and tracking progress and outcome on individual patients will be precluded.

USING SELF-REPORT FUNCTIONAL SCALES

Measurement of functional status serves the following two important and distinct purposes: (1) documentation of physical therapy outcome in *groups* of patients for quality assurance, establishment of clinical standards, or research purposes; and (2) documentation of functional level, goal setting, and measurement of functional progress and outcome in *individual* patients.

Patient Group Comparisons

Outcome assessment procedures typically focus on the measurement of function at initial assessment and at discharge to answer the question "Has this group of patients' functional status changed during the intervention period?" This information provides clinicians, administrators, and payers with data regarding physical therapists and clinic performance on groups of patients. Patients might be grouped by categories such as diagnosis, clinic, physical therapist, and demographic factors to draw conclusions about patient outcome in these groups. Where comparative data are available, such as in pooled databases, clinics and clinicians can compare outcomes to other groups of patients and clinics. When the goal of measuring functional outcome is to compare groups of patients within a clinic or between clinics with respect to functional status, demonstration of the scale's reliability and validity, including sensitivity to change, must be apparent. Validity must be established for use in the intended patient population. Condition-specific and generic measures are appropriate for between-group comparisons, whereas patient-specific scales are not.

Individual Patient Measurement and Goal Setting

Little information is available in the literature to assist physical therapists in the use of available functional scales to document function, set patient goals, and measure patient progress in individual patients. Self-report functional scales are often many pages long and require detailed calculations to score, and are therefore not suitable for clinicians to administer, score, and interpret in the clinical setting on a regular basis. In addition, clinicians must be armed with information regarding the tool's reliability, validity, and sensitivity to valid change. In this case, the information must be provided in a format that enables a clinician to answer the following questions: (1) What is the functional status of a patient at a given point in time? (2) Has a patient's functional status truly changed? and (3) Is this change important?

A self-report functional scale might be used to determine the functional status of an individual patient at a given point in time. In interpreting such a scale, however, one must recognize the inherent variability in any clinical test or measure. This variability can be attributed to the patient, examiner, instrument, or measurement process. The variability in a test or measure, the *test-retest reliability*, is usually expressed as a reliability coefficient, such as an intraclass correlation coefficient. A reliability coefficient expressed as R=0.85 can be difficult to interpret, particularly as it applies to an individual patient. Thus, for decisions on individual patients, the expression of the error in the units of the scale, that is, scale points, is important in addition to a high reliability coefficient. If the error for any given scale measure is expressed in scale points, with a given confidence associated with that error estimate, the clinician can apply this to a given patient measure. Consider an example in which the error associated with a particular 100-point scale is 11 scale points, with a 90% confidence interval. For patients who score 20/100 on this scale, the true score will be between 9 and 31 for 9 out of 10 patients. A convenient way of thinking of this statistic when interpreting a score on a single patient is that the clinician can be about 90% confident that the true score is in the range given for the confidence interval.

To determine if true change has occurred in an individual patient's functional status between an initial and follow-up point in time, one must examine the change score between the two points. In this case, however, the estimate of the error of this change score must account for potential error at both initial and follow-up assessments. This error is termed the *minimal detectable change* (MDC) and is expressed as scale points.[28,29] If, for example, the MDC for a 100-point scale is 15, a change of 15 or greater in the scale is required to be confident that true change has occurred in your patient's functional status.

Finally, clinicians need to know if change in scale scores represents an *important* functional change. The *minimal clinically important difference* (MCID) is defined as the minimal change in score, indicative of change in function, that is important to a patient.[29] The MCID is estimated for a scale from studies examining sensitivity to valid change. The MCID is an important tool for the clinician when making decisions about whether improvement or deterioration that is clinically important has occurred.

CONDITION-SPECIFIC SHOULDER SCALES

Many condition-specific functional scales relevant to patients with shoulder conditions are available. These include the Shoulder Pain and Disability Index (SPADI),[1-4] The Disabilities of the Arm, Shoulder and Hand Questionnaire,[10-12] the Upper Extremity Functional Scale (UEFS),[30] the Shoulder Questionnaire,[23] the Simple Shoulder Test,[4,31-36] the Subjective Shoulder Rating System,[4,21] the Shoulder Rating Questionnaire,[22] the Constant-Murley Assessment,[33] and the American Shoulder and Elbow Surgeons Form.[37] At present, no condition-specific functional scales that meet all of the criteria outlined for measurement of progress and outcome in both patient groups and individual patients exist. The tables in Appendix 6–A provide an overview of many of the scales, including clinical efficiency, measurement properties, and comments on current knowledge and utility of the scales. The scales selected for inclusion in the table meet one or more of the following criteria:

1. They are used commonly in clinical practice or cited often in the literature.
2. They include function items, rather than impairments only, such as pain.
3. They have at least preliminary evidence of validity.
4. They are reasonably efficient to administer and score.

The measurement properties relevant to application at an individual patient level have not been reported in the literature for any of the upper extremity or shoulder scales. The values of error associated with a single measure and the MDC have been calculated by extrapolating data from the literature, when available.

Of the self-report functional outcome measures applicable to the shoulder, the measurement properties of the SPADI have been most thoroughly documented at this time.[1-3] The SPADI does not take long to administer to patients. Scoring, however, requires conversion of visual analogue scales to numerical rating scales, thus reducing its clinical efficiency when compared to other condition-specific scales. The internal consistency of the SPADI is acceptable (0.86 to 0.95), whereas the test-retest reliability of the SPADI has been reported to be only moderate (R = 0.63 to 0.66). Possible ceiling and floor effects have been reported for the SPADI. Finally, the SPADI has been reported to be more sensitive to change than the Sickness Impact Profile for the upper extremity.[1]

The Shoulder Rating Questionnaire, the UEFS, and the DASH have been documented to have adequate internal consistency and test-retest reliability. Initial validation also has been done.[11,12,22,33] Further work is required to document the validity of these scales, including sensitivity to change and the measurement properties necessary to apply these scales at the individual patient level. The DASH and the UEFS have the potential clinical advantage of applicability to all conditions of the upper extremity.

GENERIC HEALTH STATUS OUTCOME MEASURES

Several generic health status outcome measures have been applied to a variety of patients with orthopaedic conditions. These measures include the Sickness Impact Profile (SIP),[9] the SF–12,[38] the Musculoskeletal Functional Assessment Questionnaire (MFA),[39–41] the SF–36,[5–7,42–44] and the Functional Status Index (FSI).[45] The SIP takes more than 20 minutes for patients to complete and, therefore, will not be addressed here. The SF–36 and the MFA include a variety of physical and psychosocial dimensions of health, each taking approximately 15 minutes to complete. Scoring the SF–36 and the SF–12 is relatively complex, whereas the mechanism of scoring of the FSI and the MFA is straightforward.

The SF–36 is a multidimensional generic health status instrument that includes the following eight health concept scales: (1) physical functioning, (2) role limitation (physical), (3) bodily pain, (4) general health, (5) vitality, (6) social function, (7) role limitation (emotional), and (8) mental health. In total, the instrument contains 36 items that represent a broad array of health concepts. All scales are linearly transformed to a 0 to 100 scale, with 100 indicating the most favorable health state. The measurement properties of the SF–36 have been well established on samples from diverse populations.[5–7,42–44] In orthopaedic patients, the physical function and pain dimensions appear to be most relevant, whereas the other scales pick up minimal dysfunction.[17,42,43] In addition, the SF–36 questions are more applicable to lower limb and lower back problems, possibly lacing the content validity for neck and upper extremity problems.

The reliability, validity, and sensitivity to change have been well documented for the SF–36.[5–7,17,42,43] Whereas several of the SF–36 subscales have the capacity to measure change on patients with low back and lower extremity conditions, many of the subscales do not change in outpatient musculoskeletal conditions. For example, the mental health subscale of the SF–36 does not appear to measure important changes in this patient population.[17,42–44] The SF–36 addresses many aspects of health in a wide variety of patient populations. However, attempting to measure change in orthopaedic outpatients with minimal levels of overall health dysfunction might be problematic. In a patient referred with impingement syndrome of the shoulder, questions such as "I lay in bed most of the day due to my condition" are not likely relevant to the patient's problem. Awareness of which of the subscales are sensitive to change in the patient group for which it is used is necessary, because many items in a generic health status measure will not be relevant to patients in an outpatient orthopaedic practice. Concluding that patients have not changed on many subscales of the SF–36 is possible, when, in fact, one would not expect these scales to pick up change that might be occurring in outpatients with orthopaedic conditions.

The SF–12 was designed as a shorter version of the SF–36 with the goal of reproducing the Physical Component and Mental Component summary scores of the SF–36.[38] In reporting on the reliability and validity of the SF–12, Ware et al.[38] state that the SF–12 and SF–36 always reached the same statistical conclusions about group differences for physical and mental health status. The authors caution that because the SF–12 defines fewer levels of function and pools less reliable variance, the scale might yield less reliable assignments of individuals to those levels.[38] Ware et al. conclude that "for large group studies (e.g., n=500), the difference in measurement properties between the SF–12 and the SF–36 are not as important, because confidence intervals around group averages are determined largely by the sample size."[38] Thus, the SF–36 appears to be more appropriate than the SF–12 when group sizes are less than 500, as is often the case with clinical and research data in physical therapy.

The FSI includes physical and social-role function activities. Patients rank the degree of assistance required and the degree of pain and difficulty for each activity.[45] The FSI has been documented as reliable and valid in patients with total hip replacements.[45] The sensitivity to change and application to other orthopaedic conditions has not been reported for the FSI.

The MFA, a condition-specific measure designed for patients with upper and lower extremity musculoskeletal conditions, has been shown to have acceptable reliability for application to groups, but not for use at an individual patient level.[45] Construct validity has been demonstrated for the MFA, although both ceiling and floor effects have been demonstrated for some patient groups and for several of the subcategories of the MFA.[39–41] For example, 30% of all patients scored 0 (no disability) on self care and 40% of patients with rheumatoid arthritis scored 100 (maximum disability) on the employment/work category. The existence of these ceiling and floor effects, as well as the single-group design used to demonstrate the tool's responsiveness, are of concern in using the MFA at this time.

When the intent of using a scale is to document function and measure incremental change on an individual patient level, the reliability and sensitivity to change of a tool must be superior to the measurement properties traditionally considered acceptable for tools designed for group decision making.[39,45] The generic scales reviewed here are excellent choices when the goal is group decision making, but lack adequate reliability or sensitivity to change for individual patient monitoring. In addition, the most common scale used in orthopaedic practice and research, the SF–36, is time consuming to complete and score. Therefore, generic scales should be used at admission and discharge only, rather than as tools to measure incremental change on a weekly basis. Generic scales are most appropriate for use in groups of patients in whom overall health is expected to be impacted by their condition and by physical therapy intervention. An example might be in groups of patients with chronic shoulder conditions, such as 'frozen shoulder' or arthritis.

USING PATIENT-SPECIFIC AND CONDITION-SPECIFIC FUNCTIONAL SCALES FOR INDIVIDUAL PATIENT FUNCTION, PROGRESS, AND GOAL SETTING

Clinicians can use a measure of patients' initial function to set functional goals and track patients' progress. To establish short- and long-term goals using a functional scale, the clinician uses the clinical history, objective findings, and initial score to set goals that address a change in the score. The goal for change is set at a value that is greater than the MDC for the scale. In addition, an estimate of change that is considered clinically important can be made using the MCID. For example, consider a patient with an initial PSFS score of 3/10. The true initial score, based on the error associated with a single measure, is between 1 and 5. In setting a short-term goal for a patient with a condition that is considered chronic and expected to change slowly, the clinician might select a 2-week time frame for a change in score just at the MDC of 2. In this case, the short-term goal would be "PSFS greater than or equal to 7/10." In setting a short-term goal for a patient with a more acute condition that is predicted to change quickly, a shorter time frame of 1 week, with change greater than the MDC of 2 and the MCID of 3, may be selected. In this case, the goal may be "PSFS greater than or equal to 6/10." On follow-up, progress is determined by amount of change on the scale. In cases in which improvement greater than the MDC and MCID occurs, clinicians can be confident that true (MDC) and important (MCID) change has occurred. In cases where improvement is greater than or equal to the MDC, but the change falls below the MCID, clinicians can be confident that true change has occurred, but that this change might not be clinically important. Continuation of the intervention, or discharge if goals are met, would be justified in both of these scenarios. For cases in which there is no change or the change is less than the MDC, clinicians may be confident that true change has not occurred. In this case, depending on the clinical picture and time frame since previous assessment, a change in intervention or discharge may be considered.

INCORPORATING FUNCTIONAL SCALES INTO CLINICAL PRACTICE

The following case scenario is intended to illustrate use of the PSFS and a condition-specific scale, the DASH, to track patient progress, set short- and long-term goals, and measure outcome.

CASE STUDY 6–1

Mr. P is referred to you with impingement syndrome in the right shoulder. He works on the assembly line at a local bearing factory. He routinely manipulates 2- to 5-pound tools at shoulder level throughout the day. He has had a gradual onset of superolateral region shoulder pain over the past 2 months. He is currently off work, on workers compensation. There is no previous history of shoulder pain.

Pain: Baseline pain 6/10. Main area of pain is superolateral shoulder, extending distally to wrist when pain is at its worst. Aggravating factors include working, putting on shirt, reaching overhead, throwing. Unable to sleep on shoulder. Eased with ice and rest.

Function: Off work for 1 week. Right hand dominant. Usual activities include running, recreational baseball. Unable to play ball at this time. Patient-specific functional scale score 3/10. DASH score 70/100.

General Health: Excellent.

Medications: Anti-inflammatories.

Objective examination reveals the following:

Posture: Forward head posture, protracted shoulders.

Range of Motion: Shoulder elevation limited by 10°, painful arc in abduction between 80° and 105°; painful arc in flexion 85° to 100°. Hand-behind-back full motion, pain reproduced.

Strength: Not tested at initial assessment.

Passive Mobility Testing: Passive physiological flexion and abduction lacks approximately 10° compared to left. Restricted posterior-anterior and inferior motion of GH joint (tested in elevation).

Other: Tenderness on palpation of insertion of supraspinatus. Resisted isometric shoulder abduction and lateral rotation reproduced pain.

Summary: The following functional goals and outcomes worksheet was developed to record patient-specific activities and scores, condition-specific or generic scale scores, as well as to track impairment measures and goals on a weekly basis (Fig. 6–1). The form is filled in to illustrate the use of functional scales to set goals and track patient progress for Mr. P. This form is kept in the front of all of our patients' charts in our clinic for easy reference. Short- and long-term goals were set at the first postoperative visit and tracked on the same form. The goals were set to be greater than the MDC and MCID for the PSFS. In the case of the DASH, the error associated with a single measure can be obtained from the available literature. Because the data required to calculate the MDC and MCID of the DASH are not available, this example is based on a hypothetical estimate of these values for the DASH of 15 scale points. The decision about how much greater the expected change would be than these minimal levels at 2 weeks and 4 weeks was based on clinical experience with the condition and the scales. The final goals of "PSFS greater than 9/10" and "DASH less than or equal to 15/100" were based on clinical experience and data that suggest that these are reasonable goals for this type of patient.

Functional Goal and Outcome Worksheet – Mr. P

	Date and Score (weekly)					
PATIENT SPECIFIC ACTIVITIES	7/21/98 (Initial)	7/28/98	8/5/98	8/12/98		
1. Working – manipulating tools	3	3	4	7		
2. Throwing	2	5	6	8		
3. Reaching overhead	4	6	8	10		
AVERAGE: (/10)	3	4.3	6	8.3		
ADDITIONAL ACTIVITIES:						
1. Shaving	7	8	9	10		
2. Driving	8	8	10	10		
PSFS PAIN QUESTIONS:						
PAIN LIMITATION SCORE: (No limitation=10)	4	6	7	10		
PAIN INTENSITY SCORE: (Severe pain = 10)	6	2	2	1		
CONDITION-SPECIFIC MEASURE: (DASH)	70	53	36	12		
IMPAIRMENT MEASURES: (EG. ROM, STRENGTH)						
1. Painful arc flexion	85-100°	'catch' at 90°	None			
2. Painful arc abduction	80-105°	90-100	None			
3. Limited act/pass elevation	10°	5°	full			
SHORT TERM GOALS: 2 Weeks						
1. No painful arc in flex			✓			
2. PSFS ≥ 5/10			✓			
3. DASH ≤ 40/100			✓			
4. Baseline pain ≤ 2/10		✓				
LONG TERM GOALS: 4 Weeks						
1. PSFS ≥ 9/10				✓		
2. DASH ≤ 15/100				✓		
3. Return to Work				✓		

FIGURE 6–1. Functional Goal and Outcome Worksheet. (Copyright Stratford & Brinkley, 1995.)

INCORPORATION OF FUNCTIONAL STATUS OUTCOME MEASURES IN CLINICAL PRACTICE

The following three issues affect the successful clinical implementation of self-report functional outcome measures: (1) effortless administration of the questionnaire, (2) easy interpretation of the result, and (3) efficient documentation in the medical record. It might be easiest to begin implementation of one scale initially. Many clinicians have found that the PSFS is a simple and efficient place to begin using a standard measure of functional outcome. Once clinicians are familiar with setting goals and tracking progress on a regular basis using one scale, other scales may be introduced.

To facilitate administration of the measures, a laminated copy of the PSFS and folders with condition-specific self-report scales in the assessment areas can be kept for easy access. Condition-specific scales can also be laminated, and patients can respond directly using a transparency marking pen to decrease the need to file excess paperwork and to minimize the cost of printing. Once the scale has been scored it is wiped clean and ready for re-use.

The scoring and subsequent transfer of functional scores to the medical record must be efficient. The functional goal and outcome worksheet provides an efficient method of recording the following: (1) a patient-specific measure; (2) components of the physical assessment important to a specific patient (e.g., ROM measures); (3) a pain measure; (4) a condition-specific functional measure and, if desired, an SF–36 admission and discharge score; and (5) short- and long-term goals. Having all of this information in one place in the medical record facilitates the use of functional scale scores for goal setting, determination of progress, and tracking the achievement of treatment goals. Regular weekly follow-up of all patients on these measures provides an efficient and comprehensive approach to documentation of patient progress and outcome.

USING FUNCTIONAL SCALE SCORES TO COMMUNICATE WITH REFERRAL SOURCES AND PAYERS

The documentation of initial functional status and the identification of functional goals is demanded by many payers. When functional scales with documented measurement properties are used, clinicians have a tool to justify intervention for a particular group of patients or at an individual patient level. The preeminent justification for physical therapy intervention is provided through randomized, controlled clinical trials documenting the effectiveness of the intervention. In the absence of evidence demonstrating the effectiveness of a particular intervention, however, functional scales are a powerful tool to demonstrate progress and outcome at an individual patient level to referral sources and payers. The following is a clinical example of the use of functional scale scores in communication with payers. Mrs. S is a 54-year-old woman referred for physical therapy following an open reduction and internal fixation of a humeral fracture. She has significant pain, severely restricted shoulder range of motion, and weakness. She is unable to do her regular job, which involves lifting, and has difficulty with most of her usual activities of daily living, including eating, bathing, and driving. In light of her job demands, age, and significant impairment, the physical therapist determines that she will likely not attain full function without an intensive physical therapy program of at least 12 visits over

4 or 5 weeks. Her insurance company allows five physical therapy visits. There are no randomized controlled clinical trials available to support the planned intervention of manual therapy and exercise after internal fixation of a humeral fracture. Using a functional scale with documented measurement properties, the physical therapist is able to objectively demonstrate the current low level of function and to clearly articulate the change in the level of function predicted through the short- and long-term goals. As treatment progresses, change that is greater than the MDC and the MDIC of the scale demonstrates that true and important change is occurring, justifying continuation of treatment. Communicating functional goals and improvement in numerical terms that have clinical meaning is a significant contribution to the rationalization for physical therapy intervention. In the absence of clinical trials that support the effectiveness of an intervention, this approach is effective in justifying physical therapy to referring physicians and payers.

CHAPTER SUMMARY

Self-report functional scales with documented measurement properties that are efficient to administer and score enhance clinical practice in a number of ways. Information is provided that allows comparison of the clinical outcomes of different groups of patients. Functional scales can also be used to document function, track progress, and document outcome on individual patients. This information enhances clinical decision making. Finally, functional scales provide information that is critical to the reporting of patient progress to referring physicians and payers.

REFERENCES

1. Heald, S, et al: The Shoulder Pain and Disability Index: The construct validity and responsiveness of a region-specific disability measure. Phys Ther 77:1079, 1997.
2. Roach, KE, et al: Development of a Shoulder Pain and Disability Index. Arth Care Res 4:145, 1991.
3. Williams, JW, et al: Measuring shoulder function with the Shoulder Pain and Disability Index. J Rheumatol 22:727, 1995.
4. Beaton, D, and Richards, RR: Measuring function of the shoulder. J Bone Joint Surg 78-A:882, 1996.
5. Ware Jr, JE, and Sherbourne, CD: The MOS 36–item short-form health survey (SF–36): I. Conceptual framework and items selection. Med Care 30:473, 1992.
6. McHorney, CA, et al: The MOS 36-item short-form health survey (SF–36): II. Psychometric and clinical tests of validity in measuring physical and mental health constructs. Med Care 31:247, 1993.
7. McHorney, CA, et al: The MOS 36-item short-form health survey (SF–36): III. Tests of data quality, scaling assumptions, and reliability across diverse patient groups. Med Care 32:40, 1994.
8. Patrick, DL, et al: Assessing health-related quality of life in patients with sciatica. Spine 20:1899, 1995.
9. Bergner, M, et al: The Sickness Impact Profile: Development and final revision of a health status measure. Med Care 19:787, 1981.
10. Armadio, PC, et al: Measuring disability and symptoms of the upper limb: A validation study of the DASH questionnaire (abstract). Arth Rheum 39:(9)S112, 1996.
11. Armadio, PC, et al: Development of an upper extremity outcome measure: The "DASH" (Disabilities of the arm, shoulder and hand) (abstract). Arth Rheum 39:(9)S112, 1996.
12. Hudak, PL, et al: Upper Extremity Collaborative Group. Development of an upper extremity outcome measure: The DASH (Disabilities of the Arm, Shoulder, and Hand). Amer J Industrial Med 29:602, 1997.
13. MacKenzie, C, et al: A patient-specific measure of change in maximum function. Arch Intern Med 146:1325, 1986.
14. Tugwell, P, et al: The MACTAR patient preference disability questionnaire: An individualized functional priority approach for assessing improvement in physical disability in clinical trials in rheumatoid arthritis. J Rheumatol 14:446, 1987.

15. McHorney, CA, and Tarlov, AR: Individual-patient monitoring in clinical practice: Are available health status surveys adequate? Quality Life Res 4:293, 1995.
16. Ruta, DA, et al: A new approach to the measurement of quality of life: The patient-generated index. Med Care 32:1109, 1994.
17. Chatman, AB, et al: The Patient Specific Functional Scale: Measurement properties in patients with knee dysfunction. Phys Ther 77:820, 1997.
18. Stratford PW, et al: Assessing disability and change on individual patients: A report of a patient specific measure. Physiotherapy Canada 47:258, 1995.
19. Westaway, M, et al: The Patient Specific Functional Scale: validation of its use in persons with neck dysfunction. J Orthop Sports Phys Ther 27:331, 1998.
20. Streiner, DL; and Norman, GR: Health Measurement Scales: A Practical Guide to Their Development and Use. Oxford University Press, Oxford, 1995.
21. Kohn, D, and Geyer, M: The subjective shoulder rating system. Arch Orthop Trauma Surg 116:324, 1997.
22. L'Insalata, JC, et al: A self-administered questionnaire for assessment of symptoms and function of the shoulder. J Bone Joint Surg 79-A:738, 1997.
23. Dawson, J, et al: Questionnaire on the perceptions of patients about shoulder surgery. J Bone Joint Surg 78-B:593, 1996.
24. van der Windt, DAWM, et al: The responsiveness of the shoulder disability questionnaire. Ann Rheum Dis 57:82, 1998.
25. American Psychological Association (eds): Standards for Educational and Psychological Testing. American Psychological Association, Washington, DC, 1985.
26. Stratford, PW, et al: Health Status Measures: strategies and analytic methods for assessing change scores. Phys Ther 76:1109, 1996.
27. Kirshner, B, and Guyatt, G: A methodological framework for assessing health indices. J Chronic Dis 38:27, 1985.
28. Stratford, PW, et al: Defining the minimal level of detectable change for the Roland Morris Questionnaire. Phys Ther 76:359, 1996.
29. Stratford, PW, and Binkley, JM: Applying the results of self-report measures to individual patients: An example using the Roland-Morris Questionnaire. J Orthop Sports Phys Ther. In Press.
30. Pransky, G, et al: Measuring functional outcomes in work-related upper extremity disorders. Development and validation of the Upper Extremity Function Scale. J Occup Environ Med 39:1195, 1997.
31. Winters, JC, et al: A shoulder pain score: A comprehensive questionnaire for assessing pain in patients with shoulder complaints. Scand J Rehab Med 28:163, 1996.
32. Croft, P, et al: Measurement of shoulder related disability: Results of a validation study. Ann Rheum Dis 53:525, 1994.
33. Constant, CR, and Murley, AH: A clinical method of functional assessment of the shoulder. Clin Orthop 214:160, 1987.
34. Lippitt, SB, et al: A practical tool for evaluating function: the Simple Shoulder Test. In Matsen, FA, et al (eds): The Shoulder: A Balance of Mobility and Stability. American Academy of Orthopaedic Surgeons, Rosemont, IL, 1993, p 501.
35. Rozencwaig, R, et al: The correlation of comorbidity with function of the shoulder and health status of patients who have glenohumeral joint disease. J Bone Joint Surg 80-A:1146, 1998.
36. Matsen, FA, et al: Patient self-assessment of health status and function in glenohumeral degenerative joint disease. J Shoulder Elbow Surg 4:345, 1995.
37. Richards, RR, et al: A standardized method for the assessment of shoulder function. J Shoulder Elbow Surg 3:347, 1994.
38. Ware Jr, JE, et al: A 12-item short-form health survey: Construction of scales and preliminary tests of reliability and validity. Med Care 34:220, 1996.
39. Martin, DP, et al: Comparison of the Musculoskeletal Function Assessment Questionnaire with the Short-Form-36, the Western Ontario and McMaster Universities Osteoarthritis Index, and the Sickness Impact Profile health-status measures. J Bone Joint Surg 79-A:1323, 1997.
40. Engelberg, R, et al: Musculoskeletal Function Assessment Instrument: criterion and construct validity. J Orthop Res 14:182, 1996.
41. Martin, DP, et al: Development of a Musculoskeletal Extremity Health Status Instrument. J Orthop Res 14:173, 1996.
42. Jette, DU, and Jette, AM: Physical Therapy and health outcomes in patients with spinal impairments. Phys Ther 76:930, 1996.
43. Jette, DU, and Jette, AM: Physical Therapy and health outcomes in patients with knee impairments. Phys Ther 76:1178, 1996.
44. Riddle, DL, and Stratford, PW: Use of generic versus region-specific functional status measures on patients with cervical spine disorders: A comparison study. Phys Ther 78:951, 1998.
45. Jette, AM: The Functional Status Index: reliability and validity of a self-report functional disability measure. J Rheumatol 14:15, 1987.

APPENDIX 6A: FUNCTIONAL OUTCOME MEASUREMENT SCALES

Scale	Background and Description	Measurement Properties	Comments
Patient-Specific Functional Scale[1–3]	*Developer of Measure: Stratford, P.W.* Intended patient group: All patients with musculoskeletal dysfunction Classification of measure: Self-report, patient-specific measure Conceptual framework: Conceived with individual patient decision-making in mind Time to complete (patient): Less than 5 minutes Time to score (clinician): About 10 seconds Possible scores: 0 to 10 (average of individual activity scores) Scale orientation: Higher scores represent less disability	*Traditional Expression:* Test-retest reliability: 0.84 to 0.98 Sensitivity to change: 0.51 to 0.77 (global rating); 0.54 (prognosis rating) *Clinical Expression:* Variation around a measured value (90% CI): ±2 PSFS points Minimal detectable change (90% CI): 2 PSFS points (for scale average) 3 PSFS points (for individual items) Minimal clinically important difference: 3 PSFS points	1. Measurement properties provided in a manner suitable for decision making at the level of the individual patient. 2. The PSFS completed by patients and scored by clinicians efficiently. 3. Because patients generate different activities, the PSFS not intended for comparison between patients. Therefore, recommended for clinicians as an initial step in measuring functional outcome or as a complement to condition-specific measures to assist in measuring patient progress and outcome.

146

| Shoulder Pain and Disability Index (SPADI)[4-6] | *Developer of Measure: Roach, K.E., et al.*

Intended patient group: Patients with shoulder disability

Classification of measure: Self-report, condition-specific measure

Conceptual framework: To be used in outpatient setting

Brief description: 1 page; 2 subscales, pain (5 items) and disability (8 items) scored on a 10-cm visual analogue scale of pain or difficulty that is converted to a numerical value for each subscale and total score
(Note: Williams et al.[6] converted scale to numerical.)

Time to complete (patient): About 5 minutes
Ease of scoring: Moderate
Possible scores: Pain, disability, and total score (each 0 to 100); VAS and numerical rating scoring formats
Scale orientation: Higher scores represent more disability | *Traditional Expression:*

Internal consistency: 0.86 to 0.95
Test-retest reliability: 0.64 to 0.66
Validity:
• Scale correlated adequately with Sickness Impact Profile; SF-20 and Health Assessment Questionnaire, and SF-36 and shoulder ROM.
• Scale might not adequately measure occupational and recreational disability.
• Sensitivity to Change: 1.38 (standardized response mean).

Clinical Expression (estimated from available literature)

Variation around a measured value (90% CI): ±6 SPADI points
Minimal detectable change (90% CI): ±12 points
Minimal clinically important difference: ±10 points | 1. Head-to-head comparison studies showing the SPADI comparable to other shoulder function scales.
2. More evidence related to measurement properties of scale than for other measures of shoulder disability.
3. The SPADI completed by patients and scored by clinicians efficiently. Scoring requiring conversion of visual analogue scale to numerical scale and averaging. |

Continued

APPENDIX 6A: FUNCTIONAL OUTCOME MEASUREMENT SCALES *con't*

Scale	Background and Description	Measurement Properties	Comments
Upper Extremity Function Scale[7]	*Developer of Measure: Pransky, G., et al.* Intended patient group: Patients with upper-extremity disability Classification of measure: Self-report, condition-specific measure Conceptual framework: Conceived for all patients with upper extremity disability Brief description: 1 page, 8 items, scored on a 10-point scale Time to complete (patient): Approximately 3 minutes Ease of scoring: Easy Possible scores: 8–80 Scale orientation: Higher scores represent more disability	*Traditional Expression:* Internal Consistency: 0.83 to 0.93 Test-retest reliability: Not available Validity: • Scale demonstrated to correlate with clinical findings and measures of symptom severity. • Sensitivity to Change: not available. *Clinical Expression:* Variation around a measured value (90% CI): ± 5 UEFS points.	1. Suitable for application to the entire upper extremity. 2. More evidence needed with respect to reliability and validity, including sensitivity to change. 3. Clinical expression of measurement properties not available. 4. Easy to administer and score.

Disability of Arm Shoulder Hand (DASH) [8-10]	*Developer of Measure: Institute for Work and Health, Ontario and American Academy of Orthopaedic Surgeons*	*Traditional Expression:*	1. Suitable for application to the entire upper extremity.
	Intended patient group: Patients with upper extremity disability	Internal Consistency: 0.96	2. More evidence needed with respect to reliability and validity, including sensitivity to change.
	Classification of measure: Self-report, condition-specific measure	Test-retest reliability: Not yet available	3. Somewhat less efficient to administer and score than other condition-specific scales in the clinic.
	Conceptual Framework: All patients with upper extremity disability	Validity: Not available.	
		Clinical Expression (estimated from available literature):	
	Brief description: 3 pages with optional sports/performing arts module; 30 items related to symptoms and activities, scored on a 5-point scale of severity or difficulty	Variation around a measured value (90% CI): ±10 DASH points	
	Time to complete (patient): Approximately 5 minutes		
	Ease of scoring: Moderate		
	Possible scores: 100		
	Scale orientation: Higher scores represent more disability		

Continued

APPENDIX 6A: FUNCTIONAL OUTCOME MEASUREMENT SCALES *con't*

Scale	Background and Description	Measurement Properties	Comments
Subjective Shoulder Rating System[11,12]	*Developer of Measure: Kohn, D., and Geyer, M.* Intended patient group: Patients with shoulder disability Classification of measure: Self-report, condition-specific measure Conceptual framework: All patients with shoulder disability Brief description: 1 page, 5 items, scored related to pain, motion, shoulder dislocation, and general and overhead activity; rated using descriptors that are scored to increase weighting of pain and motion, less on activity and overhead work. Time to complete (patient): 2 minutes Ease of scoring: Easy Possible scores: 100 Scale orientation: Lower scores represent higher disability	*Traditional Expression:* Internal Consistency: Not available Test-retest reliability: Not available Validity: • Correlated adequately with Constant-Murley score and a patient reported results of treatment rating (poor to excellent) in a group of surgical shoulder patients. • Low correlations with SF-36 pain and physical function and other shoulder rating scales. *Clinical Expression:* Not available.	1. Poor face validity if the goal is to measure shoulder function because of high emphasis on pain, motion, and fear of shoulder dislocation. 2. Rationale for item weighting not adequately described. 3. More evidence related to measurement properties of scale than for other measures of shoulder disability.

Shoulder Rating Questionnaire[24]

Developer of Measure: L'Insalata, J.C., et al.

Intended patient group: Patients with shoulder disability

Classification of measure: Self-report, condition-specific measure

Conceptual framework: All patients with shoulder disability able to assess symptoms and function

Brief description: 2 pages, 21 questions related to pain and function, 6 separately scored domains (global, pain, daily activities, recreation/athletic, work, satisfaction, importance) that are weighted using formula provided.

Estimated time to complete for patient: Not available

Ease of scoring: Moderate

Possible scores: 17-100

Scale orientation: Lower scores represent higher disability

Traditional Expression:

Internal Consistency: 0.86

Test-retest reliability: 0.81 to 0.96

Validity:

- Correlated adequately with Arthritis Impact Measure in a group of patients with a variety of shoulder diagnoses and with overall patient satisfaction; other measures of construct validity also demonstrated.
- Sensitivity to Change: 1.1 to 1.9 (standardized response mean), also a significant improvement demonstrated in groups of postoperative patients.

Clinical Expression:

Not available.

1. Rationale for item scoring and weighting not adequately described.
2. Formula for scoring and weighting more complex than comparable measures.
3. Further evidence required for ability of scale to measure valid change.
4. No information to date on clinical expression of measurement properties for application to individual patients.

Continued

APPENDIX 6A: FUNCTIONAL OUTCOME MEASUREMENT SCALES *con't*

Scale	Background and Description	Measurement Properties	Comments
Shoulder Questionnaire (12-item)[13]	*Developer of Measure: Dawson, J., et al., 1996* Intended patient group: Patients with shoulder disability Classification of measure: Self-report, condition-specific measure Conceptual framework: Measurement of outcome of shoulder surgery Brief description: 1 page, 12 items related to pain and function, scored on 5-point scales of severity and difficulty Estimated time to complete for patient: Not available Ease of scoring: Easy Possible scores: 12 to 60 Scale orientation: Lower scores represent lower disability	*Traditional Expression:* Internal Consistency: 0.89 Test-retest reliability: Initial evidence of test-retest reliability Validity: • Correlated adequately with Constant-Murley scores, SF-36, and Stanford Health Assessment Questionnaire. • Sensitivity to Change: 1.2 (effect size) *Clinical Expression:* Not available.	1. Further evidence required related to ability of scale to measure valid change. 2. No information to date on clinical expression of measurement properties for application to individual patients.

Simple Shoulder Test[11,14–16]

Developer of Measure: Lippitt, S.B., et al.

Intended patient group: Patients with shoulder disability

Classification of measure: Self-report, condition-specific measure

Conceptual framework: All patients with shoulder disability able to assess symptoms and function

Brief description: 12 items related to shoulder function scored by yes or no

Estimated time to complete for patient: Less than 3 minutes

Ease of scoring: Easy

Possible scores: 0 to 12

Scale orientation: Lower scores represent more disability

Traditional Expression:

Internal Consistency: Not available

Test-retest reliability: Not available

Validity:
- Scale correlated adequately with SF-36 and other condition-specific measures of shoulder function; shown to correlate negatively with comorbidity.

Clinical Expression:

Not available.

1. Reliability and internal consistency not reported to date.
2. Further evidence required related to ability of scale to measure valid change.
3. No information to date on clinical expression of measurement properties for application to individual patients.

REFERENCES

1. Chatman, AB, et al: The Patient Specific Functional Scale: Measurement properties in patients with knee dysfunction. Phys Ther 77:820, 1997.
2. Stratford PW, et al: Assessing disability and change on individual patients: A report of a patient specific measure. Physiotherapy Canada 47:258, 1995
3. Westaway, M, et al: The Patient Specific Functional Scale: validation of its use in persons with neck dysfunction. J Orthop Sports Phys Ther 27:331, 1998
4. Heald, S, et al: The Shoulder Pain and Disability Index: The construct validity and responsiveness of a region-specific disability measure. Phys Ther 77:1079, 1997.
5. Roach, KE, et al: Development of a Shoulder Pain and Disability Index. Arth Care Res 4:145, 1991.
6. Williams, JW, et al: Measuring shoulder function with the Shoulder Pain and Disability Index. J Rheumatol 22:727, 1995.
7. Pransky, G, et al: Measuring functional outcomes in work-related upper extremity disorders. Development and validation of the Upper Extremity Function Scale. J Occup Environ Med 39:1195, 1997.
8. Armadio, PC, et al: Measuring disability and symptoms of the upper limb: A validation study of the DASH questionnaire (abstract). Arth Rheum 39:(9)S112, 1996.
9. Armadio, PC, et al: Development of an upper extremity outcome measure: The "DASH" (Disabilities of the arm, shoulder and hand) (abstract). Arth Rheum 39:(9)S112, 1996.
10. Hudak, PL, et al: Upper Extremity Collaborative Group. Development of an upper extremity outcome measure: The DASH (Disabilities of the Arm, Shoulder, and Hand). Amer J Industrial Med 29:602, 1997.
11. Beaton, D, and Richards, RR: Measuring function of the shoulder. J Bone Joint Surg 78-A:882, 1996.
12. Kohn, D, and Geyer, M: The subjective shoulder rating system. Arch Orthop Trauma Surg 116:324, 1997.
13. Dawson, J, et al: Questionnaire on the perceptions of patients about shoulder surgery. J Bone Joint Surg 78-B:593, 1996.
14. Lippitt, SB, et al: A practical tool for evaluating function: the Simple Shoulder Test. In Matsen, FA, et al (eds): The Shoulder: A Balance of Mobility and Stability. American Academy of Orthopaedic Surgeons, Rosemont, IL, 1993, p 501.
15. Rozencwaig, R, et al: The correlation of comorbidity with function of the shoulder and health status of patients who have glenohumeral joint disease. J Bone Joint Surg 80-A:1146, 1998.
16. Matsen, FA, et al: Patient self-assessment of health status and function in glenohumeral degenerative joint disease. J Shoulder Elbow Surg 4:345, 1995.

Musculoskeletal Patterns of the Shoulder

Musculoskeletal Pattern D: Impaired Joint Mobility, Motor Function, Muscle Performance, and Range of Motion Associated with Capsular Restriction

Phil McClure, PhD, PT, OCS

INTRODUCTION

Limited shoulder range of motion (ROM), one of the most common problems treated by therapists, can be the result of various pathologies. This chapter deals exclusively with disorders involving limited passive motion (with or without active deficits) in contrast to conditions involving full passive motion but a limited active motion due to weakness or neurologic dysfunction.

CLASSIFICATION AND TERMINOLOGY

In 1934, Codman[1] introduced the term *frozen shoulder*, referring to this condition as "difficult to define, difficult to treat, and difficult to explain." In 1945, Neviaser[2] introduced the term *adhesive capsulitis*, describing distinct pathology reflecting glenohumeral adhesion formation and capsular contracture. Reeves[3] elaborated on the natural history of frozen shoulder and distinguished three specific and sequential phases, the painful stage, the stiff stage, and the recovery stage. More recently, Neviaser and Neviaser[4] distinguished between adhesive capsulitis and the stiff and painful shoulder. They reserve the term *adhesive capsulitis* for those conditions in

157

which limited shoulder motion is directly attributable to pathologic changes in the joint capsule. The term *stiff and painful shoulder* is used for conditions in which the motion is limited by pain and protective muscle guarding rather than by true capsular contracture.

Nash and Hazelman[5] describe the concept of *primary* and *secondary frozen shoulder.* *Primary frozen shoulder* refers to painful and limited glenohumeral movement (particularly external rotation) of unknown causes. *Secondary frozen shoulder* is defined as having the same clinical presentation but related to a particular traumatic event or disease state such as diabetes mellitus, myocardial infarction, or various neurologic disorders.

In this chapter, a simplified classification scheme of two categories relating directly to conservative treatment provided by therapists based on patient history and clinical evaluation findings are used. This classification system has been reported previously and used successfully in the treatment of limited shoulder motion (see Table 7–1).[6,7]

The first category is limited ROM resulting from *structural changes* in the periarticular tissues, regardless of specific cause. These changes include shortening of capsule, ligament, or muscle and adhesion formation. Therefore, this category includes adhesive capsulitis described by Neviaser[2,4,8] and the stiff and recovery

TABLE 7–1 Summary of Classification System for Limited Passive Glenohumeral Motion

Structural	Nonstructural
Underlying Pathology	
• Capsular & periarticular fibrosis • Anteroinferior capsular recess • Subscapular synovial recess in rotator interval • Coracohumeral ligament • Adaptive muscle shortening • Subscapularis	• Acute inflammation • Tenosynovitis • Subacromial bursitis • Myofascial trigger points
Clinical Features	
• Pain usually only at end-range • Capsular end-feel • History of trauma & immobilization • Limited motion > 3 weeks • Capsular pattern (greatest % loss of ext rot)	• Resting pain or pain before end-range • Muscle guarding end-feel • Signs of acute inflammation
Other Terms	
• Adhesive capsulitis (mid- to end stages) • Frozen shoulder (mid- to end stage) • Primary, idiopathic • Secondary, posttraumatic • Posttraumatic stiffness	• Stiff and painful shoulder • Frozen shoulder (early stage)
General Treatment Strategy	
• Controlled tensile stress to encourage biologic remodeling of shortened tissue • High-load brief stress • Low-load prolonged stress	• Pain control • Antiinflammatory agents • Muscle relaxation

stages of frozen shoulder described by Reeves.[3] These fibrotic structural changes generally result from a combination of inflammation and immobilization.[9–12] The origins of these structural changes might be associated with the healing process following some form of overt trauma (posttraumatic stiffness) or the more classic adhesive capsulitis or idiopathic, primary frozen shoulder that has an insidious onset and essentially unknown etiology.[2,13]

The second category is limited ROM due to problems with *no associated structural change* in the periarticular tissues. These nonstructural problems are associated with pain and associated protective muscle guarding to prevent painful movements.[14] Various pathologies might produce pain and subsequent muscle guarding without true, fixed contracture of the joint capsule or surrounding musculature. The stiff and painful shoulder as described by Neviaser[4] would fit in this category. Also, patients in the acute inflammatory phase of adhesive capsulitis would fit in this category because they have not yet developed the structural changes in the capsule.

Findings from the history and physical examination that lead to a hypothesis of limited passive motion due to structural changes include the following:

1. A history of trauma followed by immobilization[9–12]
2. A history of restricted motion greater than 3 weeks[9–12]
3. Loss of passive motion in a capsular pattern (for the shoulder, greatest percentage limitation of lateral rotation followed by abduction)[15]
4. A capsular end-feel (defined as a firm halt to passive movement with only a slight degree of give with further force[15])

The primary finding suggesting a nonstructural loss of motion is significant pain and a muscle guarding type of end-feel. Acute inflammation of various soft-tissue structures is probably the most common cause of nonstructural limitation of motion. Another common cause of a nonstructural limitation is myofascial trigger points that might be sensitive to stretching during passive range of motion.[16] Although the actual true pathology of trigger points remains elusive, trigger points represent irritable points in the muscle that, when treated, seem to readily allow significant changes in muscle length and ROM.

This structural-nonstructural classification system is useful to form the basis for choosing a conservative treatment strategy. Treatment of limited ROM due to structural changes as defined previously would be geared toward applying controlled tensile stress to cause elongation of the restricting tissues.[6,7,9,17–25] On the other hand, treatment of limited ROM due to nonstructural changes would be focused on relieving whatever problem was producing the pain.[4,26] For example, treatment of an acutely inflamed joint with associated pain and protective muscle action would most likely include modalities oriented to control of pain and inflammation rather than to the application of significant amounts of stress to the joint.[3,26,27] This chapter focuses on limited shoulder motion due to structural changes.

Origins and Pathology of Structural Changes

Regardless of the causes, limited motion due to structural changes eventually results in a fibrotic process consisting of adhesion formation and contracture of the glenohumeral (GH) joint capsule and surrounding periarticular soft tissues. The

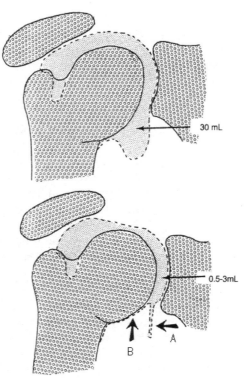

FIGURE 7–1. The normal capsule has a large inferior pouch and can accommodate at least 30 mL of fluid. In adhesive capsulitis, the inferior capsular pouch is lost due to adhesions *(A)* and the capsule may also become adherent to the humeral head *(B)*. (From Calliet, R, Shoulder pain and impairment. In Soft Tissue Pain and Disability, ed 3. FA Davis, Philadelphia, 1996, p 279.)

specific site of the pathologic contracture seems to be either the anteroinferior recess of the capsule, the tissues at the rotator interval (subscapular synovial recess of the capsule), the coracohumeral ligament, or some combination of the three[2,4,8,28,29] (Fig. 7–1 and Fig. 7–2).

Muscle also exhibits morphologic changes when immobilized in a shortened position.[30–32] Sarcomeres are lost, causing the muscle itself to become shorter.[32] The connective tissue within a muscle also undergoes adaptive shortening when immobilized in a shortened position.[33] A shortened subscapularis muscle has been implicated as a cause of limited motion in patients diagnosed with adhesive capsulitis.

IMMOBILIZATION AND ADAPTIVE SHORTENING

Although multiple initiating mechanisms have been postulated, a common feature in virtually all cases of limited motion due to structural changes is an initial period of immobility. Understanding the biologic processes responsible for structural changes in and around the joint capsule as the result of immobility forms the basis for a treatment strategy.

Under normal conditions of use, degradation and synthesis of collagen and other extracellular components of connective tissue such as glycosaminoglycans (GAGs) are

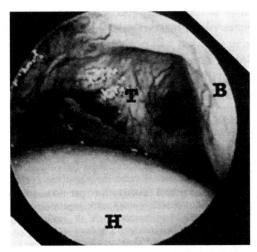

FIGURE 7–2. Hyperernic hypertrophic synovial tissue *(T)* occupying subscapular recess, Superior border *(S)* of subscapularis, biceps tendon *(B)*, humeral head *(H)*. (From Fareed, DO, and Gallivan, WR, Office management of frozen shoulder syndrome. Clin Orthop 242:177, 1989, with permission.)

balanced.[9,12,34–36] As a result, the necessary structural and mechanical characteristics of the tissue required for normal use are maintained. When the normal pattern of use is altered significantly (primarily by increased or decreased tensile loading), morphological, biomechanical, and biochemical changes occur in the periarticular tissues.[9,10,31,37,38] Frost has termed this general phenomenon *structural adaptation to mechanical usage,* and the reader is referred to his work for a more complete explanation of his theoretical model.[35]

Periarticular connective tissues are designed to withstand tensile stress. If these tissues are deprived of tensile stress by being immobilized in a shortened position, predictable changes will occur. Collagenous tissues deprived of tensile stress exhibit decreased amounts of collagen, GAGs, and water, as well as an increase in the amount of reducible cross-links.[9,12,36] Immobilized tissues also become shorter, weaker, and less stiff.[9,10,34,36,39,40] The decrease in tissue stiffness should be distinguished from an increase in joint stiffness (increased resistance to motion) found with immobilization.[10,36] Increased joint stiffness occurs despite actual weakening of periarticular connective tissues because these tissues assume a shorter length and therefore exert greater resistance to a given amount of joint motion. These detrimental changes associated with immobilization are considerably worse if the tissues have been traumatized. Immobilization alone without trauma might not produce significant clinical stiffness.

Woo et al.[36] proposed a mechanism for the development of limited joint ROM or contracture. They theorized that with immobilization, loss of GAGs and water allow the formation of new inter- and intramolecular cross-links within the periarticular connective tissue, limiting the extensibility of the tissue. Other investigators suggest that connective tissues may shorten by the process of contraction.[39] The contractile protein actin, identified in fibroblasts, has been implicated in the process of ligament contraction. Others believe the *myofibroblast,* a specialized cell that resembles a smooth muscle cell, might be the primary mediator of connective tissue contraction.[41,42]

Another mechanism by which joint motion might be limited is adhesion formation. An *adhesion* is simply scar tissue that has formed between tissues that normally move relative to one another.[2] Adhesions have been identified as an important source of limited motion in many common clinical problems.[43,44] Abnormal cross-links, periarticular tissue contraction, and adhesion formation might all play a role in formation of a joint contracture.

NONTRAUMATIC ADAPTIVE SHORTENING

The well-described wound healing process following a traumatic event clearly leads to structural changes that result in loss of motion. However, the etiology of GH joint structural changes with no clear history of a traumatic event (i.e., idiopathic or primary frozen shoulder) is less clear. Codman[1] suggested that the early precursor to these capsular changes was a rotator cuff tendinitis. Many other authors have also suggested that inflammation of the synovial tissues around the GH joint such as the subacromial bursa or the subscapularis bursa are the precursors to the GH joint synovitis. The cause of these initial inflammatory events might be repeated microtrauma or an autoimmune response. There is conflicting evidence for this idea of initial inflammatory events. Some authors have documented inflammatory changes at arthroscopy whereas others have found little evidence of inflammation but rather a fibroblastic process.[28,41] This conflict might be due to the studies involving patients at different stages of the same pathologic process.

Bunker and Anthony[41] have provided some interesting data to explain the findings of glenohumeral stiffness associated with various disease states such as diabetes mellitus, cardiac pathology, and neurologic injuries. After excising the coracohumeral ligament in 12 patients with idiopathic frozen shoulder, a tissue analysis was performed using routine histological stains and immunocytochemistry to assess the cellular nature of the tissue. They showed that a fibrotic process occurs. Smooth muscle-like cells (myofibroblasts) were identified in the capsular contracture, suggesting that they are responsible for the active contraction of the capsule. They failed to find significant evidence of inflammatory cells (leukocytes or macrophages). They suggest that adhesive capsulitis (primary frozen shoulder) is a Dupuytren's-like process, essentially a fibrotic process rather than an inflammatory process. Furthermore, they have provided data to show that patients with idiopathic or primary frozen shoulder have elevated serum lipid levels (triglycerides and cholesterol).[45] Patients with diabetes or cardiac problems and those treated with phenobarbitone postsurgically are known to have elevated serum lipid levels and an increased incidence of idiopathic frozen shoulder. These findings suggest that the elevated lipid levels might in some way be responsible for the active fibrotic process.[45] Others have suggested a collagen abnormality or microvascular change in diabetics as being responsible for the higher incidence of idiopathic frozen shoulder.[46]

Some authors have suggested an autonomic dysfunction and sympathetically maintained pain as evidenced by abnormal thermography and lower skin temperatures as a cause of idiopathic frozen shoulder.[47–49] Also, evidence exists that degenerative changes in the cervical spine might give rise to limited shoulder motion. Johnson et al.[50] documented significant loss of passive shoulder abduction initially with subsequent increases in a series of 27 patients following anterior cervical discectomy. Hargreaves et al.[51] also showed that a history of neck pain and trauma was related to the risk of frozen shoulder. These patients with frozen shoulder also have decreased cervical motion when compared to controls.

To summarize, stiffness following overt trauma can clearly be attributed to fibrosis and adhesion formation that are characteristic of the wound healing process. The capsular changes that cannot be attributed to a known traumatic event (i.e., primary, idiopathic frozen shoulder or adhesive capsulitis) might have multiple initiating causes or predisposing factors, including synovial inflammation from microtrauma or autoimmune processes, neurologic changes as a result of cervical pathology or autonomic dysfunction, abnormalities of collagen biosynthesis, and abnormal serum lipid levels. Whatever the initiating event, a common history of inflammation and immobility followed by an active period of fibrosis and capsular contracture appear to be present.

TREATMENT

Most authors agree that prevention is of the utmost importance. The early recognition of limited motion and emphasis on maintenance of motion might prevent a substantial percentage of hypomobile shoulder cases.[26] This is particularly true in patients known to be at high risk, such as those with diabetes, cardiac pathology, neurologic injury, or a history of neck pain. Several authors have argued the merits of early mobilization whenever possible following injury to prevent the tissue weakening and adaptive shortening that occur with prolonged immobilization.[12,21,24]

Medical/Surgical Treatment

Several forms of medical/surgical treatment have been studied, primarily addressing idiopathic frozen shoulder or adhesive capsulitis rather than posttraumatic stiffness. Virtually all authors recognize the value of conservative treatment. They suggest that failure of supervised, conservative treatment is a requirement prior to implementing more invasive procedures, such as corticosteroid injection, manipulation under anesthesia, hydraulic distention of the capsule, arthroscopic lysis, and debridement and open surgical capsulotomy.

Rizk et al.[52] studied the effects of four different forms of injection in 48 patients diagnosed with frozen shoulder for less than 6 months. They compared injection of intra-articular steroid and lidocaine, steroid and lidocaine into the subacromial bursa, intra-articular lidocaine only, and intrabursal lidocaine alone. They found that those treated with the steroid and lidocaine obtained better pain relief but failed to find a significant difference in motion recovery between injection methods. Bulgen et al.[53] found that patients in the early stages of frozen shoulder showed significant improvement in pain and range of motion with injections containing a steroid, although they failed to find any long-term improvements. Leffert suggested that oral anti-inflammatory agents might be just as effective in the early stages of frozen shoulder as steroid injections are.[26]

Manipulation under anesthesia remains a controversial form of treatment primarily due to the potential serious complications associated with its use. Specifically, humeral fracture, glenohumeral dislocation, rotator cuff rupture, and neurovascular injury might occur.[26] Despite these problems, judicious use of manipulation while avoiding what Neviaser[4] refers to as "superheroic force" seems to be widely accepted. Various authors report good results using manipulation under anesthesia.[2,13,54,55] However, well-controlled, randomized studies with control groups are lacking. Those advocating the use of manipulation under anesthesia seem to agree that closed manipulation might speed rehabilitation and recovery of motion even though the time required for full recovery might not be changed. There has been arthroscopic documentation that the snapping and popping heard during manipulation represents tearing of the anteroinferior capsule.[56] Ogilvie-Harris[57] found a high frequency of rupture of the subscapularis. However, others have reported no rupturing of the subscapularis muscle with closed manipulation.[32,13] Neviaser and Neviaser[4] have pointed out that postoperative care following manipulation is critical. They recommend maintaining the arm in 90° of abduction and external rotation immediately after manipulation with immediate physical therapy emphasizing internal and external rotation. They further suggest that the arm must be held in abduction for several days, and that the patient requires 3 to 5 days of hospitalization to ensure compliance and successful outcome. Continuous passive motion postoperatively may also be used. The author's experience is that this treatment is well tolerated and effective.

Pollack et al.[29] report the use of arthroscopy in conjunction with manipulation under anaesthesia. With successful outcomes in 25 of 30 shoulders, they suggest that arthroscopy is useful for identifying associated pathology such as subacromial space lesions and also for releasing the coracohumeral ligament. Ogilvie-Harris[57] report arthroscopic surgical release in patients with frozen shoulders. Although they found improved motion on successive release of the anterior capsule, they did not provide outcome data. Neviaser and Neviaser[4] felt that arthroscopy had no role in the treatment of frozen shoulder.

Hydraulic distention, which seems to have gained popularity, has been studied by several authors.[28,58–60] This treatment consists of injecting fluid under pressure into the GH joint to burst adhesions. Typically both an anesthetic and steroid are injected in conjunction with the saline solution. If the procedure is done using arthrography, a contrast material is also used. Immediate pain relief and rapid restoration of motion and function in a high percentage of patients has been reported in multiple studies.[28,58,60] Using arthroscopy, Fareed and Gallivan[28] demonstrated detachment of hyperemic synovial tissue in the interval between the subscapularis and the biceps tendon (subscapularis bursa), allowing normal motion. Rizk[60] documented the same phenomenon arthrographically by showing the subscapularis bursa filling following hydraulic distention. Active and passive mobilization is instituted immediately following hydraulic distention to maintain and improve motion. Although randomized clinical trials are lacking, the results obtained with hydraulic distention are quite favorable. This method seems to avoid some of the risks of manipulation under anesthesia.

Open surgical release appears to be less commonly performed than the procedures mentioned previously. Neviaser[4] suggests that its use be reserved for cases in which manipulation under anesthesia is contraindicated, specifically for patients with severe osteopenia or a history of humeral fracture or dislocation, and for those with recurrence following manipulation. The procedure is performed through an anterior, deltopectoral approach. Adhesions between the capsule and humeral head are dissected free, and the capsule is released on the humeral side. Postoperative care is the same as that described for manipulation under anesthesia, with the arm being held in abduction and external rotation for several days.

Conservative Treatment: Nonstructural Limitation

As mentioned previously, the treatment for nonstructural limitation of motion consists of pain control, anti-inflammatory agents, and methods to encourage muscle relaxation. It is essential to distinguish this group of shoulder problems because traditional stretching procedures will only increase pain, worsen the inflammatory process, and ultimately increase the fibrotic process. As Leffert[26] states, "For the patient with an acutely and globally painful shoulder, there is little to do but provide support with a sling for a limited time, as well as appropriate analgesics." He also recommends the use of TENS and oral anti-inflammatory agents. Even with an acutely painful shoulder, patients should be encouraged to perform gentle, pain-free motions as they are able (not stretching), rather than completely immobilizing the joint. Doing so helps to minimize the morbidity associated with immobilization.

Conservative Treatment: Structural Limitation

The primary rationale supporting conservative forms of treatment for increasing ROM is the biological principle that periarticular connective tissues will remodel over time in response to the type and amount of physical stress they receive.[9,12,17,35] *Remodeling* refers to a physical rearrangement of the connective tissue extracellular matrix (fibers, cross-links, and ground substance). Strong evidence supports the process of remodeling as being mediated by the fibroblast in response to physical forces.[9,12] Remodeling is a biological phenomenon that occurs over long periods of time rather than a mechanically induced change that occurs within minutes. The process of adaptive shortening that occurs following inflammation, injury, and immobilization in a shortened position must be reversed by the stimulus of tensile stress to shortened periarticular connective tissues and muscle.

Many authors have found that subjecting periarticular tissues to controlled tensile loading will result in adaptive changes.[17,37,38] Frost theorizes that a *minimal effective strain* exists for a given tissue. When this level of strain is exceeded, biologically mediated adaptive changes occur.[35] In general, collagenous tissues respond to increased tensile loading by increasing synthesis of collagen and other extracellular components. The collagen is oriented parallel to the lines of stress, thus increasing tensile strength. Muscles subjected to prolonged positioning in a lengthened position will become lengthened by adding sarcomeres.[32]

Studies using both animal and human models provide evidence that controlled tensile stress applied cyclically or statically leads to remodeling of periarticular tissue. Arem and Madden used a rat model to study the effects of prolonged periods of tensile stress (6 hours/day) applied for 4 weeks to healing scar tissue.[17] When the stress was applied to 3-week-old scars, the scars were markedly elongated when compared to controls. However, when the same amount of tensile stress was applied to 14-week-old scars, essentially no scar elongation was observed. These data suggest that following trauma, scar tissue formation is influenced by mechanical stress, but the scar becomes less dynamic and amenable to change over time.

HIGH-LOAD BRIEF STRESS VERSUS LOW-LOAD PROLONGED STRESS

In general, the techniques available to apply tensile stress may be categorized as either high-load brief stress (HLBS) or low-load prolonged stress (LLPS). Techniques such as traditional passive and active stretching, joint mobilization, contract-relax, or hold-relax stretching are classified as HLBS techniques because the intensity of the stress is near the maximum tolerated by the patient, but the duration for which the stress is applied is brief. Splinting, continuous passive motion (CPM), and other end-range stress methods are classified as LLPS because the intensity of stretch is significantly less than the maximum tolerable level, but the duration for which it is applied is rather long, typically hours per day. Understanding the differences in these techniques is critical to making treatment decisions related to structural shoulder stiffness.

In two clinical studies, the effects of LLPS (via prolonged positioning in a traction apparatus) have been directly compared to HLBS forms of stress for gaining ROM. Light et al.[20] studied elderly subjects with longstanding knee flexion contractures. They compared LLPS applied with a modified Buck's traction apparatus to passive stretching applied manually. Rizk et al.[22] studied subjects with adhesive capsulitis of the shoulder. They compared LLPS applied to the shoulder with a pulley system to more traditional active and passive exercises. The data from both of these studies indicated significantly more improvement in ROM for those subjects receiving the LLPS when compared to traditional HLBS methods.

The total amount of time the joint is held at or near an end-range position, or *total end-range time* (TERT),[21,61] might be the most critical variable in determining the amount of tensile stress applied to a joint with limited ROM. Flowers and Lastayo[61] studied the hypothesis that changes in ROM of structurally stiff joints are proportional to the amount of end-range time. They randomly applied static, end-range splints to patients with stiff (flexion contractures) proximal interphalangeal (PIP) joints for both a 3-day period and a 6-day period. They found that the 6-day period yielded almost double the increase in ROM compared to that of the 3-day period of splinting. Hence their data provide support for the notion that gains in ROM might be proportional to the amount of time spent at end-range. While not part of their original data analysis, the data provided by Light et al.[20] also seem to show that the mean difference between groups in ROM gains achieved was of a similar proportion (3.9:1) to differences in the amount of time spent at end-range each day (120 minutes: 30 minutes or 4:1).

In summary, the primary rationale for increasing ROM is that by holding the joint at or near its end-range over time, therapeutic tensile stress is applied to the restricting periarticular tissues and muscles. This induces remodeling of these tissues to a new, longer length, allowing increased ROM. The available evidence seems to favor LLPS methods for accomplishing this goal as compared to HLBS.

REMODELING VERSUS TRANSIENT PHYSICAL CHANGES

Remodeling can be contrasted with other processes that lead to a more transient increase in ROM. Because periarticular tissues are viscoelastic, they demonstrate the phenomena of creep, stress-relaxation, and preconditioning.[62] When noninjurious loads (i.e., loads within the elastic limit) are applied to tissues, either statically or cyclically, tissues readily demonstrate a transient lengthening (creep or preconditioning) or a decrease in the amount of force required to hold a given length (stress-relaxation). These phenomena occur within a short period of time, typically a few minutes, and are thought to be highly dependent on the viscous component of the tissue. However, unless a tissue is deformed beyond its elastic limit, and therefore injured (a truly plastic change), length increases due to viscoelastic phenomena are only temporary.[18,34,35] Controversy exists in this area because mechanical studies demonstrating creep, stress-relaxation, and preconditioning are usually performed with tissues isolated from the body, and length changes are only monitored for a short period following release of the load.[25] In these studies mechanical changes, characterized as permanent or plastic, tend to remain after forces are removed. However, when applying forces to tissues in living humans, the tissue remains in a closed, fluid-filled homeostatic biological system. Here, the contents and organization of the extracellular matrix remain under the influence of cellular control. Therefore, a purely mechanically induced change might be less likely to remain once external forces are removed. Because the periarticular tissue is innervated with nociceptors, it is unlikely that routine clinical techniques produce significant tearing of tissue because patients would not tolerate such stresses. Only while under anesthesia is there the possibility of substantial tissue tearing to achieve permanent length increases. Brand[18] has noted "any elongation of tissue accomplished by stretch will shorten again once the force is relaxed." Frank et al.[34] have similarly stated that following short term stretching procedures, "ligaments return to prestretch lengths."

Changes in ROM due to viscoelastic phenomena can be easily demonstrated with procedures that are typically applied for brief periods, such as joint mobilization and other passive stretching techniques. However, these stretching procedures share a significant drawback because they can be applied only for a short time. Therefore, tissues that have been temporarily preconditioned or "stretched out" are permitted to return to prestretch lengths. The major advantage of using LLPS techniques to increase ROM is that they allow forces to be applied for longer periods of time and are, therefore, more likely to induce a change in tissue length by remodeling.

DETERMINING THE PROPER DOSE OF STRESS: HIERARCHY OF TENSILE STRESS DELIVERY AND A CLINICAL DECISION MAKING ALGORITHM

The basic strategy in treating structural stiffness is to apply tensile stress to the tissues that are restricting motion, typically the anterior and inferior capsule and the anterior musculature in the shoulder. The total amount of stress being applied is commonly thought of as the *dose* in much the same way *dose* is used in regard to medication. In treating structural joint stiffness, the clinician must adjust the dose of tensile stress until a therapeutic result (increased ROM) is achieved. An insufficient dose of stress will have no therapeutic effect, whereas an excessive dose will produce complications such as pain and inflammation. The following three factors should be considered when calculating the dose, or total amount of stress delivered to a tissue: intensity, frequency, and duration.

The TERT, calculated by multiplying the *frequency* and *duration* of time spent at end-range daily, is a useful tool for gauging the dose of tissue stress.[21,61] For example, a patient using an end-range splinting device four sessions per day for 30 minutes each session has a TERT of 120 minutes or 2 hours. *Intensity*, the *amount* of force applied, is usually limited by the patient's pain tolerance. Because remodeling is a biologic process that occurs over long periods of time, frequency and duration of the applied stress are the key factors to maximize, whereas intensity is less important. Increasing intensity is less useful because the use of high forces might cause microtears in tissue, resulting in inflammation and subsequent fibrosis.[43] The amount of force necessary to cause tissue injury is probably dependent on the rate of application, the amount of time the force is applied, as well as the temperature and initial mechanical state of the tissue.[24] Studies on isolated tissue suggest that strains beyond 2% cause damage to connective tissues. However, it is impossible to know the degree of strain placed on a given tissue during a clinical procedure.

In making decisions about the dose of tissue stress in the management of structural joint stiffness, the various forms of stress may be considered as levels within a hierarchy of tissue stress (Fig. 7–3). Immobilization represents the total absence of tensile stress, whereas traditional active and passive exercises represent HLBS forms of treatment. The dose of stress is increased further if joint mobilization and a consistent home program are added. The highest tensile stress doses are achieved by LLPS methods because the TERT is maximized. Only manipulation under anesthesia causes abrupt physical changes in tissue length and ROM by tearing tissue. Lesser forms of tissue stress might cause microscopic tearing if done vigorously. However, these should be considered methods of inducing biological remodeling rather than causing immediate and permanent changes in length.

Therefore, the goal with each patient is to determine the therapeutic level of tensile stress. The primary factors that guide this process are *pain* and *ROM*. A significant increase in pain, reflective of an adverse reaction to tensile stress, is an indicator that the patient should be re-evaluated, and the dose of stress should be

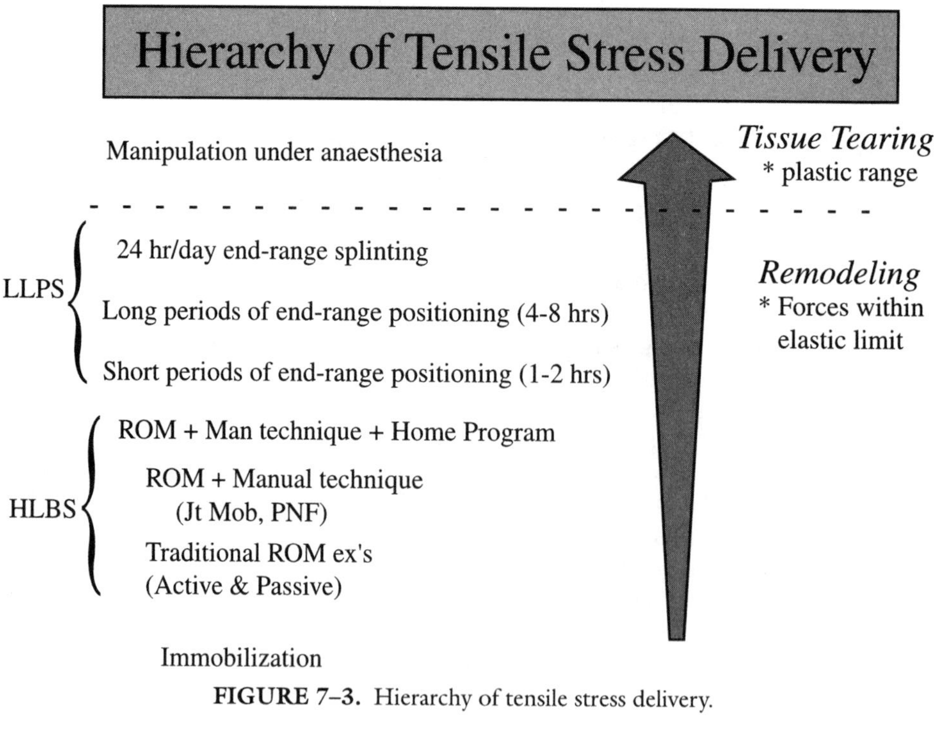

FIGURE 7–3. Hierarchy of tensile stress delivery.

decreased. Typically, with increased pain, there will also be decreased ROM. If pain is not increased following a given level of tissue stress, ROM becomes the key variable to assess. If ROM is unimproved or not progressing at an acceptable rate within a given time frame, the dose of tissue stress should be increased. If ROM is improving at a satisfactory rate, then the dose is probably correct. This clinical decision making process is presented in the algorithm shown in Figure 7–4.

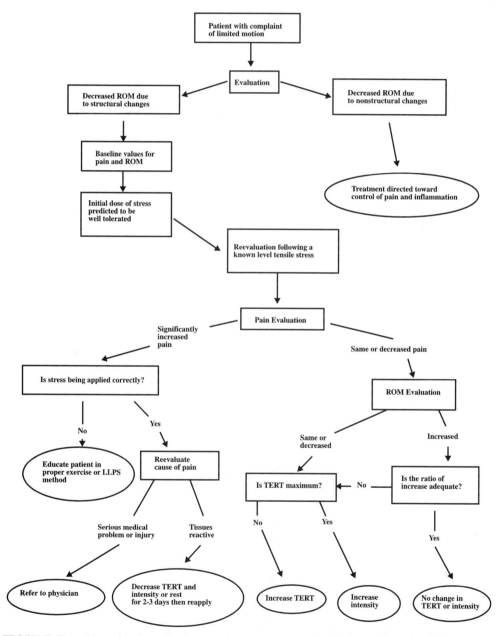

FIGURE 7–4. Algorithm for adjusting the dose of tissue stress based on pain and ROM response. (Modified from McClure, PW, et al, The use of splints in the treatment of joint stiffness: biologic rationale and an algorithm for making clinical decisions. Phys Ther 74:1101, 1994.)

The initial parameters of tensile stress (frequency, duration, and intensity) should be based on the patient's history and clinical examination. In general, the initial dose of end-range stress should be such that the therapist is confident that it will be well tolerated. Thus understressing the joint initially is preferred, with subsequent increases in the stress being added in a controlled manner. This avoids unnecessary pain and inflammation and also gives the patient a positive first experience with therapy, which improves compliance. Typically, the patient should be seen within 2 days following initiation of an exercise program so the reaction can be monitored closely. In this way, the dose of stress can be rapidly and progressively increased until a therapeutic dose is achieved.

Methods of Stress Delivery for the Stiff Shoulder

SELF-STRETCHING EXERCISES

A variety of methods are available for self-stretching, two of which are shown in Figures 7–5 and 7–6. Patients need clear guidelines regarding intensity (how vigorous), frequency (how often), and duration (how long to hold the stretch) so that the dose of stress is known and, therefore, can be adjusted as required based on the patient's response. Also using some form of mild heat to encourage muscle relaxation and preconditioning of tissue before exercise is generally beneficial.[23,25] Frequent, shorter sessions throughout a 24-hour period are preferable to single, prolonged sessions because frequent sessions have the potential to keep the tissue in a preconditioned state throughout the day. This also seems to minimize reactive inflammation. A common problem with active or active-assisted exercises is substitution at the scapulothoracic articulation in an effort to get the arm through a greater range (Fig. 7–7). This pattern of motion should be discouraged as early as possible in rehabilitation in order to prevent the formation of aberrant motor patterns that become difficult to reverse once they are established.

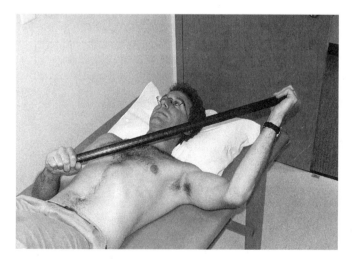

FIGURE 7–5. Self-stretch into abduction and external rotation using a cane.

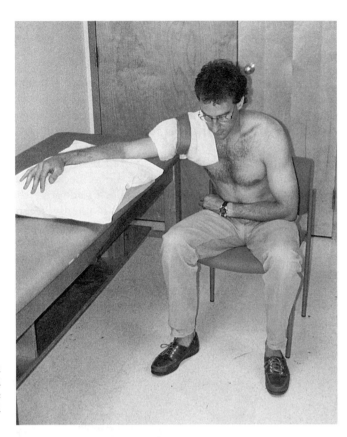

FIGURE 7–6. Self-stretch into scapular plane abduction with arm supported on table (combined with superficial heat).

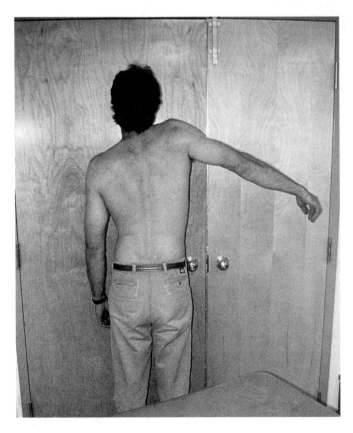

FIGURE 7–7. Substitution by excessive scapulothoracic motion during abduction.

MANUAL TECHNIQUES

Numerous manual techniques have been described for use with the shoulder, including various systems of describing the vigor or grade of technique.[63-68] For structural stiffness, high grade, end-range techniques are indicated, generally performed with the joint positioned at or near its physiological end-range position. Immediate ROM gains made with manual techniques represent transient tissue preconditioning and must be supported by other exercises and methods that can be done more frequently by the patient alone. Because the anterior and inferior capsule are known to be the most common sites of adaptive shortening, methods of anterior and inferior gliding will be used most frequently because these techniques stress the anterior and inferior capsule, respectively. Some examples of these forms of joint mobilization are shown in Figures 7–8, 7–9, 7–10, and 7–11. Traditional joint mobilization techniques may be combined with hold-relax stretching methods to maximize relaxation during the mobilization. For example, an anterior glide might be preceded by an isometric contraction (typically less than 50% maximum effort) of the shoulder internal rotators, after which the glide is performed while the muscles relax (Fig. 7–12).

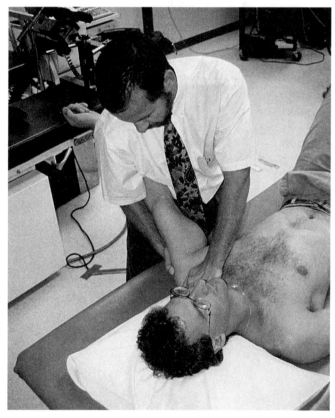

FIGURE 7–8. Anterior glide at the GH joint with patient supine and the arm at 45° with slight external rotation. The therapist's left hand stabilizes the scapula while the right hand applies an anteriorly directed force.

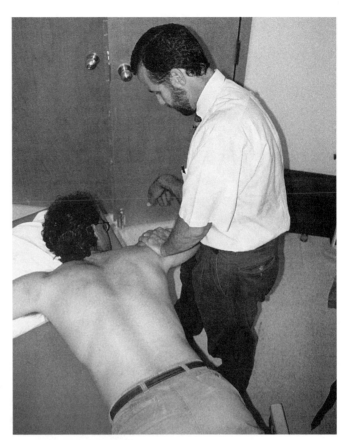

FIGURE 7–9. Anterior glide at the GH joint with patient prone and the arm at 90° with moderate external rotation.

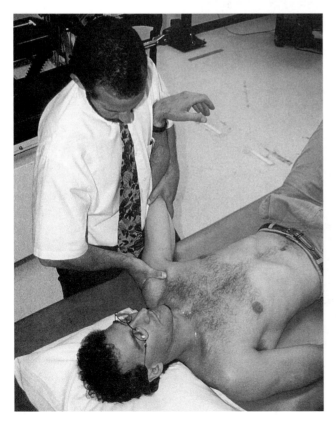

FIGURE 7–10. Inferior glide at the GH joint with the arm in 30° abduction and neutral rotation.

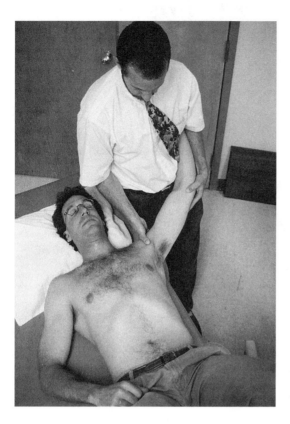

FIGURE 7–11. Inferior glide at the GH joint with the arm in 100° abduction with moderate external rotation.

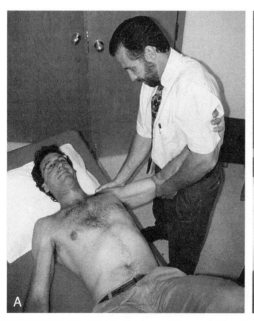
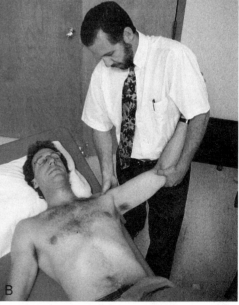

FIGURE 7–12. Hold relax stretching combined with joint mobilization. *(A)* Isometric contraction of internal rotators and horizontal adductors. *(B)* As the patient relaxes, an inferior glide is performed.

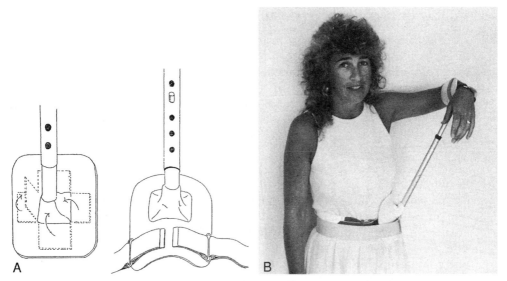

FIGURE 7–13. Abduction splint. *(A)* Attachment of adjustable aluminum rod to the waist resting pad using a cross-shaped piece of thermoplastic material. *(B)* Subject wearing shoulder elevation splint. (From McClure, PW, and Flowers, KR: Treatment of limited shoulder motion using an elevation splint. Phys Ther 72:57, 1992, p 60.)

LOW-LOAD PROLONGED STRESS METHODS

The shoulder may be held at or near end-range by methods as simple as propping the arm on pillows, a table, or the back of a couch. Continuous passive motion devices, also possibly used, are particularly helpful postoperatively because they provide a safe and predictable arc of motion that can be controlled by the patient. These factors encourage muscle relaxation. A commercial splint is available (Dynasplint Inc.) that provides a comfortable method of achieving low-load prolonged stress. However, for proper use the patient must lie supine. Rizk et al.[22] described the use of pulley traction applied to the arm via the patient's wrists to hold the arm in abduction while also imposing a distraction force. McClure and Flowers[6] have described the construction of a simple, inexpensive abduction splint that is fabricated from thermoplastic materials (Fig. 7–13).

CASE STUDY 7–1

IDENTIFICATION OF THE PATIENT'S PROBLEM

The patient, a 57-year-old female who fell, sustained a Neer two-part fracture of the humerus with avulsion of the greater tuberosity. The patient was employed as a medical secretary, and the injury was on her dominant right side. She also had a concomitant anterior dislocation, which was reduced at the time of the fall by the patient's husband, who is a physician. She was initially immobilized for 6 weeks in a sling and swathe, which held the arm in medial rotation. She was referred for physical therapy 6 weeks following the injury.

Characteristics of the Problem

Her primary problem was restricted shoulder movement with subsequent difficulty in activities that required reaching above head level. Her chief goal was to regain motion to allow independent dressing, hair care, and household activities such as cooking, cleaning, and gardening. She was not involved in athletics or other strenuous recreational activities. She did not have pain at rest.

Factors Affecting the Problem

She was unable to actively flex or abduct the arm to horizontal. Passive flexion and abduction were limited to 80° and 60°, respectively. All ROM data are presented in Table 7–2. Mild pain was elicited as the end ranges of passive motion were approached. The pain was confined to the anterolateral shoulder area, with no radiation distal to the insertion of the deltoid. Motions in all directions were limited by capsular end-feel.[15] No gross atrophy was observed, but manual muscle testing was not done for the shoulder musculature. The motions of shoulder flexion, abduction, and medial and lateral rotation were tested isometrically with the arm by the side in neutral rotation. The patient was able to produce moderate resistance to all motions without pain. The cervical spine, elbow, wrist, and digits revealed full active range of motion without gross weakness based on isometric testing. No gross deficit of sensibility was noted.

IDENTIFICATION AND IMPLEMENTATION OF A SOLUTION TO THE PROBLEM

Assessment

This patient presents with limited shoulder motion due to structural changes. Her chief complaint was limited functional ability due to the stiffness. Although some pain was present, her shoulder did not seem particularly irritable. Therefore, the basic treatment strategy was to apply progressive tensile stress to the joint until ROM and function were restored.

Treatment Progression (Table 7–2)

6 Weeks Postinjury

The stress applied during the first treatment was maintained purposefully to a minimum level to avoid any adverse reactions. Moist heat and ultrasound were performed to promote muscle relaxation and heating of the capsule respectively. The ultrasound was applied with the arm held near the end range of external rotation. Simple pendulum exercises with a 2-pound weight on the wrist were performed for 3 to 5 minutes following the ultrasound. After this, low grade anterior and inferior gliding was performed (3 minutes each) at the GH joint with the arm slightly abducted and in neutral rotation. Ice was applied following exercise to control pain and inflammation.

On evaluation the next day, the patient experienced no increased pain and her ROM was unchanged. Therefore, the vigor of the program was increased by moving to high grade (end range) anterior and inferior gliding techniques.

TABLE 7-2 Chronological Description of Treatment and Passive Range of Motion

Weeks Post Injury	TREATMENT	PROM (Degrees)		
		Flexion	Abduction[a]	Lat Rot[b]
0	Fracture/dislocation			
6	Moist heat, ultrasound, pendulum, low-grade manual therapy, ice post-exercise (visits 3×/week)	80	60	5
6 + day	Increase to high-grade manual therapy, CPM, home program (3×/day): pendulum, wand, ice	80	60	5
8	Allow gentle ADL	100	75	15
10	Reduce visits to B/W, discontinue ultrasound, add elevation splint 1 hour QID	105	85	20
12	Discontinue all treatment in clinic, continue to monitor outcome of home program, add strengthening, increase splint time to 2 hours 4×/day	130	105	40
13	No change	140	120	50
14	No change	155	145	65
15	No change	165	160	65
16	No change	165	165	70
25	Patient discharged	75	170	80

[a] Abduction measured with the arm 40° to the coronal plane
[b] Lateral rotation measured with the arm by the side

Additionally, 30 minutes of continuous passive motion oscillating in the last 20° of her available scapular plane abduction ROM was added. A home program was also instituted, consisting of pendulum exercise (3 minutes) and overhead cane stretching into flexion and abduction (3 minutes) in a supine position. This routine was performed three times per day.

8 Weeks Postinjury

At this point, there was reasonable progress with ROM and no increase in pain. The patient was encouraged to completely wean herself from use of the sling, which she did, and to begin to use her arm for light functional activities.

10 Weeks Postinjury

At this point, ROM gains were being made but not at the rate expected. Because the scar was becoming more mature, a decision was made to significantly increase the stress by adding LLPS in the form of an elevation splint (similar to that shown in Figure 7-13) that was worn for four 1-hour sessions per day. The clinic visits were reduced to two times per week. The heating modalities were discontinued because they did not seem to affect the patient's response to mobilization and exercise. Clinic visits were less frequent because the principal means of applying stress to the joint were being accomplished by the patient at home via the splint and exercise.

12 Weeks Postinjury

Considerable gains were made in passive ROM during the 2-week interval. The patient was very confident in her ability to apply and adjust the splint to maintain an end-range stress. She also was becoming more comfortable with functional use of the arm for daily activities. Although no specific deficits in muscle performance were identified through muscle testing, the patient reported that her arm fatigued easily during function activities. Therefore, a resistive exercise program for the rotator cuff (internal and external rotation and abduction) using Thera-Band™ was begun. Beginning with just 10 repetitions in each direction, she was instructed to increase the number of repetitions as she was able. Her end-range time was increased to 8 hours/day because she had only minor discomfort. Additionally, as the scar matures, more stress is required to achieve gains in ROM. Because she was achieving long end-range times at home and not having significant pain, clinic treatment was discontinued at this point. The patient was seen once a week to monitor progress.

Evaluation of the Effects of the Chosen Resolution to the Problem

At 25 weeks after the injury, the patient was discharged, having achieved near full, painless ROM and complete independence in all of her normal functional activities.

Of particular interest in this case were the relatively modest gains in ROM achieved from 6 to 10 weeks postinjury with manual therapy and traditional stretching exercises. Despite the scar being more mature at 10 weeks postinjury, increasing the end-range time by adding the splint appeared to produce significant gains in ROM. Also of interest is that gains in external rotation were concomitant with gains in scapular plane abduction even though the splint did not specifically hold the GH joint in external rotation. This suggests that holding the joint at the end range of abduction also affected the tissue(s) limiting external rotation, most likely the anterior capsule.

Adapted with permission from McClure and Flowers.[7]

CHAPTER SUMMARY

Historically, the medical model has presented a confusing array of definitions to describe the hypomobile shoulder. The reason was and remains partly due to the lack of a clear consensus concerning the etiology and pathology of the problem. Terms like *frozen shoulder* became a descriptor of a common set of signs and symptoms, rather than a precise medical diagnosis. The classification of the hypomobile shoulder with a common set of impairments described in this chapter is designed to clarify the approach to assessment and treatment regardless of the medical diagnosis. A clearly defined impairment-based classification system should improve the overall quality of care and facilitate the development of controlled outcome studies to assess the effectiveness of treatment in the hypomobile shoulder, previously confounded by mixing diagnoses.

REFERENCES

1. Codman, EA: The Shoulder. Thomas Todd, Boston, 1934, p 78.
2. Neviaser, J: Adhesive capsulitis of the shoulder. J Bone Jt Surg 27:211, 1945.
3. Reeves, B: The natural history of the frozen shoulder syndrome. Scand J Rheum 4:193, 1975.
4. Neviaser, RJ, and Neviaser, TJ: The frozen shoulder: Diagnosis and management. Clin Orthop Rel Res 223:59, 1987.
5. Nash, P, and Hazelman, BL: Frozen shoulder. Bailliere's Clin Rheum 3:551, 1989.
6. McClure, PW, and Flowers, KR: Treatment of limited shoulder motion using an elevation splint. Phys Ther 72:57, 1992.
7. McClure, PW, and Flowers, KR: Treatment of limited shoulder motion: A case study based on biomechanical considerations. Phys Ther 72:929, 1992.
8. Neviaser, IS: Adhesive capsulitis and the stiff and painful shoulder. Orthop Clin North Am 11:327, 1980.
9. Akeson, W, et al: Effects of immobilization on joints. Clin Orthop 219:28, 1987.
10. Lavigne, AB, and Watkins, RP: Preliminary results on immobilization-induced stiffness of monkey knee joints and posterior capsule. In Kenedi, RM (ed): Perspectives in Medical Engineering. MacMillan, New York, 1973.
11. Peacock, E: Comparison of collagenous tissue surrounding normal and immobilized joints. Surg Forum 963; 14:440, 1963.
12. Woo, SLY, and Buckwalter, JA: Injury and Repair of the Musculoskeletal Soft Tissues. American Academy of Orthopedic Surgeons, Park Ridge, IL, 1988.
13. Lundberg, BJ: The frozen shoulder. Acta Orthop Scand (Suppl) 119, 1969.
14. Babyar, SR: Excessive scapular motion in individuals recovering from painful and stiff shoulders: Causes and treatment strategies. Phys Ther 76(3):226, 1996.
15. Cyriax, LJ: Textbook of Orthopedic Medicine, Vol 1, Diagnosis of Soft Tissue Lesions, ed 6. Williams and Wilkins, Baltimore, 1975.
16. Travell, JG, and Simons, DG: Myofascial Pain and Dysfunction: The Trigger Point Manual. Williams and Wilkins, Baltimore, 1983.
17. Arem, AJ, and Madden, JW: Effects of stress on healing wounds: Intermittent noncyclical tension. J Surg Res 20:93, 1976.
18. Brand, PN: The forces of dynamic splinting: ten questions before applying a dynamic splint to the hand. In Hunter, JM, et al (eds): Rehabilitation of the Hand, ed 2. CV Mosby, St Louis, 1984.
19. Hepburn, GR: Case studies: Contracture and stiff joint management with dynasplint. Phys Ther 8:498, 1987.
20. Light, KE, et al: Low-load prolonged stretch vs. high-load brief stretch in treating knee contractures. Phys Ther 64:330, 1984.
21. McClure, PW, et al: The use of splints in the treatment of joint stiffness: Biologic rationale and an algorithm for making clinical decisions. Phys Ther 74:1101, 1994.
22. Rizk, TE, et al: Adhesive capsulitis: A new approach to its management. Arch Phys Med Rehabil 64:29, 1983.
23. Sapega, AA, et al: Biophysical factors in range of motion exercise. Phys Sports Mod 9:57, 1981.
24. Tillman, LJ, and Cummings, GS. Biologic mechanisms of connective tissue mutability. In Currier, DP, and Nelson, RM (eds): Dynamics of Human Biologic Tissues, FA Davis, Philadelphia, 1992.
25. Warren, CG, et al: Heat and stretch procedures: An evaluation using rat tail tendon. Arch Phys Med Rehabil 57:122, 1976.
26. Leffert, RD: The frozen shoulder. Inst Course Lec AAOS 34:199, 1985.
27. Michlovitz, SL: Cryotherapy: The use of cold as a therapeutic agent. In Michlovitz, SL, (ed): Thermal Agents in Rehabilitation. FA Davis, Philadelphia, 1986, p 87.
28. Fareed, DO, and Gallivan, WR: Office management of the frozen shoulder syndrome. Clin Orthop Rel Res 242:177, 1989.
29. Pollock, RG, et al: The use of arthroscopy in the treatment of resistant frozen shoulder. Clin Orthop and Rel Res (304):30, 1994.
30. Gossman, MR, et al: Review of length-associated changes in muscle: experimental evidence and clinical implications. Phys Ther 62:1799, 1982.
31. St. Pierre, D, and Gudiner, PF: The effect of immobilization and exercise on muscle function: A review. Physiother Can 39:24, 1987.
32. William, PE, and Goldspink, G: Changes in sarcomere length and physiological properties in immobilized muscle. J Anat 127:459, 1978.
33. Williams, PE, and Goldspink, G: Connective tissue changes in immobilized muscle. J Anat 138:343, 1984.
34. Frank, C, et al: Normal ligament properties and ligament healing. Clin Orthop 196:15, 1985.
35. Frost, HM: Skeletal structural adaptations to mechanical usage: Part 4. Mechanical influences on intact fibrous tissues. Anat Rec 226:433, 1990.
36. Woo, SLY, et al: Connective tissue response to immobility: Correlative study of biomechanical and biochemical measurements of normal and immobilized rabbit knees. Arth & Rheum 18:257, 1975.

37. Laros, GS, et al: Influence of physical activity on ligament insertions in the knees of dogs. J Bone Jt Surg 53A:275, 1971.
38. Tipton, CM, et al: Influence of exercise on strength of medial collateral knee ligaments of dogs. Am J Physiol 218:894, 1970.
39. Dohners, LH, et al: The relationship of actin to ligament contraction. Clin Orth Rel Res 210:246, 1986.
40. Noyes, FR: Functional properties of knee ligaments and alterations induced by immobilization. Clin Orth Rel Res 123:210, 1973.
41. Bunker, TD, and Anthony, PP: The pathology of frozen shoulder: A Dupuytren-like disease. J Bone Jt Surg (Br Vol) 77(5):677, 1995.
42. Gabbiani, G, et al: Presence of modified fibroblasts in granulation tissue and their possible role in wound contraction. Experimentia 27:549, 1971.
43. Brand, P: Clinical Mechanics of the Hand. CV Mosby, St Louis, 1984, p 68.
44. Enneking, WF, and Horowitz, M: The intraarticular effects of immobilization on the human knee. J Bone Jt Surg (Am) 54:973, 1972.
45. Bunker, TD, and Elser, CN: Frozen Shoulder and Lipids. J Bone Jt Surg (Br Vol) 77(5):684, 1995.
46. Stam, HW: Frozen shoulder: A review of current concepts. Physiotherapy 80(9):558, 1994.
47. Jeracitano, D, et al: Abnormal temperature control suggesting sympathetic dysfunction in the shoulder skin of patients with frozen shoulder. Br J of Rheum 31(8):539, 1992.
48. Middleditch, A, and Jarman, P: An investigation of frozen shoulder using thermography. Physiother 70:433, 1984.
49. Waldberger, M, et al: The frozen shoulder: Diagnosis and treatment. Prospective study of fifty cases of adhesive capsulitis. Clin Rheum 11(3):364, 1992.
50. Johnson, J, et al: Outcome following anterior cervical discectomy without fusion. J Ortho Sports PT (abst) 23:67, 1996.
51. Hargreaves, C, et al: Frozen shoulder and cervical spine disease. Br J Rheum 28:78, 1989.
52. Rizk, TE, et al: Corticosteroid injections in adhesive capsulitis: investigation of their value and site. Arch of Phys Med and Rehab 72(l):20, 1991.
53. Bulgen, DY, et al: Frozen shoulder: prospective clinical study with an evaluation of three treatment regimens. Ann Rheum Dis 43:353, 1984.
54. Lloyd-Roberts, GC, and French, PR: Perarthritis of the shoulder. A study of the disease and its treatment. Br Med J 1:1569, 1959.
55. Uitvugt G, et al: Arthroscopic observations before and after manipulations of frozen shoulder. Arthroscopy. 9(2):181–185, 1993.
56. Ogilvie-Harris, DJ, et al: The resistant frozen shoulder: Manipulation versus arthroscopic release. Clin Orthop and Rel Res 319:238, 1995.
57. Ogilvie-Harris, DJ, and Wiley, AM: Arthroscopic surgery of the shoulder. J Bone Jt Surg 68B:201, 1986.
58. Ekelund, AL, and Rydell, N: Combination treatment for adhesive capsulitis of the shoulder. Clin Orthop and Rel Res (282):105, 1992.
59. Gavant, ML, et al: Distention arthrography in the treatment of adhesive capsulitis of the shoulder. J of Vasc and Interven Radiol 5(2):305, 1994.
60. Rizk, TE, et al: Treatment of adhesive capsulitis with arthrographic capsular distention and rupture. Arch of Phys Med and Rehab 75:803, 1994.
61. Flowers, KR, and Lastayo, P: Effect of total end range time on improving passive range of motion. J Hand Ther 7: 150, 1994.
62. Fung, YC: Biomechanics, Mechanical Properties of Living Tissues. Springer-Verlag, New York, 1981.
63. Kaltenborn, FM: Mobilization of the Extremity Joints. Olaf Noris Bokhandel, Oslo, Norway, 1980.
64. Kisner, C, and Colby, LA: Therapeutic Exercise: Foundations and Techniques. FA Davis, Philadelphia, 1985.
65. Maitland, GD: Peripheral Manipulation, ed 2. Butterworths, London, 1977.
66. Mennell, JM: Joint Pain. Little Brown, Boston, 1964.
67. Wadsworth, CT: Manual Examination and Treatment of the Spine and Extremities. Williams and Wilkins, Baltimore, 1988.
68. Wooden, MJ: Mobilization of the upper extremity. In Donatelli, R, and Wooden, MJ (eds): Orthopedic Physical Therapy. Churchill Livingstone, New York, 1989.

CHAPTER 8

Musculoskeletal Pattern E: Impaired Joint Mobility, Muscle Performance, and Range of Motion Associated with Ligament or Other Connective Tissue Disorders

Todd S. Ellenbecker, MS, PT, SCS, CSCS

INTRODUCTION

Shoulder instability is characterized by symptoms that develop from the inability of the neuromuscular system to compensate for excessive ligamentous laxity. According to the APTA's *Guide to Physical Therapist Practice*,[1] shoulder instability is classified under musculoskeletal practice pattern E. This practice pattern describes impaired joint mobility, muscle performance, and range of motion associated with ligament or other connective tissue disorders.[1]

This chapter reviews the common classification systems used to define glenohumeral instability and discusses how instability can lead to specific tissue pathology. The chapter also presents an evaluation process that identifies the degree of glenohumeral (GH) joint instability, specific tissue pathology, and the common impairments to be addressed in rehabilitation.

181

DEFINITIONS

Several operational definitions are presented to increase the clinician's understanding of the unstable shoulder. Important to clarify are the difference in meaning between laxity and instability and the meaning of translation. *Laxity* is defined as the amount of movement of the humeral head relative to the glenoid when stress is applied.[2] Increased laxity might lead to hypermobility, but this condition is not an impairment. *Instability* is defined as excessive, symptomatic laxity or translation of the humeral head relative to the glenoid, and the inability of the individual to maintain the humeral head centered within the glenoid fossa.[2] Humeral head *translation* is defined as the motion of the center of the humeral head relative to the face of the glenoid fossa.[2] When evaluating a patient's shoulder, significant laxity or humeral head translation might be present. However, if no symptoms or functional limitations exist, the term *unstable* is not used.[2,3]

Maintaining the humeral head within the glenoid fossa under stressful, dynamic conditions while allowing a large excursion of range of motion is challenging. A healthy shoulder should inherently possess a fine balance between stability and mobility, particularly with high levels of athletic or ergonomic function.

CLASSIFICATION OF INSTABILITY

Several terms or schemes have been used to better understand or classify shoulder instability. While considerable overlap among terms and classification schemes exists, the importance of understanding the full spectrum of instability in the human shoulder is imperative for successful evaluation and management.

Macrotraumatic Versus Microtraumatic Instability

The terms *macro-* and *microtraumatic* instability attempt to classify the shoulder instability by referring to the specific etiology. *Macrotraumatic instability* typically occurs from a single traumatic event, such as a fall on an outstretched arm, that the patient can recall. This incident often results in a complete dislocation of the humeral head from the glenoid.[4] This type of instability is the most easily diagnosed, but can leave the patient with substantial limitations and disability if mismanaged. *Microtraumatic instability* differs from macrotraumatic instability because it does not occur from one isolated event. Microtraumatic instability is usually because of an accumulation of repeated stresses imparted to the shoulder during overhead activities such as baseball pitching, swimming, or tennis serving.[4] These repeated microtraumatic events lead to labral and capsular attenuation. In the presence of poor dynamic stabilization and faulty mechanics, this can lead to an unstable shoulder.

AMBRII Versus TUBS

Matsen et al.[5] present a different classification scheme for unstable shoulders that incorporates the mechanism of injury, direction of instability, and involved tissue pathology. They describe an *AMBRII* syndrome as an **A**traumatic onset of **M**ultidirectional instability that is accompanied by **B**ilateral laxity or hypermobility. **R**ehabilitation is the primary course of treatment used to restore GH joint stability, but if an operation is necessary, a capsulorraphy is performed that tightens the **I**nferior capsule and the rotator **I**nterval.[6]

The second category in the classification described by Matsen et al.[5] is *TUBS*, which means instability occurring from a **T**raumatic event, producing **U**nidirectional anterior instability with a **B**ankart lesion, and resulting in **S**urgery. The GH joint has lost the stabilizing effect of the anterior inferior glenohumeral ligament complex when the arm is in abduction, extension, and external rotation. Compromise of the anterior glenoid labrum results in less congruency of the glenoid fossa, also possibly predisposing the joint to instability. The TUBS or "torn loose" situation, which is in direct contrast to the "born loose" AMBRII syndrome, allows for classification based on patient history, mechanism of injury, and clinical examination.

Additional Factors

The degree of humeral head translation is also important in understanding the degree and classifying the type of instability. Joint instability in the shoulder can range between complete dislocation to subtle subluxation of the humeral head. A complete dislocation, which involves disassociation of the humeral head from the glenoid fossa, often requires manual reduction. Subluxation involves translation of the humeral head beyond physiological limits, followed by self-reduction.

Also of relevance to the unstable shoulder is whether the condition is acute, chronic, or volitional. The patient with an acute dislocation of the GH joint might receive a different surgical and rehabilitative approach than a patient with chronic instability—possibly experiencing hundreds of episodes of instability. The ability to volitionally or voluntarily sublux or dislocate the shoulder is also an important issue in classifying the unstable shoulder.[7] Volitional or voluntary instability represents the ease with which a patient can sublux or dislocate the shoulder. This information provides both an indication of the degree of instability, as well as insight into the chronicity of the disability.

CLINICAL ASSESSMENT OF IMPAIRMENTS ASSOCIATED WITH INSTABILITY

A detailed physical examination is used to classify the shoulder as unstable. While subjective reports of previous dislocations or feelings of shifting in the arm clearly indicate shoulder joint instability, subtle symptoms such as fatigue or "dead arm," anterior shoulder pain, or impingement type sensations might also suggest instability. A complete and thorough history is necessary. Particular emphasis is placed on activity or sports-specific movement patterns producing the symptoms. Knowledge of the mechanics of a specific sport activity might give the clinician insight into the loads, forces, and muscle activation patterns inherent in that activity. This information might assist in detecting tissue pathology and planning the physical examination.

Objective Evaluation

Whereas it is beyond the scope of this chapter to completely outline the entire evaluation process, special tests used to determine joint mobility require a review. See Chapter 5 for a complete review of the shoulder examination.

HUMERAL TRANSLATION TESTS

The most important tests that identify shoulder joint instability are humeral head translation tests.[8,9] The classic test to identify the unstable shoulder, the apprehension sign, involves the combination of abduction and external rotation. This test does not attempt to measure how mobile the humeral head is relative to the glenoid. Rather, it gauges the patient's response to a provoking movement pattern.[10]

Clinical application of humeral head translation tests can be achieved using the load and shift test, or supine anterior and posterior drawer test (see Chap. 5). These tests attempt to measure the amount of excursion of the humeral head relative to the glenoid with the application of stress. Harryman et al.[11] documented in-vivo the human GH joint laxity in normal, healthy subjects using a three-dimensional (3D) spatial tracking system. They found a mean of 7.8 mm of anterior humeral head translation and 7.9 mm of posterior translation. Inferior translation is typically evaluated using a multidirectional instability (MDI) sulcus sign. In this test, the examiner attempts to displace the humeral head inferiorly relative to the glenoid. Harryman et al.[11] found a mean of 10 mm of inferior displacement in-vivo.

Attempting to quantify the exact movement of the humeral head in millimeters is not always clinically accurate.[12] Altchek[13] has proposed a grading scheme using the glenoid rim as a reference (Table 8-1). A grade I+ translation involves translation within the glenoid, but not up onto the glenoid rim. A II+ translation involves movement of the humeral head up onto and over the glenoid rim with spontaneous reduction on removal of the anterior or posterior force. A grade III+ involves complete dislocation without reduction and is seldom applied in the clinical setting (Fig. 8-1).

Use of anterior, posterior, and inferior humeral head translation tests allows the examiner to determine the direction and extent of increased translation using the contralateral extremity as a baseline. Care must be taken in interpreting the findings of translation testing. Differences in humeral head translation of up to one grade between extremities has been reported consistently in normal, uninjured athletic subject populations.[14] Additionally, translation of up to II+ is often found in shoulders of healthy, uninjured subjects.[14] Therefore, the clinical finding of increased humeral head translation coupled with patient symptoms are required to label the shoulder as unstable.

TABLE 8–1 Grading of Humeral Head Translation Tests

Grade	Glenohumeral Joint Translation
I+	Humeral head translates within the glenoid and up the glenoid slope but not over the rim
II+	Humeral head rides up and over the glenoid rim but spontaneously reduces when stress is removed
III+	Humeral head rides up and over the glenoid rim and remains dislocated on removal of stress

(Adapted from Altchek et al.[13]: Arthroscopic labral debridement: A three-year follow-up study. Am J Sports Med 20(6):702, 1992.)

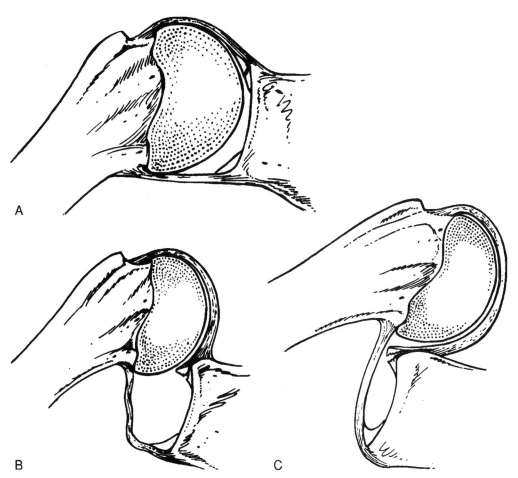

FIGURE 8–1. Humeral head translation. *(A)* Grade I+. *(B)* Grade II+. *(C)* Grade III+. (Adapted from Altchek, DW, et al.: Arthroscopic labral debridement. A three year follow-up study. Am J Sports Med 20(6):702, 1992, with permission.)

The direction or pattern of hypermobility is important in diagnosing GH joint injury and in formulating the appropriate exercise and stabilization programs. Hawkins et al.[15] found a consistent pattern of humeral head translation in patients with anterior, posterior, and MDI when compared to uninjured controls. Patients with anterior instability were found to have greater anterior and inferior humeral head translation than uninjured controls. Additionally, patients with posterior instability were found to have increased posterior humeral head translation. Patients with MDI had greater anterior, posterior, and inferior translation than control subjects in the study. This group comprised the greatest challenge with regard to nonoperative or operative stabilization.[15]

Classification of patients into one of two categories, unidirectional or multidirectional, is possible with a structured musculoskeletal evaluation using humeral head translation tests. Patients with unidirectional instability typically have increased or excessive humeral head translation in one primary direction. Patients classified as having MDI typically demonstrate excessive inferior translation identified with the MDI sulcus sign and increased translation in an anterior and/or posterior direction.[16]

Patients with excessive joint laxity or a connective tissue disorder such as Ehlers-Danlos syndrome are likely to have MDI.[16]

SUBLUXATION-RELOCATION TEST

Another test to identify the unstable shoulder is the subluxation-relocation test.[17] In this test, the examiner abducts the patient's shoulder to 90° and externally rotates the shoulder to 90°. The examiner then exerts a small anteriorly directed force, attempting to sublux the shoulder anteriorly (Fig. 8–2A). A report of pain is considered a positive subluxation part of the test. The examiner then switches his or her hand onto the anterior aspect of the humeral head and presses in a posterior direction, attempting to relocate the humeral head (Fig. 8–2B).[17] This test is used to determine subtle anterior instability and is useful for application to patients with unidirectional anterior instability and secondary impingement. A critical evaluation of the subluxation-relocation test has been performed by Speer et al.,[18] who examined the effectiveness and accuracy of the subluxation-relocation test in 100 patients undergoing arthroscopic shoulder surgery. They reported questionable sensitivity and accuracy of the subluxation-relocation test when the response of pain alone was considered (less

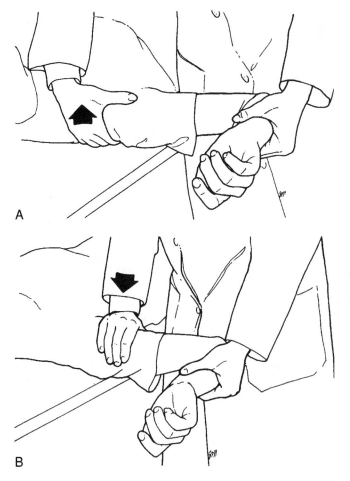

A

B

FIGURE 8–2. Jobe subluxation/relocation test. *(A)* Subluxation. *(B)* Relocation. (Adapted from Jobe, FW, and Bradley, JP: Diagnosis of shoulder injuries. Clin Sports Med 8:3, 1989, p 427, with permission.)

than 50% accuracy), and improved accuracy (greater than 80%) when the response of apprehension alone was considered. Increasing the amount of external rotation to the patient's end range that increases the stress to the anterior capsule and more closely approximates the position inherent to overhead sport activities is a suggested modification for improving the accuracy of the subluxation-relocation test.[18–21]

ADDITIONAL EVALUATION PROCEDURES

Additional evaluation procedures, such as the Kibler lateral scapular slide test and the scapular assistance test,[20] are used to identify impaired scapular stabilization. According to Kibler,[20] bilateral asymmetries of one to 1 to 1.5 cm between the inferior angle and the corresponding vertebral spinous process are considered to indicate deficiencies in dynamic muscular stabilization. Additionally, in the scapular assistance test, the clinician mechanically assists moving the inferior angle of the scapula outward into protraction and upward rotation while the patient is actively elevating the arm. Negation of impingement type symptoms indicates a lack of proper scapular control. Thus, exercises to strengthen the muscles that dynamically stabilize the scapula are emphasized during rehabilitation. The proprioceptive and kinesthetic function of the shoulder also should be assessed in the unstable shoulder. Impaired afferent activity, evidenced by a reduction in proprioceptive and kinesthetic function, has been reported in the shoulders of patients who have suffered an anterior GH joint dislocation, as well as following acute muscular fatigue.[22,23] Clinical tests used to measure the proprioceptive and kinesthetic ability of the shoulder are outlined in Chapter 5. These tests commonly consist of angular reproduction and threshold to sensation of movement maneuvers and protocols.[23,24]

ROLE OF GLENOHUMERAL JOINT INSTABILITY IN ROTATOR CUFF INJURY

Injury to the rotator cuff has traditionally been attributed to GH joint impingement and the progression of impingement through the stages described by Neer.[25] Clinical findings among younger, more active patients with shoulder instability have led researchers and clinicians to the current understanding of the important role that instability plays in rotator cuff injury.[17,19,26,27] The inferior glenohumeral ligament is the primary restraint against anterior humeral head translation with the shoulder in 90° of GH joint abduction.[28] Attenuation of the anterior glenohumeral capsular complex and the anterior labrum with repeated overhead activity involving external rotation and abduction can cause excessive anterior translation of the humeral head.[17,19,27] This increased anterior humeral head translation can create excessive contact between the rotator cuff and biceps tendon and the undersurface of the acromion[17] (Fig. 8–3). This type of impingement, termed *secondary impingement*, occurs because of the primary underlying instability of the GH joint. Rotator cuff lesions in patients with secondary impingement observed on the bursal (superior side) of the rotator cuff result from mechanical abrasion and compression of the cuff against the acromion.[29,30] See Chapter 9 for a detailed discussion of impingement.

Also, tensile overload is another factor relating rotator cuff pathology to GH joint hypermobility. In the shoulder with inherent hypermobility, the rotator cuff tendons

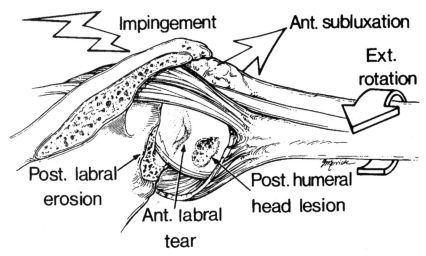

FIGURE 8–3. Secondary impingement. (Adapted from Jobe, FW, and Bradley, JP: Diagnosis of shoulder injuries. Clin Sports Med 8:3, 1989, p 430, with permission.)

are subjected to large intrinsic eccentric loads during overhead activities such as throwing or swinging a tennis racquet.[26] These repetitive eccentric loads can lead to overload failure of the tendons, possibly progressing to rotator cuff tears on the undersurface (articular side) of the tendon.[31] Histologic study of the rotator cuff tendons by Nakajima et al.[31] has shown that the undersurface or articular side of the supraspinatus tendon is less resistant to tensile loading, as opposed to the superior or bursal side of the tendon, which can tolerate greater tensile loading. This lack of tensile strength of the undersurface of the supraspinatus tendon, coupled with the high stresses (as high as 1090 Newtons) needed to resist GH joint distraction during the deceleration and follow-through phases of the throwing motion, often results in overuse injury.

Analysis of outcomes following arthroscopic partial rotator cuff debridement suggests a correlation between instability and rotator cuff pathology. Payne et al.[32] studied 43 athletes under age 40 who each underwent arthroscopic treatment for a partial tear in the rotator cuff. In one group of 14 patients who had acute, traumatic onset of shoulder symptoms, but did not have increased humeral head translation or labral lesions, successful outcomes occurred in 86%, with 64% returning to full preinjury sports levels. A second group of 29 overhead athletes had insidious development of rotator cuff symptoms. Many of these athletes had increased humeral head translation and labral tears. Successful outcomes were reported in 66% of the patients in this group, with only 45% returning to preinjury sports levels. These results indicate that functional outcomes are less successful when a patient has combined instability and rotator cuff pathology.

Other chapters in this text further define the relationship between increased humeral head translation and rotator cuff pathology. When evaluating the unstable shoulder, clinicians should understand the increased demand that glenohumeral laxity places on the rotator cuff in the human shoulder. When the rotator cuff muscles fail to control the laxity, the pattern of instability develops. Use of tests outlined in Chapter 5 can identify involvement of the rotator cuff clinically. See Chapter 5 for a more complete description of the tests used to delineate rotator cuff pathology.

ROLE OF HYPERMOBILITY ON THE GLENOID LABRUM

The glenoid labrum serves several important functions including deepening the glenoid fossa to enhance concavity and serving as the attachment for the important glenohumeral capsular ligaments. Injury to the glenoid labrum can compromise concavity, compressing the GH joint by as much as 50%.[5] In the patient with generalized joint hypermobility and increased humeral head translation, the glenoid labrum is subjected to increased shear forces, possibly becoming attenuated or compressed; thus limiting the ability to stabilize the humeral head within the glenoid.[19] Using the example of the throwing athlete, large anterior translatory forces are present (up to 50% of body weight) during arm acceleration of the throwing motion while the arm is in a position of 90° of abduction and external rotation.[33] This position places tremendous stress on the anterior capsular structures and the glenoid labrum. Further stresses are imparted to the posterior rotator cuff as it resists approximately 1090 Newtons of distraction force as the humeral head is pulled anteriorly in the direction the ball has been thrown.[34]

An important component of the hypermobile shoulder is the status of the glenoid labrum. Detachment of the anterior-inferior labrum from the glenoid is called a Bankart lesion[35] (Fig. 8–4). This detachment decreases GH joint stability by interrupting the continuity of the glenoid labrum and compromising the glenohumeral capsular ligaments.[36] Detachment of the anterior inferior labrum increases both anterior and inferior humeral head translation, commonly observed in patients with GH joint instability.[36]

An additional labral lesion described in the hypermobile shoulder is the *SLAP lesion*. SLAP lesions are defined as **S**uperior **L**abral lesions that are both **A**nterior and **P**osterior.[37] SLAP lesions have been classified into four main types by Snyder.[37] One of the consequences of a SLAP lesion is the frequent involvement of the insertion of the biceps tendon or biceps anchor.[37,38] This compromise of both the integrity of the superior labrum and loss of the biceps anchor leads to substantial losses in the static

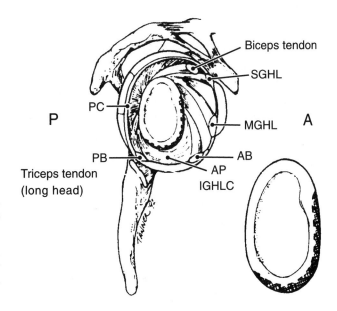

FIGURE 8–4. Glenoid labrum, glenohumeral capsular ligaments, and site of Bankart lesion. (Adapted from Speer, KP, et al.: Biochemical evaluation of a Bankart Lesion. J Bone Joint Surgery 76A(12):1819, 1994, p 1821 with permission.)

stabilizing elements in the human shoulder. Cheng and Karzel[39] further illustrated the effects of a SLAP lesion by experimentally creating a labral detachment in the 10 o'clock to 2 o'clock position in cadaver shoulders. They found an 11% to 19% decrease in the shoulder's ability to withstand rotational force, as well as a 100% to 120% increase in the stress on the anterior inferior glenohumeral ligament. Their findings demonstrate the increased load on ligamentous structures in the presence of labral pathology.

The role of the labrum in the hypermobile shoulder was clinically illustrated by Altchek et al.[13] in a 3-year follow-up of patients following arthroscopic labral debridement. Forty overhead athletes underwent surgery following labral injury. Of these patients, 72% initially noted a significant relief of symptoms during the first year following surgery. At a 2-year follow-up however, only 7% of the patients reported significant symptomatic relief, with a consistent generalized deterioration occurring over time. These authors concluded that arthroscopic labral debridement is not an effective long-term solution for labral pathology. The authors of this study postulated that the underlying instability or hypermobility of the shoulder that often leads to labral injury must be addressed to effectively return function and symptomatic relief to the patient.

The role between GH joint instability and both rotator cuff and labral pathology highlights the importance and need for a comprehensive evaluation. The detection of specific tissue pathologies occurring with GH joint instability allows the clinician to determine if the patient is a candidate for nonoperative rehabilitation. It also helps the clinician develop specific rehabilitative strategies. The use of various techniques to improve the dynamic stability of the GH joint is indicated in the unstable shoulder even in the presence of rotator cuff and labral pathology.[27]

Clinical tests used to identify glenoid labrum pathology are outlined in Chapter 5. Use of tests such as the crank test, clunk test, and O'Brien's active compression test are indicated to identify glenoid labrum pathology in the human shoulder.[40] All of these tests approximate the GH joint, attempting to trap the labrum between the humeral head and glenoid to reproduce patient symptoms. See Chapter 5 of this text for a more complete discussion of the tests indicated to identify glenoid labrum pathology.

STATIC AND DYNAMIC GLENOHUMERAL JOINT STABILIZERS

To effectively evaluate and treat a hypermobile shoulder, the clinician must be familiar with both the static and dynamic stabilizers of the GH joint.

Static Stabilizers

The static stabilizers of the GH joint are generally described as the (1) joint geometry, (2) negative intraarticular pressure, (3) glenoid labrum, and (4) capsular ligaments. Joint geometry refers to the outline and osseous components of the proximal humerus and glenoid fossa. Important to joint biomechanics is the concept of the scapular plane.[40] The scapular plane has been described as the plane 30° to 45° anterior to the frontal or coronal plane of the body. The scapular plane position places the GH joint in an optimum position with respect to osseous congruity between the humeral head and glenoid. It also minimizes bony impingement.[41] Several osseous characteristics of the GH joint contribute to the enhanced stability reported in the scapular plane.[41] These characteristics include the 30° retrotorsion angle of the articulating portion of the humeral head relative to the distal shaft of the humerus, coupled with a 30° anterior angulation of the glenoid fossa. These are examples of the static osseous parameters of the human shoulder that provide enhanced stability by increasing osseous contact in the scapular plane.[41] This scapular plane position is often advocated for exercise, immobilization, surgical treatment, and rehabilitation.[26,27,42]

Negative intra-articular pressure formed by the sealed GH joint capsule is another mechanism that serves to provide static stability to the shoulder.[43] Kumar and Balasubramanium[43] presented evidence that the vacuum effect created by a sealed GH joint capsule was one of the main static stabilizers for inferior translation of the GH joint. Increases in inferior translation following venting or releasing the capsule have been reportedly caused by loss of intra-articular pressure.

The labrum, which is an important influence on shoulder stability discussed previously in this chapter, has an intimate relationship with the capsular ligaments. The GH joint capsular ligaments attach to the peripheral surface of the labrum. O'Brien et al.[28] have provided a detailed description of the glenohumeral capsular ligaments. The anatomical orientation of these structures produces stabilizing influences against anterior humeral head translation depending on the degree of elevation. The superior glenohumeral ligament is primarily effective during the first 30° of abduction. The middle glenohumeral ligament is most effective at limiting anterior translation at mid-range (30° to 60°) levels. The inferior glenohumeral ligament possesses a unique hammocking-type effect on the humeral head. At 90° of shoulder abduction and 90° of humeral external rotation, the inferior glenohumeral ligament supports the anterior inferior aspect of the humeral head, preventing anterior translation. The position of the inferior glenohumeral ligament changes with internal rotation of the humerus in 90° of abduction such that it can also effectively limit posterior translation of the humeral head.[28]

This ligamentous structure provides essential stability to the abducted shoulder. Bigliani et al.[44] reported that the strength of the inferior glenohumeral ligament is only 15% that of the human anterior cruciate ligament (ACL). Therefore, the combination of the tremendous repetitive forces imparted to the anterior capsular structures and the lack of tensile strength of the glenohumeral ligaments often lead to acquired GH joint instability in the overhead athlete.

Dynamic Stabilizers

The primary dynamic stabilizers of the GH joint are the four rotator cuff muscles and the long head of the biceps.[45,46] The rotator cuff provides exceptional dynamic stability to the GH joint in the following four primary ways: (1) providing passive bulk, (2) developing muscle tensions that compress the joint surfaces together, (3) moving the humerus with respect to the glenoid to produce tightening of the static restraints; and (4) limiting the arc of motion via muscle tensions.[45] The study by Blaiser and colleagues[45] demonstrates the important role that the rotator cuff plays in compressing the humeral head within the glenoid, ultimately providing stability to the GH joint. Tension simulated experimentally within any of the rotator cuff tendons resulted in a measurable and significant contribution to anterior GH joint stability.[45]

Because of the intimate association with the superior labrum and close proximity to the humeral head, the biceps brachii long head tendon provides both anterior and superior stability to the GH joint.[46–48] Kumer et al.[46] showed a 16% increase in proximal humeral head migration when the biceps long head tendon was absent, whereas Pagnani et al.,[48] and Rodosky et al.[49] have shown that increased anterior translation of the humeral head occurs with biceps tendon and superior labral deficiencies.

NONOPERATIVE TREATMENT OF THE UNSTABLE SHOULDER

Primary treatment goals for the patient with GH joint instability include optimization of the dynamic stabilizers and protection of the static stabilizers of the GH joint.

Submaximal Exercise

The first limiting factor that must be addressed is pain and/or inflammation in the shoulder. Modalities such as interferential electrical stimulation and ultrasound are applied to increase local blood flow and to assist in the healing process.[50] Often,

STAGES:

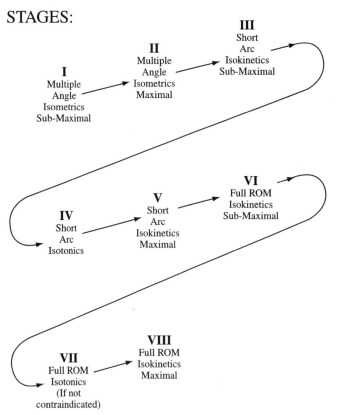

FIGURE 8–5. Davies resistive exercise progression. (From Davies, GJ: A compendium of isokinetics in clinical usage. S & S Publishers, LaCrosse, Wisc., 1984, p 243, with permission.)

one of the most important early applications in the treatment of the hypermobile shoulder is the use of submaximal exercise.[51] Intramuscular laser-doppler flowmetry has been used to measure blood flow in the supraspinatus muscle during isometric contractions at 20%, 30%, and 50% of maximal voluntary contraction levels.[51] Results showed increased intramuscular blood flow during the contractions, as well as a reactive hyperemia for a period of 1 minute after exercise. Therefore, the use of submaximal exercise in the stabilizing musculature of the GH joint is indicated for muscular re-education and strengthening and also improvement of local blood flow.[51]

Progression of resistive exercise follows the Davies resistive exercise progression (Fig. 8–5). Progression from multiple angle isometrics applied via the pain-free range of motion for internal and external rotation to isotonic internal and external rotation with either manual resistance for greater control or light weights and rubberized tubing are indicated. The patient should avoid using positions that compromise stability until adequate motor control is attained. Manual resistance to the scapula in the patterns of protraction and retraction (Fig. 8–6) are also an important part of early treatment to ensure that the musculature controlling the movements of the scapula are recruited in a low-resistance high-repetition format.

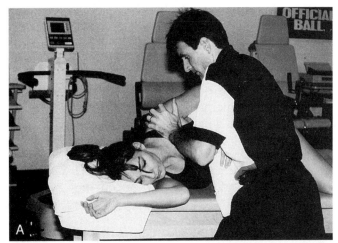

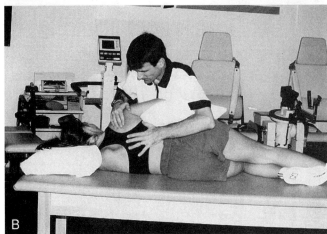

FIGURE 8–6. Sidelying scapular protraction and retraction. *(A)* Protraction. *(B)* Retraction.

Range of motion of the hypermobile shoulder must be closely monitored and evaluated early in treatment to determine the optimal type of intervention. In most cases of GH joint instability, gross range of motion of the shoulder is not restricted, particularly in the shoulder with a generalized increase in joint laxity and in those with MDI.[52,53] Careful evaluation and documentation of range of motion is necessary, particularly rotational range of motion with the shoulder abducted 90°. Significant differences in internal rotation range of motion have been reported using a specific procedure to stabilize the scapula as compared to a procedure with no scapular stabilization.[54,55] Care must be taken to measure internal rotation (Fig. 8–7) with the scapula stabilized to determine the amount of humeral excursion.[54,56]

Measurement of shoulder internal rotation using the Appley's scratch test (see Chap. 5) is not recommended because this maneuver involves a composite motion of several joints and does not isolate internal rotation of the shoulder.[56] Use of this motion alone might not accurately represent the amount of GH joint internal rotation and the amount of posterior capsular tightness.

In most unstable shoulders, gentle maintenance of joint arthrokinematics via passive range of motion in the available range is indicated, without further stress being imparted to the capsulolabral tissues of the shoulder. Application of accessory joint mobilization might increase joint play and stress on the static stabilizers, possibly further increasing mobility and perpetuating the instability of the patient's shoulder.

Occasionally, specific limitations in GH joint range of motion are identified during evaluation of the patient with an unstable shoulder. One specific indication of an application for joint mobilization would be in the patient with subtle anterior instability with limited internal rotation of the shoulder, often by as much as 10° to 20° when compared to that of the contralateral shoulder. The use of posterior glide mobilization to mechanically stretch the posterior capsule and improve internal rotation range of motion is indicated (Fig. 8–8). The rationale for the use of this type of specific mobilization is best illustrated in a cadaveric study in the human shoulder by Harryman et al.[57] A posterior capsular shift, performed in cadaver specimens, resulted in a significant increase in anterior shear forces and anterior humeral head translation with cross arm adduction and flexion movement patterns. The restriction in the posterior capsule coupled with certain movement patterns created an increase in

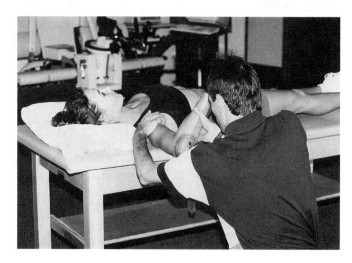

FIGURE 8–7. Shoulder range of motion measurement using isolated technique with scapular stabilization.

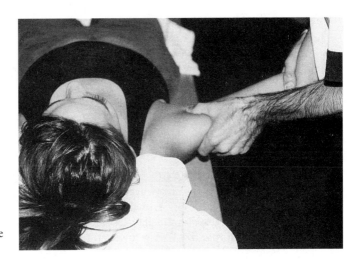

FIGURE 8–8. Posterior glide mobilization technique.

anterior movement of the humeral head. Additionally, increased superior translation of the humeral head was also documented earlier in the range of motion of elevation with tightness of the posterior capsule. Therefore, using measurement methods that allow the clinician to document posterior capsular restriction and the careful use of specific joint mobilization is a critical part in the early treatment of patients with GH joint hypermobility.

Progressive Exercises

As patients progress in their tolerance to submaximal resistive exercise for the internal and external rotators, additional exercises are added to improve the dynamic stabilization of the scapulothoracic (ST) and GH joints. Exercises that produce the highest relative electromyography (EMG) activation levels in the rotator cuff musculature are emphasized. These exercises are also designed to minimize the contribution from muscles, such as the deltoid and pectoralis major, that produce translational patterns (anteriorly and superiorly directed shear forces), which are less desirable to GH joint function.[42,58–61] Figure 8–9 lists exercises that are commonly used to elicit increased levels of posterior rotator cuff EMG activation.[58–61] GH joint protection principles, listed in Table 8–2, include exercise ranges of motion that minimize the effects of impingement. Strategies include keeping the shoulder below 90° of elevation, as well as placing the arm in front of the scapular plane to minimize stress to the anterior capsular ligaments.[29] A low-resistance, high-repetition format is followed with sets of 15 repetitions or more to foster local muscular endurance.[62]

In addition to traditional exercises that focus on the rotator cuff, additional exercises are performed to strengthen the biceps, using the pattern of elbow flexion, with varying positions of forward flexion, abduction, and scapular plane elevation. Increased biceps activity has been reported in shoulders of throwing athletes with instability when compared to normal throwers. This suggests that the long head of the biceps has a stabilizing effect on the GH joint.[63]

Scapular stabilization exercises are also emphasized in an effort to improve dynamic stability of the shoulder joint. Exercises including seated rows, wall pushes,

1. SIDE-LYING EXTERNAL ROTATION:
Lie on uninvolved side, with involved arm
at side with a small pillow between arm and
body. Keeping elbow of involved arm bent
and fixed to side, raise arm into external
rotation. Slowly lower to starting position,
and repeat.

2. SHOULDER EXTENSION:
Lie on table on stomach with involved arm
hanging straight to the floor. With thumb
pointed outward, raise arm straight back into
extension toward your hip. Slowly lower arm
and repeat.

3. PRONE HORIZONTAL ABDUCTION:
Lie on table on stomach with involved arm
hanging straight to the floor. With thumb
pointed outward, raise arm out to the side
parallel to the floor. Slowly lower arm, and
repeat.

4. SUPRASPINATUS - "EMPTY CAN":
Stand with elbow straight and thumb
pointed down toward ground. Raise
arm to shoulder level at 30° angle to
body. Slowly lower arm and repeat.

5. 90/90 EXTERNAL ROTATION:
Lie on table on stomach with shoulder
abducted to 90° and arm supported on
table with elbow bent at 90°. Keeping
the shoulder and elbow fixed, rotate
arm into external rotation, slowly
lower to start position and repeat.

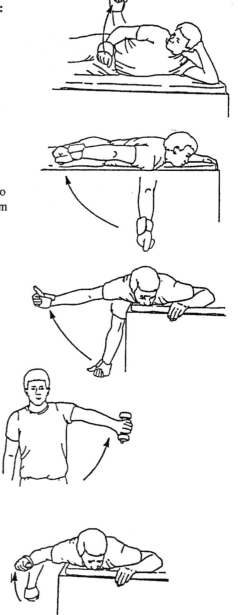

FIGURE 8–9. Rotator cuff strengthening exercises. (Courtesy of Physiotherapy Associates. Scottsdale Sports Clinic, Scottsdale, Ariz.)

upper extremity plyometric chest passes using a medicine ball, and closed chain
upper extremity step-ups (Fig. 8–10) are all recommended.[64,65] Particular emphasis is
placed on balancing the force couples of the shoulder. A force couple exists when two
muscles work together exerting forces along different lines to enable a particular
motion to occur.[66] These muscles can be agonist-antagonist pairs. Often they are

TABLE 8–2 Glenohumeral Joint Protection Principles

Goal	Application
Avoidance of impingement positions	Keep humerus below 90° elevation
Decrease in stress on anterior capsule	Keep arms anterior to scapular plane
Avoidance of tendon overload and improvement of local muscular endurance	Use a low-resistance high-repetition format (i.e., 3 sets, 15 reps)

synergistic muscles. In addressing scapular stability, strengthening the serratus anterior and lower trapezius muscles becomes important because they work together to produce upward rotation of the scapula during elevation of the humerus. They also work to provide a stabilizing influence for the scapula against the thoracic wall to prevent winging and loss of control.[20]

Use of closed kinetic chain exercise is of extreme importance for strengthening the hypermobile shoulder. The inherent benefits of the closed chain environment, including muscular cocontraction, cohesion of joint surfaces, and multijoint training, make these exercises an excellent choice for patients with this impairment. Performance of closed chain exercises such as the step-ups and push-ups with a plus are utilized along with quadruped exercises with manual resistance application using a modification of a rhythmic stabilization technique (Fig. 8–11).[65] Additional benefits of the closed chain exercises and the use of rhythmic stabilization are in the provision of proprioceptive stimulus. Because deficits in proprioceptive function have been documented in the unstable shoulder, the inclusion of exercises that increase afferent neural activity and challenge the proprioceptive and kinesthetic awareness of the patient with GH joint instability are indicated.[24,67,68] Limited published information exists regarding the use of closed kinetic chain exercise in the upper extremity. Some studies suggest that the use of closed kinetic chain testing and training for the upper extremity might produce unique activation and strength patterns, and thus might be

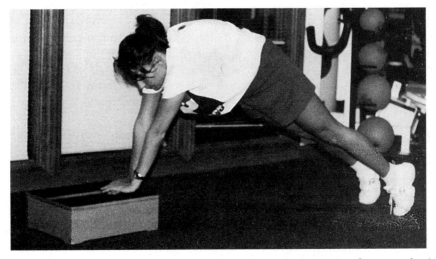

FIGURE 8–10. Closed chain upper extremity step-ups with protraction for strengthening the serratus anterior.

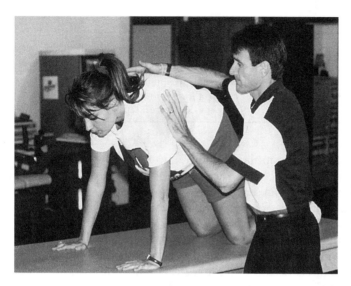

FIGURE 8–11. Modified rhythmic stabilization technique in quadriped with manual resistance application. A protracted scapular position is used to increase serratus anterior activation.

an important adjunct in rehabilitation of the GH joint.[67,68] Further research is clearly needed before a more definitive statement can be made regarding the role of the closed chain environment in shoulder rehabilitation.

Additional strengthening is used both in the clinic and at home using rubberized tubing or Thera-Band. The pattern of internal and external rotation with the arm held in slight abduction and horizontal flexion (scapular plane) is applied, with emphasis on both the concentric and eccentric phases of the exercise (Fig. 8–12). Recent research by Bridgett[69] demonstrated significant internal and external rotation strength improvements following a 6-week training program with Thera-Band. Additional support for the use of rubberized tubing for strengthening comes from an EMG study verifying high levels of rotator cuff activation with the pattern of internal and external rotation.[70] In addition to providing significant strength improvements, Treiber et al.[71] found internal and external rotation strengthening with rubber tubing to produce improvements in tennis serving velocity when compared to a control group. Whereas evidence exists confirming the efficacy of internal and external rotation training with Thera-Band, improvements in rotator cuff strength were not demonstrated in a 6-week training study using the proprioceptive neuromuscular facilitation (PNF) diagonal 2 flexion pattern.[72] Therefore, extensive use of the patterns listed in this chapter are emphasized based on their demonstrated effect on either rotator cuff activation or rotator cuff strength production.

Progression of the patient with a hypermobile shoulder consists of the above mentioned exercise patterns and methods, but also includes the use of isokinetic testing and training. Following the progression from submaximal to maximal exercise intensity, the patient is placed primarily in the scapular plane, 30° to 45 ° of abduction, to perform internal and external rotation training in what has been termed the modified base position (Fig. 8–13).[73] Precursors to isokinetic training recommended by this author include the ability to perform the isotonic rotator cuff exercises in a pain-free fashion using a 2.5-pound weight, or external-internal rotation resistance using medium level rubber tubing.

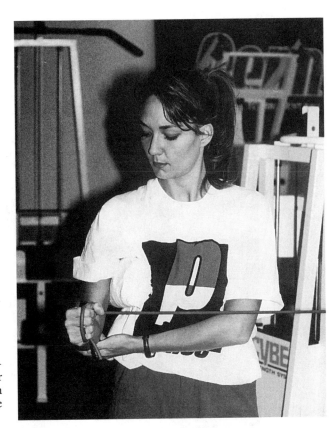

FIGURE 8–12. External rotation exercise with the shoulder stabilized in slight abduction with the use of a towel roll and the contralateral extremity.

In addition to the inherent benefits of using the accommodative resistance afforded in the isokinetic environment,[73] isokinetics is used for testing to determine not only strength, but also muscle strength balance. Of particular importance in the patient with anterior unidirectional instability is the integrity and function of the external rotators.[74] Analysis of the isokinetic testing data includes bilateral comparison of internal and external rotation strength and also focuses on the external-internal unilateral strength ratio. Recommended ratios for the normal population based on descriptive studies are 66% to 70%.[73,75] External to internal rotation ratios on the higher end of this normal range are desirable because of the benefits of a posterior dominant shoulder and increased external rotation strength relative to the internal rotators.[42,73,74] Alterations of this normal external-internal rotation balance have been reported in patients with impingement and instability, as well as in athletic populations such as elite junior tennis players, and in professional baseball pitchers.[76–79] This alteration is proposed because of the excessive internal rotation strength development inherent with performance of overhead unilaterally dominant movement patterns without concomitant external rotation strength development.[42,80]

Continued emphasis on improving local muscular endurance continues with isokinetic training. Sets with 15 to 20 repetitions are used for both internal and external rotation. Results from recent research have shown an increase in fatigue in the

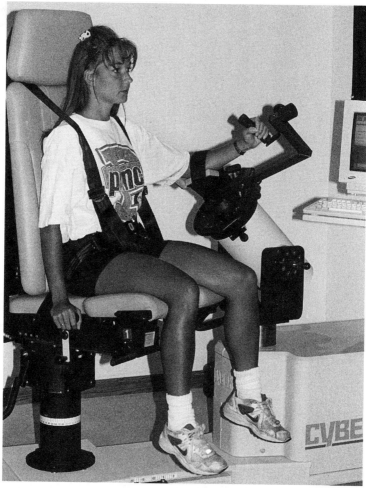

FIGURE 8–13. Modified based testing and training position on the NORM isokinetic dynamometer. (Cybex, Ronkonkoma, New York.)

external rotators as compared to the internal rotators over 20 repetitions in elite junior tennis players.[81] This fatigue, coupled with the common finding of relative external rotation muscular imbalance on the injured extremity, provides the rationale for extensive, endurance-oriented external rotation strengthening.

Further rationale for emphasis on rotational strengthening comes from a training study by Quincy and Davies.[82] They reported an overflow of strength to flexion-extension and abduction-adduction following 6 weeks of internal and external rotation isokinetic training with no overflow of strength when flexion-extension or abduction-adduction training took place. Therefore, training the internal and external rotator musculature produces an overflow of strength to other functional patterns of movement.[82]

Progression from the initial position of rotational training with minimal to moderate (30° to 45°) scapular plane elevation to a position of more function (80° to 90°) is used during isotonic and isokinetic exercises when working with the

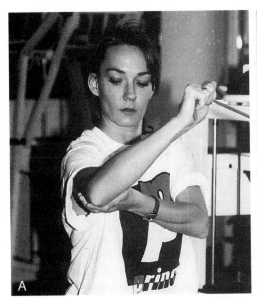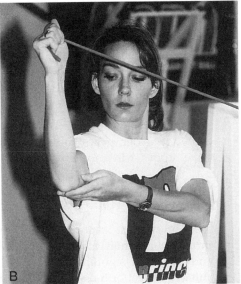

FIGURE 8–14. Ninety degree (90°) abducted external rotation exercise in the scapular plan with Thera-band rubber tubing. *(A)* Start position. *(B)* End position.

hypermobile shoulder in an individual who requires function in this position (Fig. 8–14). This progression in various positions of elevation results from the different effects of the length tension relationship inherent to muscle,[62] and the specificity of function principle described in the shoulder by Basset et al.[21] Use of the scapular plane training position with 80° to 90° of GH joint abduction is recommended because of the inherent osseous congruity, length tension enhancement, and avoidance of subacromial impingement.[41,42,73]

An aspect critical to the complete rehabilitation of the hypermobile shoulder is functional performance evaluation. Placement of the shoulder in loaded positions of shoulder horizontal abduction beyond the coronal plane increases stress to the anterior capsule and can cause increased anterior humeral head translation.[83] For example, overhead throwing or the tennis serve where sequential segmental rotation occurs, if mistimed, will lead to excessive angulation of the GH joint into horizontal abduction, creating anterior shoulder pain.[83] Use of standard video to provide feedback to the patient is important to assist with biomechanical intervention. Referral to appropriate biomechanical authorities of that particular sport or ergonomic activity is also indicated when specialized intervention is required.

CASE STUDY 8–1: REHABILITATION OF THE SHOULDER IN AN ELITE JUNIOR TENNIS PLAYER

PATIENT PROFILE

The patient is a 16-year-old right-handed elite tennis player who has been playing competitive tennis for 7 years. Nationally ranked as a junior, she has recently begun playing professional tournaments. She uses a two-handed backhand and has had the same coach for the past 4 years. Her primary goal is to return to tennis play as quickly as possible to avoid missing additional tournaments and jeopardize her ranking.

PRIMARY COMPLAINT

The patient's primary complaint is anterior shoulder pain with overhead activity. She denies any radiation of symptoms distally or any paresthesias in her distal upper extremity.

EXAMINATION

The patient reports pain that started last week while playing in a professional tennis tournament in Mexico. She played three matches in 2 days and served a significant amount, developing a region of discomfort in the anterior aspect of the shoulder. She denies any previous shoulder injuries other than transient soreness over the past several years, in a global location about the shoulder, which disappeared with rest and ice. She has had no elbow problems or any central spinal disorders.

History

The patient reports that the pain is most pronounced at impact and during the follow-through phase after impact. She denies any change in serving mechanics, racquet type, or string tension. She does report an increased schedule of junior amateur and professional tournaments over the past 3 months. She is able to hit forehands and backhands without any pain but has reproduction of the symptoms with forehand volleys, serves, and overheads. She practices in excess of 4 to 5 hours per day when not competing. She has not played tennis for 48 hours since defaulting her match in Mexico because of a severe elevation of symptoms during play. The pain is only present during, and for several hours following, tennis play. She rates the pain a level (2/10) at rest, and (8/10) with overhead tennis activity. She denies any problems sleeping unless she lies directly on her right shoulder. She has been given oral antiinflammatory medications by her orthopaedic surgeon, which she is taking as prescribed. She has no other medical complications and is not taking any other medications.

Tests and Measures

Observation

The patient stands and is observed from the posterior view to have the dominant right shoulder approximately 1 inch lower than the nondominant left. A mild thoracic scoliosis is noted in the Adam's position. Scapular winging at rest, noted in the right scapulothoracic region, is more pronounced with provocation produced by placing pressure through the hands, with the elbows locked in extension with the shoulders at 90° of flexion, and at waist level with the forearms supinated and elbows flexed. Placement of the hands on the hips shows moderate atrophy in the infraspinous fossa of the right shoulder with no other atrophy noted in the periscapular musculature.

The Kibler Lateral Scapular Slide Test

	Left	Right
Kibler 1 (at rest)	6.0 cm	6.5 cm
Kibler 2 (hands on hips)	7.2 cm	7.8 cm
Kibler 3 (90° abd)	10.2 cm	11.4 cm

Active Range of Motion

	Left	Right
Shoulder flexion	180	178
Shoulder abduction	180	180
Shoulder external rotation	105	125
Shoulder internal rotation	65	25

Manual Muscle Testing

	Left	Right
Shoulder flexion	5/5	5/5
Shoulder abduction	5/5	5/5
Empty can (supraspinatus)	5/5	5−/5
Neutral external rotation	5/5	4+/5
Neutral internal rotation	5/5	5/5
90° Abduction w/ external rotation	5/5	5−/5
90° Abduction w/ internal rotation	5/5	5/5
Elbow flexion	5/5	5/5

Special Tests

Cervical spine clearing tests are negative for shoulder pain provocation. The patient has a positive impingement sign of the right shoulder with Neer's and Hawkins' testing, and a negative cross arm impingement test. A (1+) MDI sulcus sign is present bilaterally, with (2+) anterior humeral head translation on the right shoulder at 45°, 60°, and 90° of GH joint abduction, and (2°) anterior humeral head translation testing on the left shoulder. Posterior humeral head translation is (1°) bilaterally. Labral testing is negative bilaterally. A (+) subluxation relocation test is present only on the right shoulder.

Palpation

Tenderness is present directly over the greater tuberosity and biceps tendon anteriorly, as well as over the infraspinatus just inferior and distal to the posterolateral aspect of the acromion. No tenderness is present over the acromioclavicular joint. Scapular trigger points at the superior angle and along the medial border are mildly tender.

EVALUATION

Evaluation revealed impingement secondary to GH joint instability, with rotator cuff weakness and GH joint internal rotation range of motion loss. These impairments would be classified as pattern E, according to the *Guide to Physical Therapist Practice*.[1]

INTERVENTION

Initial Phase

Treatment during this first phase focuses primarily on decreasing pain and inflammation of the involved structures. Electric stimulation and ultrasound with phonophoresis, with heat and ice were applied to the right shoulder in an attempt to increase local blood flow and to provide an analgesic effect.

Range of motion of the shoulder is performed using physiological movement patterns and gentle stretching to prevent loss of motion. Care is taken not to stress the anterior capsule, which demonstrated excessive laxity on initial exam. External rotation stretching is therefore not used or recommended. The use of accessory mobilization is strictly avoided in an anterior direction because of the patient's hypermobility and instability. The use of posterior glide mobilization is indicated because of the loss of internal rotation range of motion on the dominant arm. Posterior capsular tightness has been shown to accentuate anterior translation and superior migration, and hence, use of the posterior glide mobilization and cross arm adduction soft-tissue stretching are both applied to address the posterior capsule.[57]

The general underlying theme of this phase is to protect the injured structures from stress but not function. The patient is instructed to rest from tennis activity for 2 weeks to allow for healing and optimal application of treatment. The patient is encouraged to use the extremity for ADLs but to avoid exertional, pain-provoking activity.

Movement and gentle resistive exercise to the areas directly surrounding the injured area are of critical importance during initial treatment. In a sidelying position, manual resistance to the ST joint using the movement patterns of protraction-retraction and elevation-depression are initiated to work the musculature that stabilizes the scapula during functional activities. The presence of scapular winging on this patient provides rationale for emphasis on the serratus anterior muscle. Scapular asymmetry documented using the Kibler lateral scapular slide test dictates the inclusion of exercises to address these important muscles.[20] Additional resistive exercise is imparted to the biceps and triceps and distal forearm and wrist musculature. Submaximal isotonics to promote local muscular endurance (three sets of 10 to 15 repetitions) are used for the elbow, forearm, and wrist, providing a strengthening stimulus while not stressing the GH joint. A submaximal manual resistive exercise for the shoulder internal and external rotators is also initiated using a subpain threshold intensity level to begin working the rotator cuff. Again, an extremely low-resistance, and relatively high-repetition format is followed. The upper body ergometer is used to begin working the scapular musculature and to provide range of motion to the GH joint.

Reassessment

After two treatments during 1 week, the patient's pain levels have decreased to 0/10 at rest, and 4/10 with movement. The patient has not played tennis. Pain is no longer reproduced with impingement testing. The patient now has 35° of internal rotation in the dominant shoulder.

Total Arm Strength Phase

As the pain and inflammation decreased in the injured structures, additional rehabilitation commenced with an emphasis on restoring strength and muscular endurance. The use of isotonic exercise using movement patterns eliciting high muscular activity levels in the posterior rotator cuff are applied. The patterns applied are sidelying external rotation, prone extension with external rotation (ER), prone horizontal abduction with ER, and prone ER. These movement patterns have been subjected to EMG research and elicit greater rotator cuff activity relative to the surrounding musculature when compared to other more traditional, home fitness movement patterns.[58–60] These exercises are performed using a low resistance level, 1 to 2 pounds initially, using three sets of 10 to 15 repetitions.

Scapular training continues using rhythmic stabilization in both open and closed kinetic chain situations: seated rowing, shoulder shrugs with retraction, and a closed chain exercise pressing into a Swiss ball while performing clockwise and counter-clockwise circles. The body blade is also used for stabilization. Care is taken to place the GH joint in noncompromising positions during scapular muscle training to prevent aggravation of the primary involved structures.

Eccentric training of the rotator cuff and scapular muscles is initiated at this time by using slow movement cadences in the previously mentioned exercises, as well as through the use of rubber tubing for internal and external rotation. Care is taken to isolate the movement pattern of internal-external rotation. Plyometric upper extremity movement patterns, such as a chest pass with a medicine ball against a plyoback trampoline system are also used.[64] Biceps strengthening is also used with isotonic and rubber tubing resistance because of the stabilizing influence of the long head of the biceps on the GH joint.[46,47]

After 2 weeks of training using the above exercise program, the patient has progressed to using a 3-pound weight with the rotator cuff movement patterns and can tolerate medium (blue Thera-tube) resistance for rotational movements. At this point, she is placed on the Cybex isokinetic dynamometer in the modified base position for internal and external rotation. Training speeds range between 210° and 300° per second using 15 to 20 repetitions to encourage local muscular endurance. After two to three training sessions using four to five sets through the velocity spectrum listed previously, the patient undergoes isokinetic testing.

Reassessment

Isokinetic testing is performed at 90°, 210°, and 300° per second using five maximal concentric repetitions at each speed. Bilateral comparisons (represented as a percentage of the injured side compared to the uninjured side) showed 10% to 15% deficits in external rotation strength, with 20% to 22% greater internal rotation strength on the right dominant arm. External-internal rotation (ER/IR) ratios ranged between 50% to 55% and are well below the desired 66% standard.[73,75,79] Alteration of this ER/IR ratio has been reported in patients with impingement and GH joint instability.[76] The patient now has negative impingement signs and 40° of internal rotation range of motion measured with 90° of abduction.

Continued Treatment

Based on the patient's current signs and symptoms, she has progressed in her therapy program and is allowed to begin groundstroke activity (forehands and backhands) on the tennis court. Groundstroke activity for 20 to 30 minutes is initially followed by the addition of volleys after two to three sessions of groundstrokes if symptoms allow. Interval sport return programs are normally followed on alternate days to allow recovery between sessions. The patient continues formal rehabilitation on a twice per week basis because of the muscular imbalances measured isokinetically, as well as the obvious need for dynamic stabilization resulting from the patient's underlying GH joint laxity. Similar procedures continue as described previously with the addition of internal-external rotation training with the shoulder in 90° of GH joint abduction. Rubber tubing and isokinetic training with 90° of abduction will attempt to prepare the shoulder more specifically for the stresses of overhead activity in tennis and ADLs. More aggressive closed-chain exercises are employed using a BAPS board and Swiss ball, as well as a 6-inch step for serratus anterior strengthening in a modified push-up position.

OUTCOME

This patient returned to professional tennis play and is currently asymptomatic. She was discharged from formal physical therapy with 40° of internal rotation range of motion, and equal external rotation strength measured isokinetically with 90° of abduction. Her ER/IR strength ratios ranged from 60% to 64%. She continued to demonstrate passive (2+) anterior translation at discharge, but had a negative subluxation relocation test on the right shoulder. She was placed on a home maintenance program using the rotator cuff strengthening patterns with rubber tubing and light weights. She underwent a video analysis of her stroke technique prior to discharge. Her stroke mechanics were technically efficient and optimal with the exception of her open stance forehand. A technical flaw on her forehand consisted of premature rotation of the pelvis and trunk that produced a "lagging behind" phenomenon of the shoulder and might have provided greater stress to the anterior structures of the shoulder. Her coach worked on optimizing the segmental rotation of her pelvis, trunk, and upper body to reduce this lagging phenomenon.

CHAPTER SUMMARY

Rehabilitation of the patient with GH joint hypermobility requires several key interventions, with particular emphasis on enhancing dynamic stabilization of the GH joint. Identification of GH joint hypermobility is of critical importance because application of mobilization and extensive range of motion interventions are usually contraindicated, possibly jeopardizing the nonoperative rehabilitation outcome. Knowledge of the specific exercise movement patterns that both protect the static stabilizers and recruit the appropriate dynamic stabilizing musculature is of primary importance. Lastly, the use of methods that improve scapular stabilization and provide strengthening for the entire upper extremity kinetic chain cannot be overlooked or de-emphasized. A balance of both isolated, focused muscular strength and endurance training, as well as the use of patterns that produce cocontraction and stabilization of adjoining segments, forms the basis of the exercise prescription outlined in this chapter.

REFERENCES

1. Guide to Physical Therapist Practice. Part One: Description of patient/client management and Part Two: Preferred practice patterns. Phys Ther 77:1163, 1988.
2. Matsen, FA, et al: Practical Evaluation and Management of the Shoulder. WB Saunders, Philadelphia, 1994.
3. O'Driscoll, SW: A traumatic instability: Pathology and pathogenesis. In Matsen, FA, et al (eds): The Shoulder: A Balance of Mobility and Stability. American Academy of Orthopaedic Surgeons, Rosemont, IL, 1993.
4. Cofield, RK, and Irving, JF: Evaluation and classification of shoulder instability. With special reference to examination under anesthesia. Clin Orthop Rel Res 223:32, 1987.
5. Matsen, FA, et al: Mechanics of glenohumeral joint instability. Clin Sports Med 10(4):783, 1991.
6. Lippitt, SB, et al: Diagnosis and management of AMBRII syndrome. Tech Orthop 6:61, 1991.
7. Maruyama, K, et al: Trauma-instability-voluntarism classification for glenohumeral joint instability. J Shoulder Elbow Surg 4:194, 1995.
8. McFarland, EG, et al: Posterior shoulder laxity in asymptomatic athletes. Am J Sports Med 24(4):468, 1996.
9. Gerber, C: Clinical assessment of instability of the shoulder with special reference to anterior and posterior drawer tests. J Bone Jt Surgery 66-B(4):551, 1984.
10. Hoppenfeld, S: Physical Examination of the Spine and Extremities. Prentice Hall, London, 1976.
11. Harryman, DT, et al: Laxity of the normal glenohumeral joint: In-vivo assessment. J Shoulder Elbow Surg 1:66, 1992.
12. Ellenbecker, TS, et al: Quantification of anterior translation of the humeral head in the throwing shoulder. Am J Sports Med 28:161, 2000.
13. Altchek, DW, et al: Arthroscopic labral debridement: A three year follow-up study. Am J Sports Med 20(6):702, 1992.
14. Lintner, SA, et al: Glenohumeral joint translation in the asymptomatic athlete's shoulder and its relationship to other clinically measurable anthropometric variables. Am J Sports Med 24(6):716, 1996.
15. Hawkins, R, et al: Translation of the glenohumeral joint with the patient under anesthesia. J Shoulder Elbow Surg 5(4):286, 1996.
16. Zarins, B, et al: Shoulder instability: Management of failed reconstructions. Instructional Course Lectures. American Academy of Orthopaedic Surgeons, Rosemont, IL, 1996.
17. Jobe, FW, and Kvitne, PS: Shoulder pain in the overhead or throwing athlete. Orthop Rev 18(9):963, 1989.
18. Speer, KP, et al: An evaluation of the shoulder relocation test. Am J Sports Med 22:177, 1994.
19. Kvitne, KS, et al: Shoulder instability in the overhand or throwing athlete. Clin Sports Med 14(4):917, 1995.
20. Kibler, WB: The role of the scapula in athletic shoulder function. Am J Sports Med 26(2):325, 1998.
21. Bassett, RW, et al: Glenohumeral muscle force and moment mechanics in a position of shoulder instability. J Biomechanics 23:405, 1990.
22. Smith, R, and Brunulli, J: Shoulder kinesthesia after anterior glenohumeral joint dislocation. Phys Ther 69:106, 1989.
23. Voight, ML, et al: The effects of muscle fatigue and the relationship of arm dominance to shoulder proprioception. J Orthop Sports Phys Ther 23:348, 1996.
24. Davies, GJ, and Dickhoff-Hoffman, S: Neuromuscular testing and rehabilitation of the shoulder complex. J Orthop Sports Phys Ther 18:449, 1993.
25. Neer, CS: Impingement lesions. Clin Orthop 173:70, 1983.

26. Nirschl, RP: Shoulder tendonitis. In Pettrone, PP (ed): Upper Extremity Injuries in Athletes. American Academy of Orthopaedic Surgeons Symposium. Mosby, Washington, DC, 1988.
27. Wilk, KE, and Arrigo, C: Current concepts in the rehabilitation of the athletic shoulder. J Orthop Sports Phys Ther 18:365, 1993.
28. O'Brien, SJ, et al: The anatomy and histology of the inferior glenohumeral ligament complex of the shoulder. Am J Sports Med 18:449, 1990.
29. Neer, CS: Anterior acromioplasty for the chronic impingement syndrome in the shoulder. A preliminary report. J Bone Jt Surg 54A:41, 1972.
30. Fukada, H, et al: Pathology and pathogenesis of bursal side rotator cuff tears viewed from en bloc histologic sections. Clin Orthop 254:75, 1990.
31. Nakajima, T, et al: Histologic and biomechanical characteristics of the supraspinatus tendon. Reference to rotator cuff tearing. J Shoulder Elbow Surg 3:79, 1994.
32. Payne, LZ, et al: Arthroscopic treatment of partial rotator cuff tears in young athletes: A preliminary report. Am J Sports Med 25(3):299, 1997.
33. Bratatz, JR, and Gogia, PP: The mechanics of pitching. J Orthop Sports Phys Ther 9:56, 1987.
34. Blackburn, TA: Throwing injuries in the shoulder. In Donatelli, R (ed): Physical Therapy of the Shoulder, Churchill Livingstone, New York, 1987.
35. Bankart, ASB: Recurrent of habitual dislocation of the shoulder joint. Br Med J 2:1132, 1923.
36. Speer, KP, et al: Biomechanical evaluation of the a simulated Bankart Lesion. J Bone Jt Surg 76A(12):1819, 1994.
37. Snyder, SJ, et al: SLAP lesions of the shoulder. Arthroscopy 6:274, 1990.
38. Urban, WP, and Babom, DNM: Management of superior labral anterior to posterior lesions. Oper Tech in Orth 5(3):223, 1995.
39. Cheng, SC, Karzel, RP: Superior labrum anterior posterior lesions of the shoulder: Operative techniques and management. Operative techniques in sports medicine 5(4):249, 1997.
40. O'Brien, SJ, et al: The active compression test: A new and effective test for diagnosing labral tears and acromioclavicular joint abnormalities. Am J Sports Med 26:610, 1998.
41. Saha, AK: Mechanism of shoulder movements and a plea for the recognition of "zero position" of glenohumeral joint. Clin Orthop Rel Res 173:3, 1983.
42. Ellenbecker, TS: Rehabilitation of shoulder and elbow injuries in tennis players. Clin Sports Med 14(l):87, 1995.
43. Kumar, VP, and Baslasubrasmanian, P: The role of atmospheric pressure in stabilizing the shoulder. An experimental study. J Bone Jt Surg 67B:719, 1985.
44. Bigliani, LU, et al: Tensile properties of the inferior glenohumeral ligament. J Orth Res 10(2):187, 1992.
45. Blaiser, RB, et al: Anterior shoulder stability: Contributions of rotator cuff forces and the capsular ligaments in a cadaver model. J Shoulder Elbow Surg 1:140, 1992.
46. Kumar, VP, et al: The role of the long head of the biceps brachii in the stabilization of the head of the humerus. Clin Orthop 244:172, 1989.
47. Itoi E, et al: Stabilizing function of the biceps in stable and unstable shoulders. J Bone Jt Surg 75-B:546, 1993.
48. Pagnani MJ, et al: Effect of the long head of the biceps and superior labral lesions on glenohumeral translation. Trans Orthop Rev Soc 19:649, 1994.
49. Rodosky, MW, et al: The role of the long head of the biceps muscle and superior labrum in anterior stability of the shoulder. Am J Sports Med 22(l):121, 1994.
50. Griffin JE, and Karselis, TC: Physical Agents for Physical Therapists, ed 2. Charles C. Thomas, Springfield, IL, 1987.
51. Jensen, BR, et al: Intramuscular laser-doppler flowmetry in the supraspinatus muscle during isometric contractions. Eur J Appl Physiol 71:373, 1995.
52. Finsterbush, A, and Pogrund, H: The hypermobility syndrome: musculoskeletal complaints in 100 consecutive cases of generalized joint hypermobility. Clin Orthop 168:124, 1982.
53. MaHon, WJ, and Speer, KP: Multidirectional instability: Current concepts. J Shoulder Elbow Surg 4:54, 1995.
54. Ellenbecker, TS, et al: Glenohumeral joint internal and external rotation range of motion in elite junior tennis players. J Orthop Sports Phys Ther 24(6):336, 1996.
55. Ellenbecker, TS, and Davies, GJ: A comparison of three methods of internal rotation range of motion measurement in patients with glenohumeral joint instability and impingement. Unpublished Data, 1997.
56. Mallon, WJ, et al: Use of vertebral levels to measure presumed internal rotation at the shoulder. A radiographic analysis. J Shoulder Elbow Surg 5:299, 1996.
57. Hanyman, DT, et al: Translation of the humeral head on the glenoid with passive glenohumeral motion. J Bone Jt Surg 72-A(9):1334, 1990.
58. Blackburn, TA, et al: EMG analysis of posterior rotator cuff exercises. Athletic Training 25:40, 1990.
59. Ballantyne, BT, et al: Electromyographic activity of selected shoulder muscles in commonly used therapeutic exercises. Phys Ther 73:668, 1993.
60. Townsend, K, et al: Electromyographic analysis of the glenohumeral muscles during a baseball rehabilitation program. Am J Sports Med 19:264, 1991.

61. Malanga, GA, et al: EMG analysis of shoulder positioning in testing and strengthening the supraspinatus. Med Sci Sports Exerc 28(6):661, 1996.
62. Fleck, S, and Kraemer, W: Designing Resistance Training Programs. Human Kinetics, Champaign, IL, 1987.
63. Glousnnn, R, et al: Dynamic electromyographic analysis of the throwing shoulder with glenohumeral joint instability. J Bone Jt Sur 70-A:220, 1988.
64. Cordasco, FA, et al: An electromyographic analysis of the shoulder during a medicine ball rehabilitation program. Am J Sports Med 24(3):386, 1996.
65. Moesley, JB, et al: EMG analysis of the scapular muscles during a shoulder rehabilitation program. Am J Sports Med 20:128, 1992.
66. Inman, VT, et al: Observations on the function of the shoulder joint. J Bone Jt Surg 26:1, 1944.
67. Ellenbecker, TS, and Roetert, EP: A bilateral comparison of upper extremity unilateral closed chain stance stability in elite junior tennis players and professional baseball pitchers. Med Sci Sports Exerc 28(5):S 105, 1996.
68. Ellenbecker, TS, and Mattalino, AJ: Comparison of open and closed kinetic chain upper extremity tests in patients with rotator cuff pathology and glenohumeral joint instability. J Orthop Sports Phys Ther 25(l):84, 1997.
69. Bridgett, PB: The effect of a six week training program using Thera-Band elastic resistance on shoulder internal and external rotator performance and unilateral antagonistic ration. Unpublished Masters Thesis, Kirksville College of Osteopathic Medicine, Phoenix, 1998.
70. Hintermeister, RA, et al: Electromyographic activity and applied load during shoulder rehabilitation exercises using elastic resistance. Am J Sports Med 26(2):210, 1998.
71. Treiber, FA, et al: Effects of Thera-Band and lightweight dumbbell training on shoulder rotation torque and serve performance in college tennis players. Am J Sports Med 26(4):510, 1998.
72. Bleacher, J: The effects of a six week home exercise program using Thera-Band elastic resistance in a diagonal two flexion pattern to train the external rotators of the shoulder. Unpublished Masters Thesis. Kirksville College of Osteopathic Medicine, Phoenix, 1998.
73. Davies, GJ: A Compendium of Isokinetics in Clinical Usage. S&S Publishers, LaCrosse, WI, 1984.
74. Cain, PR, et al: Anterior stability of the glenohumeral joint: A dynamic model. Am J Sports Med 15(2):144, 1987.
75. Ivey, FK, et al: Normal values for isokinetic testing of shoulder strength. Med Sci Sports Exerc 16:127, 1984.
76. Warner, JP, et al: Patterns of flexibility, laxity, and strength in normal shoulders, shoulders with instability and impingement. Am J Sports Med 18:366, 1990.
77. Ellenbecker, TS: Shoulder internal and external rotation strength and range of motion in elite junior tennis players. Isok Exerc Sci 2:1, 1992.
78. Ellenbecker, TS, et al: Concentric versus eccentric isokinetic strengthening of the rotator cuff. Objective data versus functional test. Am J Sports Med 16:64, 1988.
79. Ellenbecker, TS, and Mattalino, AJ: Concentric isokinetic shoulder internal and external rotation strength in professional baseball pitchers. J Orthop Sports Phys Ther 25(5):323, 1997.
80. Rhu, KN, et al: An electromyographic analysis of shoulder function in tennis players. Am J Sports Med 16:481, 1988.
81. Ellenbecker, TS, and Roetert, EP: Isokinetic muscular fatigue testing of shoulder internal and external rotation in elite junior tennis players. J Orthop Sports Phys Ther 29(5):275, 1999.
82. Quincy, R, et al: Isokinetic exercises: the effects of training specificity on shoulder power. Presentation at the NATA National Meeting, June, 2000.
83. In Jobe, FW, et al: The shoulder in sports. In Rockwood CA, and Matsen, FA (eds): The Shoulder, ed 2. WB Saunders, Philadelphia, 1998.

CHAPTER 9

Musculoskeletal Pattern F: Impaired Joint Mobility, Motor Function, Muscle Performance, and Range of Motion Associated with Localized Inflammation

Karen J. Mohr, PT, SCS
Diane R. Moynes Schwab, MS, PT
Brian J. Tovin, MMSc, PT, SCS, ATC, FAAOMPT

INTRODUCTION

According to practice pattern F of the *Guide to Physical Therapist Practice,* localized inflammation in the shoulder includes bursitis, capsulitis, osteoarthritis, synovitis, and tendonitis.[1] Impairments commonly associated with soft-tissue inflammation include impaired joint mobility (including hyper- and hypomobility), motor function, muscle performance, and range of motion. An important issue to remember is that inflammation might alter muscle performance, motor control, and range of motion. Conversely, these impairments might precipitate or perpetuate inflammation. Therefore, when treating patients who present with soft-tissue inflammation in the shoulder, clinicians should understand the relationship between inflammation and impairments that result in loss of function. This relationship between tissue pathology and impairments is reciprocal and often depends on the causes.

Inflammation of soft tissues in the shoulder might result from either macrotrauma or microtrauma. Macrotrauma injuries result from a single episode involving large external forces. Examples of macrotrauma in the shoulder include falling directly on the shoulder or on an outstretched arm, receiving a blow to the shoulder, or dislocating the glenohumeral (GH) joint. Microtrauma injuries, often referred to as *overuse injuries,* occur as a result of repetitive stress to tissues. Repetitive stresses cause microtrauma to the tissue that extends beyond the ability of the tissue to repair itself.[2]

Whereas macrotrauma injuries to the shoulder might result in fractures or dislocations, microtrauma caused by repetitive compressive and tensile stresses usually results in soft-tissue injuries. In cases of macrotrauma, symptomatic management and antiinflammatory treatments are used initially. As the tissues heal, each resulting impairment is addressed. In cases of microtrauma, the clinician must first decide if the microtrauma is solely the result of overuse or if the microtrauma is the result of both overuse and physical impairments. If the microtrauma is only the result of overuse, then activity modification might be the mode of treatment. If the cause of the microtrauma is physical impairments, each impairment must be addressed through treatment intervention.

The most common area in which impairments can lead to microtrauma is the subacromial space. For example, impairments such as a weak rotator cuff, a tight posterior capsule, or poor neuromuscular control can lead to mechanical irritation from the impingement of soft-tissue structures (including the tendons of the rotator cuff, the subacromial bursa, and the joint capsule) between the greater tuberosity and the acromion. The common response to the mechanical irritation or microtrauma is soft-tissue inflammation and/or degeneration.

Stages of connective tissue healing include the inflammatory phase, fibroplasia, and maturation.[3] These stages are discussed briefly in this chapter, and they are discussed in greater detail in Chapter 12. In addition, the stages of chronic inflammation and tissue degeneration are reviewed. Discussion of these topics is followed by a detailed review of impingement syndrome at the shoulder. The review of shoulder impingement includes common mechanisms of soft-tissue injury, the disablement model (relationship between impairments, tissue pathology, and loss of function), methods of examination, and principles and procedures of treatment intervention. At the end of the chapter is a case study illustrating the practice pattern for a patient with inflammation as a result of impingement.

CONNECTIVE TISSUE HEALING

The following review of connective tissue healing has been adapted from Greenfield and Johanson.[4]

Acute and Chronic Inflammation

Following injury to soft tissue, initial vasoconstriction and homeostasis is followed within minutes by local vasodilation and increased capillary pressure. This response is mediated by histamine and prostaglandins, leading to the transudation of fluid. As the endothelial cells in the capillaries separate, larger macromolecules of protein leak into the interstitial space, resulting in a thick, viscous fluid referred to as exudate. Fluid pressure around the free nerve endings in the surrounding tissue results in increased pain, loss of motion, and muscle inhibition.

As inflammation continues, leukocytes such as neutrophils migrate to the injured tissues. The neutrophils initiate degradation of the surrounding tissue through activation of proteolytic enzymes contained within their lysosomes. After a few days, neutrophils are replaced by monocytes, which develop into macrophage cells. Macrophage cells contain proteolytic enzymes, which digest cellular debris and connective tissue fragments.

The inflammatory process typically lasts from 1 day to 2 weeks following injury. Chronic inflammation occurs when the initial inflammatory response does not fully resolve, possibly lasting several months. The cause of chronic inflammation is often attributed to repeated episodes of tissue irritation and microtrauma. Subacromial impingement is an example of a condition that can lead to chronic inflammation if not treated appropriately. As a result of chronic inflammation, the tissue contains a combination of chronic inflammatory cells (lymphocytes, monocytes, and macrophages) as well as fibroblasts and immature collagen. Chronic inflammation typically involves tissue degeneration and cell atrophy. Degenerated tissue is more vulnerable to repetitive stress, possibly resulting in mechanical fatigue or failure.

FIBROPLASIA

In the normal acute inflammatory response, endothelial and fibroblast cells that migrate to the injured area within a few days produce capillary buds and collagen. Possibly lasting up to 6 weeks after the injury, this stage is characterized by the formation of a functional scar. Immature (type III) collagen initially laid down by the fibroblasts is slowly converted to mature collagen (type I) by the formation of strong covalent cross-links between collagen fibrils and fibers. Proteoglycan molecules and water slowly increase the ground substance matrix of the connective tissue, improving the viscoelastic nature of the tissue. *Viscoelasticity,* the normal response of connective tissue to stretch, is characterized by an initial elastic response, and is followed by a plastic deformation. *Creep,* the process describing the plastic deformation of connective tissue, is the ability of connective tissue to stretch with low loads over time. The ability of connective tissue to creep under load improves the strength and ductility of the tissue.

MATURATION

Over the period of a year, the repaired connective tissue slowly regains mechanical strength as the collagen fibers arrange along the lines of normal stress patterns for a given tissue. This alignment restores normal function within the tissue, including normal extensibility and tensile strength necessary for full function.

Summary of Connective Tissue Healing

After soft-tissue injury, stages of connective tissue healing must occur to restore healthy and functional tissue. During rehabilitation, the clinician must understand the time frames of soft-tissue healing and control the stresses and strains during exercise to prevent further injury or delay healing. If repetitive stress continues unabated or impairments are not addressed, chronic inflammation and gradual tissue degeneration might result.

Common shoulder impairments, including altered motor control and altered range of motion, can perpetuate inflammation. Impingement syndrome is a common inflammatory condition of the shoulder that results from different impairments. The

TABLE 9–1 Neer's Stages of Impingement

Stage	Tissue Pathology	Prognosis
I	Rotator cuff edema and hemorrhage	Reversible; treatment with anti-inflammatories and activity modification
II	Fibrosis and tendinitis of rotator cuff or the long head of the biceps	Possibly reversible; treatment with anti-inflammatories, activity modification, range of motion, flexibility, and strengthening
III	Partial or complete tear of the rotator cuff	Usually irreversible; surgery indicated with failed rehabilitation

remainder of this chapter addresses the causes of shoulder impingement and methods for examining and treating the associated impairments.

CLASSIFICATION OF IMPINGEMENT

Classification of impingement is based on the degree of tissue pathology as indicated by Neer's three stages of impingement (Table 9–1).[5] *Stage I* impingement, usually observed in younger patients, consists of reversible rotator cuff edema and hemorrhage. In *Stage II* impingement, fibrosis and tendinitis of the rotator cuff or long head of the biceps usually exists, but this condition might be reversible. In *Stage III* impingement, a partial or complete tear occurs in the rotator cuff. This is usually irreversible.

Although this descriptive classification system might help guide medical management, the implications for rehabilitation are less apparent. Other classification schemes for shoulder impingement are based more on pathomechanics than on tissue pathology.

Primary Impingement

Primary impingement of the shoulder occurs when the superior aspect of the rotator cuff is abraded by the surrounding bony and soft-tissue structures resulting from decreased subacromial space (Fig. 9–1). Encroachment of the rotator cuff can lead to pain and excessive wear. Both static and dynamic factors contribute to this condition.

OUTLET VERSUS NONOUTLET PRIMARY IMPINGEMENT

When Neer[6] originally described his theory of impingement in 1972, his description of rotator cuff impingement was based on findings and observations in an older nonathletic population. He delineated the causes of primary impingement as either *outlet* or *nonoutlet* (Table 9–2). *Outlet impingement* is attributed to mechanical changes in the outlet of the coracoacromial arch, through which the rotator cuff passes. In this condition, impingement of the rotator cuff might be the result of abnormal acromial morphology (abnormal acromial tilt or slope), the coracoacromial ligament, or acromioclavicular joint arthritis.[6–11] A tight posterior capsule, which

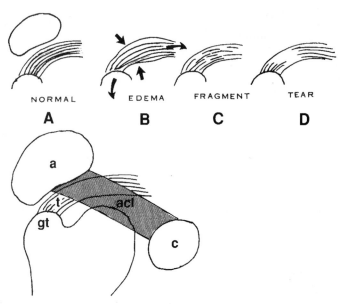

FIGURE 9–1. Impingement of subacromial space. Sequence of tendon degeneration. The large figure depicts the tendon *(t)* attaching to the greater tuberosity *(gt)* of the humeral head. It passes under the acromiocoracoid ligament *(acl)*, which attaches from the coracoid process *(c)* to the acromion *(a)*. The sequence of deterioration goes from *(A)* normal to *(B)* edema as a result of compression forces (straight arrows and traction forces (curved arrows). The edematous stage progresses to *(C)* fragmentation of the collagen fibers until *(D)* some tearing results. Tearing may be partial or total. The straight arrows show the compression occurring between the greater tuberosity and the acromion and the coracoacromial ligament. (From Calliet, R: Shoulder Pain, ed 3. FA Davis, Philadelphia, 1991, p 62, with permission.)

TABLE 9–2 Classification of Impingement

Classification	Location	Type	Causes
		Neer	
1. Outlet	Subacromial space	Primary	1. Abnormal acromial morphology
			2. Coracoacromial ligament
			3. Tight posterior capsule
2. Nonoutlet	Subacromial space	Primary	1. Poor motor control
			2. Rotator cuff weakness
			3. Rotator cuff fatigue
			4. Thickened rotator cuff or bursa
			5. Tight posterior capsule
		Jobe	
1. External	Subacromial space	Primary	1. Abnormal acromial morphology
			2. Coracoacromial ligament
			3. Tight posterior capsule
			4. Impaired motor control
			5. Rotator cuff weakness
			6. Rotator cuff fatigue
			7. Thickened rotator cuff or bursa
			8. Tight posterior capsule
2. Internal	Posterior rim of the labrum	Secondary	1. Glenohumeral instability
			2. Impaired motor control

could force the head of the humerus anteriorly and narrow the subacromial space, might also be a cause of outlet impingement.

Nonoutlet impingement syndrome is defined as rotator cuff pathology resulting from abnormal proximity to an otherwise normal outlet.[6] Proposed causes of nonoutlet impingement include poor motor control (abnormal scapular motion, loss of humeral head depression, loss of the glenohumeral fulcrum), rotator cuff weakness or fatigue, loss of the normal suspensory mechanism of the shoulder, and a thickened rotator cuff or bursa.[7,8,12–14]

INTERNAL AND EXTERNAL IMPINGEMENT

In an alternative classification system, Jobe[15] divides impingement syndrome into two categories based on age and the presence of instability (Table 9–2). *External impingement* consists of bursal-side rotator cuff irritation resulting from decreased space between the rotator cuff and the acromion without the presence of instability (Fig. 9–2). This condition, attributed to static and dynamic factors, is similar to both

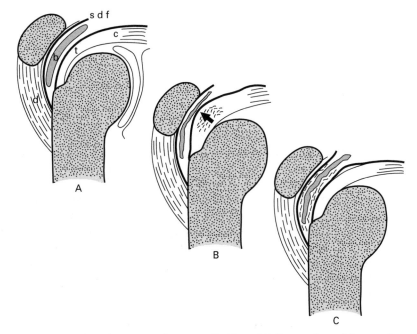

FIGURE 9–2. External impingement. Acute tendinitis and inflammation of the contiguous tissues due to external impingement. *(A)* The tissues contained between the rotator cuff *(c)* and its tendons *(t)*, and the subdeltoid fascia *(sdf)* lining the undersurface of the deltoid muscle *(d)*. The subdeltoid fascia is rich in blood vessels and sympathetic nerves that originate in the stellate ganglia. Between the subdeltoid fascia and the fascia covering the cuff is loose connective tissue within which is located the subdeltoid bursa *(b)*. *(B)* Acute bulging of the tendon compresses and causes inflammation and swelling of the fascial tissues and the bursa. This is the acute mechanical phase during which there is severe pain and mechanical limitation of motion. *(C)* The bulging of the tendon has subsided, but the resultant fascia and bursal inflammation persists, causing stiffness of the shoulder. A can go to B then to C and reverse through the entire phase back to A. The tendon remains frayed, and degenerative changes remain. (From Calliet, R: Shoulder Pain, ed 3. FA Davis, Philadelphia, 1991, p 69, with permission.)

outlet and nonoutlet impingement syndrome as described by Neer. Mechanical changes such as bursitis, tendonitis, and changes in the acromion (spurs, abnormal shape, abnormal slope) are conditions that statically decrease the space available to the rotator cuff. These mechanical changes are similar to the reported causes of Neer's outlet impingement.[5-10]

Muscle weakness or fatigue of the rotator cuff can cause motor control problems around the shoulder girdle such as loss of scapulohumeral muscle synergy. These impairments might also contribute to the loss of subacromial space by allowing the humeral head to migrate superiorly during glenohumeral abduction, thus decreasing the available subacromial space.[6-8] Similar to Neer's nonoutlet classification, external impingement caused by impaired motor control might respond well to traditional rehabilitation.

In Jobe's classification, treatment for external impingement focuses on restoring normal subacromial space. If the causes of external impingement are due to static factors (or outlet problems), rehabilitation might not be highly successful. Clinicians can strengthen the rotator cuff, improve motor control, and stretch the posterior capsule, but little can be done to change the geometry of the subacromial space. In cases in which rehabilitation is unsuccessful for external impingement and instability is not present, an acromioplasty and debridement of the subacromial space might be indicated.

In contrast, *internal impingement* involves a different portion of the rotator cuff than does external impingement (Fig. 9–3).[15] Additionally, internal impingement is caused by instability and is, therefore, classified as secondary impingement.

Secondary Impingement

Impingement syndrome is now recognized as a condition found in both older and younger patients with varying levels of activity.[15] Frequently, in the case of the younger athletic individual with a history of repetitive overhead activity, the impingement is secondary to glenohumeral instability. Jobe[15] describes internal impingement as an impairment that develops secondary to instability. Impingement in these patients results from the undersurface of the posterior rotator cuff compressing against the posterior superior surface of the glenoid and labrum, causing fraying and tearing (Fig. 9–3). In this condition, rotator cuff fatigue prevents adequate control of the humeral head, particularly during overhead movements. This repetitive microtrauma has a cumulative effect on the anterior capsule, leading to increased anterior translation of the humeral head. The end result is instability with secondary impingement of the rotator cuff musculature.

Jobe[15] has also introduced a classification system that groups patients by shoulder impairments and tissue pathologies observed in different age groups (Table 9–3). This classification system describes four different groups and emphasizes the relationship between instability and impingement.

GROUP I

Group I consists of both athletic and nonathletic patients over the age of 35. Two different subgroups exist within Group I as defined by the level of instability. The first subgroup has isolated primary subacromial impingement without any instability,

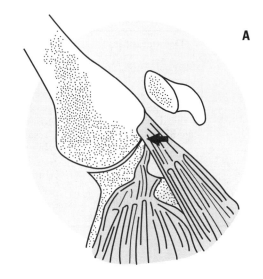

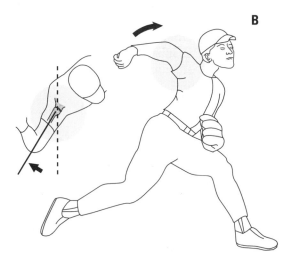

FIGURE 9–3. Internal impingement. *(A)* Schematic. *(B)* Pathologic pitching mechanism from a side view and an overhead view.

possibly also referred to as *classic supraspinatus outlet* or *external rotator cuff impingement* as described previously. The second subgroup consists of those patients with posterior impingement of the undersurface of the rotator cuff or internal impingement with instability.

GROUP II

Group II consists of overhead athletes younger than 35 years of age with impingement of the rotator cuff secondary to subtle instability. The instability is the result of the repetitive nature of an overhead sport and its cumulative effect on the anterior shoulder structures. Patients will usually have positive impingement tests as well as a positive relocation test. Arthroscopic examination of these patients will

TABLE 9–3 Jobe's Impingement-Instability Classification

Group	Demographics	Causes	Tissue Pathology
Ia	Athletes and nonathletes over age 35	Primary outlet or external impingement	Rotator cuff tendonitis
Ib	Athletes and nonathletes under age 35	Internal impingement with instability	Rotator cuff tendonitis
II	Overhead athletes under age 35	Secondary impingement resulting from instability from repetitive overuse	Fraying of the posterior aspect of the rotator cuff
III	Athletes or nonathletes under age 35	General ligamentous laxity	Rotator cuff tendonitis
IV	Athletes or nonathletes under age 35	Single traumatic episode of anterior dislocation	Possible labral tear. No impingement signs

demonstrate intraarticular pathology that is consistent with their physical exams. The undersurface of the rotator cuff will be frayed, and when the arm is placed in a position of 90° of abduction and maximal rotation, the frayed portion of the rotator cuff will impinge on the posterior superior glenoid and labrum. Although arthroscopic examination might reveal some fraying on the posterior aspect of the rotator cuff, the subacromial space usually has a pristine appearance.[16] These findings indicate that the subacromial space is not the source of the symptoms in this group. Because the instability will continue to persist, surgical treatment with an acromioplasty will be unsuccessful.[17]

GROUP III

Patients that are in Group III are also younger than 35 years of age and present with generalized ligamentous laxity during physical examination. Other findings include excessive recurvatum at the elbow and knee and the ability to touch the thumb against the radial forearm.

GROUP IV

Group IV includes patients under the age of 35 who have experienced singular traumatic events resulting in anterior glenohumeral dislocation. These patients might have required manual relocation of the joint or might have experienced spontaneous reduction. In this group of patients, signs of impingement are not typically present.

Successful treatment for patients with impingement secondary to instability must address the instability. Any physical or surgical treatment that only considers the impingement might fail because the cause of the impingement will still persist. Although age alone is not an indicator of the cause of shoulder pain, instability should be suspected and ruled out in patients under 35 years of age presenting with shoulder impingement. This chapter only discusses treatment for primary mechanical impingement of the subacromial space without the presence of instability. See Chapter 8 for treatment for instability.

EXAMINATION

History

An accurate history can help determine whether impingement exists and the possible reasons for it. A thorough history will also guide the physical evaluation and help in treatment selection.

A patient with impingement syndrome might report pain and difficulty with certain movements, particularly with overhead activities. A report of pain located in the subacromial area during overhead sports activity should clue the examiner to assess motor control and instability during the physical examination. Conversely, a patient who presents with pain in the subacromial space during an overhead activity such as painting a ceiling might only need symptomatic management and activity modification. Previous episodes of shoulder pain, previous treatments, and previous medical management with oral or injectable nonsteroidal anti-inflammatory drugs (NSAIDs) needs to be documented.

Observation and Active Range of Motion

Patients should be observed with both shoulders freely visible. Observation during overhead elevation might reveal obvious or subtle alterations in the normal scapulohumeral rhythm on the involved side. Although total range of motion might be relatively undisturbed, a painful arc might be present between approximately 75° and 120° of elevation.

Posture

Because of the interrelationship between impaired posture and impingement syndrome, practice pattern B (impaired posture) is discussed in this chapter. Patients with impingement syndrome often have postural impairments including a forward head posture, internal rotation of the shoulders, and increased thoracic kyphosis (Fig. 9–4). These postural impairments are associated with weakness of the interscapular musculature and tightness of the anterior chest musculature. Observation of joint geometry might reveal the head of the humerus positioned anteriorly in the glenoid fossa. This glenohumeral malalignment can be attributed to either a tight posterior capsule or a hypermobile anterior capsule. These postural impairments decrease the subacromial space and predispose the GH joint to impingement.

Passive Range of Motion

Objective measurements of available passive motion might show some slight restriction at the end range of elevation, internal rotation (above 90° elevation), and horizontal adduction (above 90° elevation). A painful arc might be present between 75° and 120° elevation. The amount of restriction in range of motion will depend on the amount of inflammation, level of pain, and type of impingement. An impingement

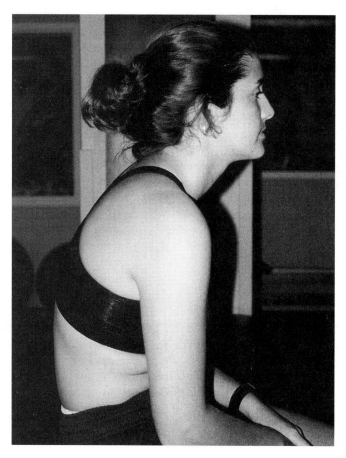

FIGURE 9–4. Forward head posture.

secondary to instability might not demonstrate a restriction in passive range of motion. However, decreased accessory motion in the posterior direction from a tight posterior capsule may be detected. Conversely a patient with an "outlet" impingement will usually present with restricted range of motion resulting from anatomical blockage.

Palpation

Palpation might reveal tenderness in several locations. Anteriorly, the patient might complain of tenderness over the long head of the biceps or the supraspinatus tendon. To facilitate palpation of the long head of the biceps, the shoulder is placed in 15° to 20° of external rotation to expose the bicipital groove. Palpation of the supraspinatus tendon is facilitated by placing the patient's hand behind the back while sitting or standing, and palpating slightly anterior and inferior to the tip of the anterior acromion (Fig. 9–5). To palpate the posterior rotator cuff muscles, the patient is placed prone on elbows with the shoulder in horizontal adduction and external rotation (Fig. 9–6). The examiner palpates inferior to the posterior aspect of the acromion.

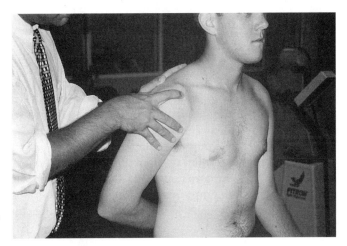

FIGURE 9–5. Palpation of supraspinatus tendon.

Resisted Muscle Testing

Integrity of the rotator cuff is difficult to assess by physical exam alone. Strength testing of the supraspinatus or other rotator cuff muscles is often weak and painful, but this result is not indicative of rotator cuff pathology. Resisted tests of other muscles in the shoulder girdle might reveal weakness, but this apparent weakness might be the result of disuse or pain inhibition rather than musculotendinous pathology. Discomfort might have led to a generalized reduction in activity in the affected extremity and a subsequent disuse weakening of the girdle musculature. Shoulder extensor and adductor muscle groups are usually spared.

Special Tests

The most commonly used clinical tests for impingement have been described by Neer[5] and Hawkins.[18] The Neer impingement sign is performed by passively elevating the affected shoulder while fixing the scapula. This position theoretically

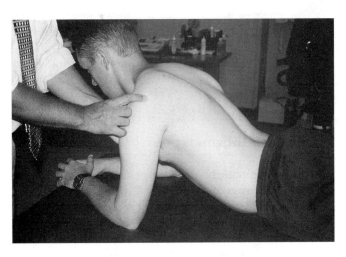

FIGURE 9–6. Palpation of posterior rotator cuff.

compresses the rotator cuff against the coracoacromial arch, causing pain. This test is a relatively nonspecific test and might be positive in conditions other than subacromial impingement.

The Hawkins sign is considered to be a more specific test for subacromial impingement. This test is performed by passively elevating the arm to 90° and then adducting and forcibly internally rotating it against a fixed scapula. If impingement is present, the symptoms will be reproduced with this maneuver. Other tests used to diagnose impingement are presented in Chapter 5.

The injection test might be the most definitive test for mechanical impingement. A positive test involves relief of pain after the injection of lidocaine into the subacromial bursa. Relief of symptoms suggests that pathology within the subacromial space is responsible for the symptoms. Although this test confirms the presence of inflamed tissues, an analgesic injection cannot distinguish the cause of the impingement.

PROGRESSION OF IMPINGEMENT SYNDROME

After the early stages of impingement, mechanical irritation might lead to rotator cuff tendonitis, shoulder bursitis, and inflammation of the capsule itself. In older patients, this process might proceed more quickly. Older patients might also have symptoms of underlying osteoarthritic joint changes in the cervical spine, thoracic spine, or GH joint. Patients with chronic impingement (practice pattern F) might develop adhesive capsulitis (practice pattern D). For this reason, impingement syndrome must be identified and treated as early as possible.

INTERVENTION

After a diagnosis of mechanical impingement and the contributing impairments are identified, intervention can be initiated. Patients who have impingement resulting from bony abnormalities or irreversible soft-tissue thickening might require surgical intervention. However, some of these patients might respond to conservative management. The decision to operate should not be made exclusively according to x-ray findings.

The goals of treatment for primary subacromial impingement are to address any impairment that might be contributing to the functional limitations caused by the impingement. Impairments that can be addressed in rehabilitation include eliminating inflammation, restoring range of motion, restoring scapulohumeral rhythm, increasing strength and endurance of the rotator cuff and scapular musculature, and restoring muscle flexibility.

Eliminating Inflammation

Activity modification is imperative for eliminating inflammation. Rather than implement a program of total rest, the patient should modify or eliminate activities that exacerbate the symptoms. The patient's physician will usually prescribe an NSAID. Additionally, modalities can be used to further decrease pain and inflammation. Phonophoresis and iontophoresis might help manage inflammation. The application of ice following exercise sessions might also help reduce inflammation.

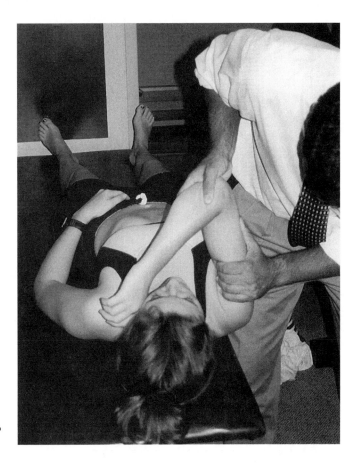

FIGURE 9–7. Stretching to the posterior capsule.

Improving Range of Motion and Joint Mobilization

Some patients with mechanical impingement also present with capsular restrictions that impede full range of motion. A tight posterior capsule can cause impingement by forcing the head of the humerus anteriorly and disrupting normal arthrokinematic motion. If this is the case, capsular stretching must be initiated to restore normal mobility (Fig. 9–7). Joint mobilization for patients with impingement can be instrumental for successful treatment. Clinicians must be careful to avoid exacerbating the inflammation when using manual therapy techniques. Chapter 13 addresses the issues involved when using manual therapy techniques for the shoulder.

Promoting Flexibility

In addition to restoring normal osteokinematic and arthrokinematic motion, muscle imbalances resulting from tightness must be addressed. If joint mobility and muscle flexibility are not addressed prior to strengthening, impingement of the subacromial tissues might continue to persist. Patients with impingement often have tightness of the anterior chest musculature, specifically the pectoralis minor, and weakness of the posterior musculature. Over time, these impairments can cause

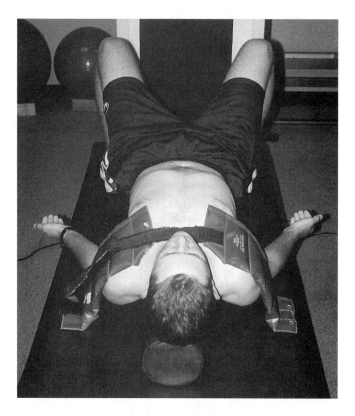

FIGURE 9–8. Static stretch to anterior chest musculature.

rounding of the shoulders. Rounding of the shoulders includes protraction of the scapulae and internal rotation of the humerus. This position of the shoulder girdle creates a narrowing of the subacromial space. Elevation of the arms with the shoulder girdle in this position can result in subacromial impingement. Many stretching exercises exist for stretching the anterior chest musculature, but some stretches cause increased stress to the anterior capsule of the GH joint. Figure 9–8 depicts one method of stretching that avoids stressing the anterior capsule. Restoring joint and soft-tissue mobility around the shoulder girdle facilitates pain-free strengthening for patients with impingement syndrome.

Implementing Exercises

A strengthening program is an important part of treatment, but each exercise should only be performed within a pain-free range of motion. As the pain-free range of motion increases, the arc of exercise is increased. Early exercise should focus on the scapular and rotator cuff muscles to enhance proximal stability of the shoulder girdle. The role of the scapular muscles, including trapezius, levator scapulae, rhomboids, serratus anterior, and pectoralis minor, is to position the scapula for optimal contact between the glenoid fossa and the humerus during arm elevation. If scapulohumeral rhythm is altered, subacromial space can be compromised and impingement might result.

Electromyographic research has been helpful in identifying the most effective exercises for targeting specific muscles.[19,20] Rowing, horizontal shoulder abduction, and shoulder extension in the prone position are excellent exercises for recruiting all portions of the trapezius, levator scapulae, and rhomboids. Elevation in the plane of the scapula, and flexion and scaption are also effective for most of the scapular muscles. However, these exercises are more challenging and should only be performed with controlled range of motion to avoid impingement. Additionally, the shoulder shrug, the press-up, and the push-up with scapular protraction added at the top of the motion (push-up with a plus) should be used for strengthening the serratus anterior, pectoralis minor, levator scapulae, and upper trapezius. These exercises are listed in Chapter 8. Early in the program, the push-up may be done on the knees and forearms. As patients improve, they can progress to push-ups on knees and hands and eventually to a traditional push-up position. During this exercise, care should be taken to prevent the humerus from moving past neutral horizontal abduction to avoid increased stress on the anterior stabilizing structures and subacromial space. Throughout the strengthening program for the scapular muscles, emphasis should be placed on symmetrical scapulohumeral rhythm.

ROTATOR CUFF STRENGTHENING

Rotator cuff strengthening is the cornerstone of the rehabilitation program for patients with impingement syndrome. Strengthening should begin with internal and external rotation exercises with the arm at the side and the elbow flexed to 90°. A towel roll or small pillow can be placed between the upper arm and thorax to keep the shoulder in slight abduction. This position puts the shoulder in a loose packed position with minimal tension on the joint capsule. Additionally, this position has been shown to maximize blood flow to the rotator cuff tendons.[21] A rotator cuff machine or elastic tubing can be used as resistance. If the patient is too weak or experiences pain with resistance, strengthening can be initiated with isometrics and progressed to isotonics. If external rotation is limited or painful, the arc of motion should be adjusted to ensure a pain-free range.

As the patient's symptoms decrease and strength increases, a free-weight program can be initiated with a continuation of scapular and rotator cuff exercises. For internal rotation, the patient is positioned on the involved side with a towel roll or bolster under the lateral chest wall to decrease the joint compression forces. If pain occurs during this exercise, the clinician might consider limiting the amount of external rotation. For external rotation, the patient is positioned on the uninvolved side with a towel roll between the trunk and distal humerus so that the arm is in slight abduction. This exercise is initiated with light weights; 1 pound is not uncommon even for athletes. During a free-weight program, the patient initially performs two sets of ten repetitions and progresses by increasing the number of repetitions as tolerated.

When the patient can perform two sets of twenty repetitions without pain or difficulty, the weight is increased by 1 pound and the number of repetitions is decreased to 10 per set. The patient works back up to two sets of twenty repetitions as strength improves.

SCAPULAR STRENGTHENING

Extension exercises can also be initiated early in the rehabilitation program. These exercises normally are performed with the patient prone. Alternately, these exercises can be done with the patient standing and bending at the waist with support provided by the uninvolved extremity. Patients do not commonly experience pain during these exercises, so they usually can be progressed quickly. The first exercise is done with the patient positioned in prone position with the shoulder off the table, the elbow extended, and the arm perpendicular to the floor. The arm is then lifted to 90° of horizontal abduction. Care is necessary to ensure that the humerus does not extend past the plane of the body, which could place too much stress on the anterior structures. The second exercise is performed from the same starting position. The arm is lifted into extension until the humerus is level with the trunk. Extending the arm beyond the trunk can cause the humeral head to sublux forward in the GH joint. Initially, two sets of ten repetitions of these exercises are performed and progressed as outlined previously. The weight of the arm might be used for resistance initially, with a progression to hand weights once the patient is able to complete two sets of twenty repetitions.

DELTOID STRENGTHENING

Once the scapular and rotator cuff muscles have sufficient strength and endurance, elevation exercises should be incorporated. These exercises are often started with just the weight of the arm as resistance. Additionally, many patients cannot perform the full arc of motion for these exercises and, therefore, begin with a pain-free range of motion. These exercises should be done in front of a mirror for visual feedback in order to prevent abnormal scapulohumeral rhythm.

The first elevation exercise is forward flexion, performed with the patient standing, feet shoulder width apart, elbows extended, and palms facing each other. The arms are lifted forward as far as possible in a pain-free range of motion. A mirror should be used to ensure symmetrical upper extremity movement and that the upper trapezius is not overactive, resulting in shrugging the shoulder. The therapist should observe posteriorly for symmetrical scapulohumeral rhythm while the arms are raised and lowered.

Abduction, the next elevation exercise, should be done in the same position as the previous exercise. The scapulae should be adducted, the elbows extended, and the arms lifted out to the side in a palms down position. The arms should be elevated to a maximum of 90°. If the patient experiences pain, the exercise arc should be modified. The patient should be observed for scapular symmetry, minimal upper trapezius activity, and sufficient horizontal abduction to place the humerus behind the scapular plane throughout the motion.

The final elevation exercise is scaption, or elevation in the scapular plane. This exercise is performed with the patient standing, the elbows extended, and the shoulders internally rotated so that the thumbs point toward the floor. The arms are elevated to 90° in the scapular plane. Because this position can cause impingement if the mechanics are not correct, the patient must have adequate scapulohumeral rhythm. As the shoulder fatigues, the patient might substitute with shoulder shrugging, loss of internal rotation, and elevation beyond 90°. Additionally, the patient might use momentum to throw the arm up to 90° in order to compensate for the loss of upper extremity control. These substitution patterns must be avoided. Scaption is usually the most challenging elevation exercise for a patient, so progress might be slower. Once these exercises can be performed without difficulty, military presses can be added with the hands and arms in front of the trunk.

TRUNK AND THORAX MUSCLE STRENGTHENING

Finally, exercises for pectoralis major and latissimus dorsi can be incorporated into the strengthening program. These exercises should only be attempted after sufficient scapular and rotator cuff muscle strength and endurance has been achieved. The press-up, bench press, and latissimus pull-down are all good exercises to strengthen these muscles.[20]

Although these exercises focus on strengthening within a pain-free range of motion, each patient should also begin endurance exercises early in the program. An arm ergometer can be used with the seat adjusted to prevent the patient from reaching overhead. Initially, the program should have a short duration and intensity and allow for frequent rest. Duration and intensity should be increased regularly as tolerated by the patient. Most patients are able to pedal the ergometer for at least a minute.

FUNCTIONAL EXERCISES

For athletic patients, the final phase of the supervised rehabilitation program should include sport-specific training. This progression should begin with low intensity activity (tossing, easy swing, slow swim, work hardening) and be increased as tolerated. Activity modification might also be needed. For example, swimmers might need to use swim fins to help propel themselves through the water and decrease the amount of stress on the shoulder. Emphasis on good biomechanical form is imperative.

When the patient is pain-free and has full range of motion, strength, and good endurance, a home program should be implemented to include a reasonable number of exercises and instructions for avoiding a reoccurrence of mechanical impingement. The three elevation exercises—flexion, abduction, and scaption—and the rotator cuff exercises with elastic band resistance, as well as one or two exercises for the scapular muscles, should be the foundation for the home program. Patients can do these exercises with minimal equipment and minimal time commitment.

CASE STUDY 9–1

HISTORY

KA is a 19-year-old female college volleyball player who presents with a chief complaint of right shoulder pain with overhead movements, particularly while playing volleyball and lifting weights. She states that she had not experienced shoulder symptoms while playing high school volleyball, but also states that she had never practiced or lifted as many weights as she is doing now. She states that she is unable to perform at a competitive level because of her symptoms. The primary area of her symptoms includes the subacromial region. She denied any numbness, tingling, or upper extremity weakness. She was evaluated by the team orthopaedist. X-rays were negative and a systems review was unremarkable. She was diagnosed with impingement syndrome. KA was placed oral antiinflammatories and referred for physical therapy.

TESTS AND MEASURES

Observation reveals the patient sitting with a forward head posture, including rounded shoulders, internal humeral rotation, scapular protraction, and increased thoracic kyphosis. Although active range of motion does not reveal any restriction, the patient reports pain at the end range of elevation. In addition, excessive upward rotation of the scapula is noted above 120° of elevation. Passive range of motion produces pain when overpressure is applied at the end range of elevation. A restricted posterior glide is noted during accessory testing. Isometric muscle testing reveals weakness with resisted external rotation and weakness with pain during resisted supraspinatus testing. Tightness of the pectoralis minor is noted during flexibility testing. Impingement tests are positive. Palpation reveals tenderness over the tendon of the supraspinatus.

EVALUATION

The history, review of systems, and tests and measures indicate that KA would be classified in practice pattern F: impaired joint mobility, motor function, muscle performance, and range of motion associated with localized inflammation.

DIAGNOSIS

KA demonstrates impaired muscle performance, motor function, and joint mobility resulting in subacromial impingement. These findings suggest a nonoutlet type of impingement, because no physical changes were noted in the subacromial space. Specific goals include restoring normal scapulohumeral rhythm, increasing the endurance of the rotator cuff and scapular stabilizers, stretching the posterior capsule, and stretching the anterior chest musculature.

PROGNOSIS

KA should return to her prior level of activity within 2 to 3 months, provided the impairments are resolved within this time frame.

INTERVENTION

First 2 Weeks

Treatment focuses on management of the inflammation and symptoms using oral antiinflammatories, cryotherapy, ultrasound, iontophoresis, and activity modification. Manual therapy techniques are introduced to stretch the posterior capsule and the anterior chest musculature. Strengthening exercises below 90° of shoulder elevation are included toward the end of the first 2 weeks. Initially, strengthening exercises focus on the rotator cuff and scapular musculature. These exercises include prone exercises for shoulder extension, horizontal abduction, and rowing. Internal and external rotation with the elbow at the side is added in side lying and standing positions.

Weeks 2 to 6

Control of inflammation and flexibility continue during this time period, but the treatment begins to focus on strengthening and endurance exercises. Both free-weights and resistive tubing are used to continue strengthening the rotator cuff and scapular musculature. Eccentric external rotation exercises are introduced, but the patient does not elevate above 90°.

Weeks 6 to 10

The criteria for progression during this time period is normal scapulo-humeral rhythm during elevation, good scapular control as evidenced by the absence of winging, and no symptoms. During this phase of rehabilitation, rotator cuff strengthening is progressed to 90° of abduction, and the patient initiates full-range deltoid strengthening. Fast-twitch, fatigue exercises are also implemented using resistive tubing for patterns that reproduce volleyball movements. As the patient progresses, she performs some volleyball drills with the team, but without forceful overhead movements.

Weeks 10 to 12

Sport specific activities, such as hitting a volleyball, are introduced at this time. The patient continues all strengthening exercises and returns to weight-lifting with the team. By 3 months, the patient has returned to full competitive volleyball.

CHAPTER SUMMARY

When treating a patient with an inflammatory condition, the clinician must identify impairments that might have predisposed the patient to the inflammation. In the case of impingement, many impairments can lead to this condition. The clinician must first decide whether the patient is a suitable candidate for rehabilitation. Patients with outlet impingement might require surgery to restore the subacromial space. Patients with impingement secondary to instability will need a treatment program that focuses on dynamic stability around the shoulder girdle. Early recognition and treatment of the impairments causing inflammatory conditions of the shoulder can prevent further tissue pathology, such as adhesive capsulitis. Treatment should focus on restoring full, pain-free range of motion, scapulohumeral rhythm, and strength of the scapular and rotator cuff muscles.

REFERENCES

1. Guide to Physical Therapist Practice. Part One: Description of patient/client management and Part Two: Preferred practice patterns. Phys Ther 77:1163, 1998.
2. Herring, SA, and Nison, KA: Introduction to overuse injuries. Clin Sports Med 6:225, 1987.
3. Michlovitz, L: Thermal Agents in Rehabilitation, ed 2. FA Davis, Philadelphia, 1990, p 1.
4. Greenfield, BH, and Johanson, M: Evaluation of overuse syndromes. In Donatelli, RA (ed): The Biomechanics of the Foot and Ankle. FA Davis, Philadelphia, 1996, p 191.
5. Neer, CS II: Impingement lesions. Clin Orthop 173:70, 1983.

6. Neer, CS II: Anterior acromioplasty for the chronic impingement syndrome of the shoulder. A preliminary report. J Bone Jt Surg 54A:41, 1972.
7. Bigliani, LU, et al: The morphology of the acromion and its relationship to rotator cuff tears. Orthop Trans 10:228, 1996.
8. Ianotti, JP: Rotator cuff disorders: Evaluation and treatment. American Academy of Orthopaedic Surgeons Monograph Series, 1991.
9. Matsen, FW, and Arntz, CT: Subacromial impingement. In Rockwood, CA, and Matsen, FA (eds): The Shoulder, WB Saunders, Philadelphia, 1990.
10. Morrison, DS, and Bigliani, LU: The clinical significance of variations in acromial morphology. Orthop Trans 11:234, 1987.
11. Zuckerman, JD, et al: The influence of coracoacromial arch anatomy on rotator cuff tears. J Shoulder Elbow Surg 1:4, 1992.
12. Mudge, MK, et al: Rotator cuff tears associated with os acromiale. J Bone Jt Surg 66A:427, 1984.
13. Neer, CS II: Shoulder Reconstruction. WB Saunders, Philadelphia, 1990.
14. Neer, CS II: The relationship between the unfused acromial epiphysis and subacromial impingement lesions. Orthop Trans 7:138, 1983.
15. Jobe, CM, et al: Anterior shoulder instability, impingement, and rotator cuff tear. In Jobe, FW (ed): Operative Techniques in Upper Extremity Sports Injuries. Mosby-Year Book, St. Louis, 1996.
16. Montgomery, WH, and Jobe, FW: Functional outcomes in athletes after modified anterior capsulolabral reconstruction. Am J Sports Med 22(3):352, 1994.
17. Tibone, JE, et al: Shoulder impingement syndrome in athletes treated by an anterior acromioplasty. Clin Orthop 198:134, 1985.
18. Hawkins, RJ, and Hobeika, PE: Physical examination of the shoulder. Orthopedics 6:1270, 1983.
19. Moseley, JB, et al: EMG analysis of the scapular muscles during a shoulder rehabilitation program. Am J Sports Med 20(2):128, 1992.
20. Townsend, H, et al: Electromyographic analysis of the glenohumeral muscles during a baseball rehabilitation program. Am J Sports Med 19(3):381, 1991.
21. Rathbun, JB, and Macnab, I: The microvascular pattern of the rotator cuff. J Bone Jt Surg 52(3):540, 1970.

CHAPTER 10

Referred Pain Syndromes of the Shoulder: An Integration of Musculoskeletal Patterns D and G and Neuromuscular Pattern D

Susan Stralka, PT
Brian J. Tovin, MMSc, PT, SCS, ATC, FAAOMPT

INTRODUCTION

The upper one-quarter of the body includes the cervical and thoracic spines, the shoulder girdle, and the upper extremity (see Chap. 1). The relationship between the soft tissues, muscles, and nerves creates an interdependent system where movement in one joint often results in concurrent movement in other joints. For example, unilateral elevation of the upper extremity results in thoracic side bending and cervical rotation (see Box 1–1). Movements of the upper extremity also require that the brachial plexus and related nerve roots can freely glide in their nerve beds.[1] Because of these structural relationships, injury or altered mechanics in one area might adversely affect other areas.

Postural changes such as forward head posture and rounded shoulders are associated with muscle imbalances around the shoulder girdle. These postural changes might affect normal patterns of movement.[2] Postural impairments and related muscle imbalances have been associated with cervical pathology, neural compression syndromes, entrapment syndromes, and adverse neural tension syndromes. Shoulder pain also might result from nerve involvement referring problems to the shoulder.

Common areas of nerve involvement that can refer symptoms to the shoulder include the cervical nerve roots as they exit the neural foramen, the thoracic outlet, entrapment of the dorsal scapular nerve by the middle scalene, entrapment of the suprascapular nerve in the suprascapular notch, and stretching of the brachial plexus nerve bed.[3–9] Any of these conditions can compromise muscle function and alter normal shoulder mechanics. If left untreated, the progression of impaired motor control can lead to subacromial impingement, glenohumeral (GH) joint instability, or a painful and stiff shoulder.[10] Therefore, the successful treatment of patients with shoulder girdle pain requires a comprehensive understanding of upper quarter structure and function and how specific impairments are associated with specific signs and symptoms.

Patients that are referred with a diagnosis of shoulder pain require an examination of the entire upper one-quarter of the body. The examination should consider all impairments of the shoulder girdle, the cervical and thoracic areas, the entire upper extremity, and related medical conditions that can refer pain to the shoulder. The preferred practice patterns related to this chapter include musculoskeletal practice pattern G, which lists impairments related to spinal disorders, and neuromuscular practice pattern D, which lists impairments related to peripheral nerve injuries.[11] Reflex sympathetic dystrophy, classified under musculoskeletal practice pattern D, is also discussed in this chapter because this condition often involves shoulder symptoms.

An essential element of these practice patterns involves an examination to identify contributing or predisposing conditions to injury, or to rule out secondary sources of pain. For the shoulder, these conditions include, but are not limited to, cervical referred pain, myofascial pain syndromes, thoracic outlet syndrome, peripheral entrapment neuropathies, adverse neural tension, and reflex sympathetic dystrophy. This chapter presents various conditions that refer symptoms to the shoulder or predispose the shoulder to injury. The etiology and progression of each condition, associated impairments, and examination and treatment procedures for each condition are reviewed. A case study is presented at the end of the chapter to illustrate the principles of evaluation and treatment for a patient with thoracic outlet syndrome.

CERVICAL SPINE REFERRED PAIN

The cervical spine and shoulder have an intimate anatomical, biomechanical, and neural relationship. Because symptoms in the C5 to C6 dermatome are often involved with cervical and shoulder symptoms, the clinician must distinguish the source of the symptoms. Injury to the cervical spine can involve structures that refer pain to the shoulder. Pain arising from the cervical spine may be classified as either *neurogenic* or *spondylogenic.*[4] Neurogenic pain is classified as pain that results from direct irritation of the spinal nerves. The signs and symptoms of neurogenic pain include sharp, burning pain that is often accompanied by tingling (paraesthesia) or numbness (anesthesia). The pain can be referred along the nerve distribution and in the related dermatome.

Conversely, *spondylogenic pain,* arising from the vertebral axis caused by mechanical irritation of the various soft tissue structures, ligaments, and facet joints, is described as a diffuse, dull ache. Spondylogenic pain can be either regional (local) or referred to distal sites. By injecting saline into the facet joint, Hirsch[12] produced pain in the back and upper thigh. Mooney and Robertson[13] reproduced anterior thigh pain with lumbar facet injections. Although the pain patterns overlapped considerably and differed in location from the conventional dermatomes, these studies indicated that pain distributions from facet joints were found to approximate that of a segmental plan.

Each spinal segment is innervated by nociceptors that arise from the related spinal nerve of that segment. A full review of spinal neurology is beyond the purview of this chapter, although sources are available for a comprehensive review of spinal neurology.[14] As the mixed spinal nerve emerges from the intervertebral foramina, it immediately branches into the recurrent meningeal (sinuvertebral) nerve, which receives input from the gray rami communicans. This nerve, now a mixture of sensory and sympathetic nerves, returns back through the intervertebral foramina to innervate the dura mater, walls of the blood vessels, periosteum, ligaments, uncovertebral joints, and the outer one-third of the intervertebral discs (annular fibers). In addition, Mooney[13] was able to isolate a sensory nerve from the mixed spinal nerve that innervates the facet joint capsule.

Cervical discs (anterior-lateral portion) can refer pain to the medial border of the ipsilateral scapula.[15] This pattern of interscapular pain is referred to as *Cloward's area*, which maps the areas of symptoms that are observed when cervical disc pathology exists. Herniation of the posterolateral aspect of the disc can also refer pain to the scapula and posterior shoulder region. Specific provocation tests for the cervical spine must be performed during an upper quarter screening to differentiate between the causes of shoulder and cervical pain. Cervical facet joints can also refer symptoms to the shoulder, but the findings from the history and physical examination are different from a patient with disc pathology.[16] These differences are delineated in the following section.

Examination

HISTORY

Typically, cervical disc pathology is associated with an insidious onset or a history of trauma. Patients present with complaints of pain in the cervical spine and possibly referred pain to the scapular area, shoulder, and upper extremity. Pain resulting solely from the disc is usually a dull ache. Maneuvers that suddenly increase intradiscal pressure, such as a Valsalva maneuver, might increase this dull ache. Prolonged positioning of the cervical spine, such as when seated at a low desk or table or seated too far from the table, usually aggravates symptoms. These positions induce craning of the neck, producing a functional forward head position. Conversely, facet joint involvement usually is associated with a sudden onset of trauma, sleeping in the wrong position, or turning the head quickly. The patient usually presents with unilateral pain that might be felt in the neck or the posterior portion of the shoulder, scapula or interscapular regions. Pain is generally not referred to the anterior shoulder or below the elbow. Symptoms of neurogenic pain are absent.

POSTURE

Normal posture might be defined as a state of musculoskeletal equilibrium that supports the supporting musculoskeletal tissue from progressive deformity and injury.[17] Patients with cervical pathology might have postural impairments such as a forward head posture, decreased cervical lordosis, rounded shoulders, scapular protraction, and increased thoracic kyphosis.[9] These impairments might cause a narrowing of the intervertebral disc space and the neural foramen, and excessive loading of the facet joints. Changes in stress within the intervertebral disc and neural arches might result in horizontal intradiscal tears, most commonly seen at the C5 to C6 and C6 to C7 segments. Degeneration of the disc leads to bone reabsorption and the development of osteophytic spurs along the uncovertebral joints and the posterior facet joints.[18] Encroachment of these structures can lead to localized symptoms or referred symptoms to the shoulder. Degeneration of the midcervical spine might produce friction of the nerve roots in the intervertebral foramina, leading to nerve root irritation and neurogenic pain.[3]

RANGE OF MOTION

Although some pain and restricted movement might occur with forward and backward bending, patients with facet involvement will usually have the greatest restriction and symptoms with unilateral movements such as side-bending and rotation. If impingement of the synovial joint capsule exists, a block (sudden restriction) might be noted during active rotation and side-bending to the ipsilateral side. Patients with disc pathology might have equal limitation at the end range of each movement. If the disc is compressing a nerve root, the patient might report referred neurogenic pain to the upper extremity during movements that encroach the nerve root.

RESISTED MUSCLE TESTING

Resisted testing will usually be strong and painless for all muscles of the shoulder girdle, unless nerve root compression exists. If a nerve root or roots are compressed, all the muscles innervated by the nerve might have weakness.

PALPATION

Patients with cervical pathology will typically present with myofascial trigger points in the suboccipital, upper trapezius, levator scapula, paraspinal, and scalene musculature. Decreased intervertebral mobility and tenderness might be detected with posterior-anterior (PA) mobilization. Intervertebral mobility is usually restricted, and pain is elicited with central PA mobilizations in patients with disc involvement (Fig. 10–1). Conversely, unilateral intervertebral restriction and pain is noted in patients with facet involvement (Fig. 10–2).

SPECIAL TESTS

Patients with cervical pathology or facet joint involvement might have a positive quadrant test, which involves positioning the head in combined ipsilateral extension, side-bending, and rotation or flexion, side-bending, and rotation (Fig. 10–3). The extension quadrant compresses the posterior structures, including the facet joints, and places tensile forces on the anterior structures such as the anterior annular fibers of the disc and the anterior longitudinal ligament. If the nerve root is irritated, the extension quadrant reduces the intervertebral foramina on the side of the test, encroaching the

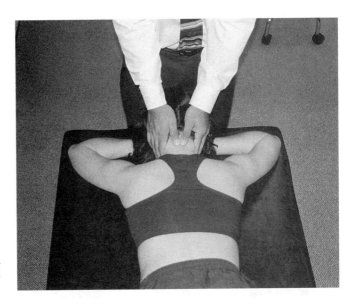

FIGURE 10–1. Central PA mobilization of the cervical spine.

involved nerve root, and reproducing neurogenic pain. The flexion quadrant compresses the anterior structures and places tensile forces on the posterior structures (Fig. 10–4). Patients with cervical pathology might also have a positive upper limb tension test and positive thoracic outlet tests (discussed later in the chapter).

Intervention

Although specific tissue pathology might be detected, physical therapy intervention must address the presenting impairments. Treatment usually involves correcting impaired posture, restoring intervertebral mobility, and improving soft tissue mobility around the cervical and upper thoracic spine. Specific treatments include joint

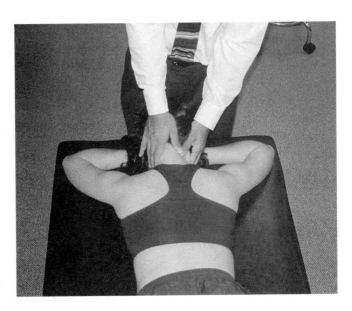

FIGURE 10–2. Unilateral PA mobilization on the right side of the cervical spine.

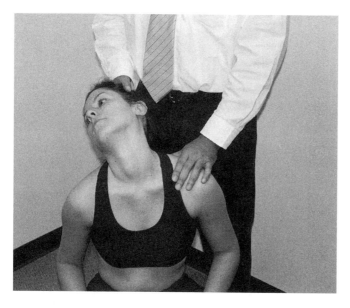

FIGURE 10–3. Extension quadrant.

mobilization or manipulation, mechanical traction, soft tissue mobilization and stretching, neural mobilization (Figs. 10–5 to 10–8) and postural correction.

MYOFASCIAL PAIN SYNDROMES

An upper quarter screening for a patient presenting with shoulder pain must include assessment of the myofascial structures. These structures can refer symptoms to the shoulder, particularly when muscle imbalances exist. Muscle imbalances are usually related to postural impairments, possibly leading to adaptive myofascial

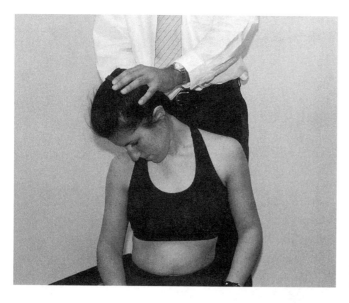

FIGURE 10–4. Flexion quadrant.

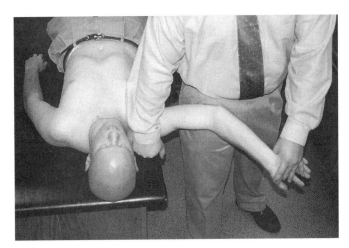

FIGURE 10–5. ULTT 1: Median nerve dominant utilizing shoulder.

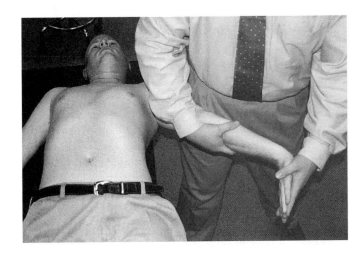

FIGURE 10–6. ULTT 2a: Median nerve dominant utilizing shoulder grade depression and external rotation.

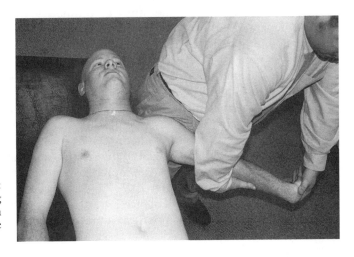

FIGURE 10–7. ULTT 2b: Radial nerve dominant using shoulder girdle depression plus internal rotation of the shoulder.

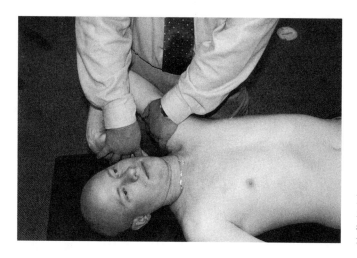

FIGURE 10–8. ULTT 3: Ulnar nerve dominant utilizing shoulder abduction and elbow flexion.

shortening, altered shoulder kinematics, and decreased muscle efficiency, or muscular trigger points.

The impact of muscle imbalances on muscle function has been studied by Janda[19] who observed that postural (musculoskeletal) imbalances produce a chain of muscle reactions. In the presence of a forward head posture and rounded shoulders, excessive scapulae protraction with downward rotation of the inferior angle of the scapula, increased thoracic kyphosis, and internal positioning of the GH joints results. According to speculation by Janda,[19] these postural changes alter the length tension relationship of various muscles around the scapula and GH joint. This posture results in adaptive muscle shortening with loss of extensibility to passive stretch of the subscapularis, teres major, latissimus dorsi, pectoralis major, and minor muscles. Conversely, the rhomboids and lower trapezius, serratus anterior muscle, and the external rotator muscles (teres minor and infraspinatus) become lengthened (over-stretched) and less able to generate tension (weaker). Because the pectoralis minor attaches to the coracoid process of the scapula, the humerus internally rotates in this position, causing shortening of the glenohumeral ligament, subscapularis, and anterior shoulder capsule.

Scapulohumeral rhythm also might be altered with impaired posture because of length-tension changes in the muscle, ultimately affecting muscle performance. Scapulohumeral rhythm is discussed in detail in Chapter 2. A muscle imbalance develops because of tight muscles inhibiting the antagonist. For example, weakness of the lower trapezius and serratus anterior are the result of shortening of both the levator scapulae and upper trapezius. Adaptive shortening of the teres major muscle might lead to inhibition of the rhomboid muscles, whereas shortening of the glenohumeral internal rotators (subscapularis) might inhibit external rotators (teres minor and infraspinatus). Subsequently, weakness of the rotator cuff muscles and axioscapular muscles occurs, altering the force couple of the GH joint and scapulothoracic (ST) joint. (Control of the scapula and humerus are primarily dictated by a series of force couples.[17] A comprehensive explanation of force couples at the shoulder is discussed in Chapter 2.)

Axioscapular muscle imbalances, particularly with weakness of the serratus anterior and lower trapezius muscles, can result in an unstable base of support for the humerus. Inefficient rotator cuff muscle function during humeral elevation impairs the control of the humeral head within the glenoid fossa. In addition, sufficient elevation by the acromion to provide adequate clearance of the greater tuberosity of the humerus might not occur. The end result of these muscle imbalances might be a painful stiff shoulder, primary impingement syndrome at the GH joint, thoracic outlet syndrome (TOS), or myofascial pain syndromes.

Muscular trigger points are commonly observed in patients with muscle imbalances and postural impairments. According to Travell and Simons,[20] a myofascial trigger point is a hyperexcitable tender point within a taut band of a muscle. Upon palpation of an active trigger point, the examiner will elicit a twitch response of the involved muscle. One principle characteristic of trigger points is the referral of symptoms to another part of the body. The pain referral pattern resulting from an active trigger point is consistent for the involved muscle and has been outlined by Travell and Simons[20] in their myofascial trigger point textbook. However, referred pain patterns from active myofascial trigger points do not follow traditional dermatomal patterns. This referral of pain, or even numbness and tingling, makes the source of the problem hard to find.

Examination

HISTORY

The most common complaint associated with trigger points is pain described as a deep ache, a burning sensation, or a numb feeling. Common areas of trigger points for the shoulder girdle include, but are not limited to, the upper trapezius, levator scapula, and rhomboids. The symptoms are usually brought on with prolonged slumped positions such as sitting at a computer. However, an *active trigger point*, by definition, refers pain at rest.[20]

POSTURE

Several postural impairments are associated with myofascial pain syndromes. A forward head posture and rounded shoulders are the most common postural impairments associated with myofascial trigger points. During the examination, these impairments should be manually corrected by the therapist to determine the extent of adaptive myofascial shortening. In older patients who have had these postural impairments for several years, aggressive stretching, mobilization, and a comprehensive home stretching and strengthening program are needed.

RANGE OF MOTION

Patients with myofascial pain might have restricted cervical range of motion, particularly with forward bending and side-bending, because of the hypomobility of the suboccipital, levator scapula, and upper trapezius musculature. Restriction of the anterior chest and internal rotator musculature might limit glenohumeral extension, horizontal abduction, and external rotation. Rounded shoulders and internal rotation of the GH joints might limit end-range elevation.

RESISTED MUSCLE TESTING

Although pain might be elicited with resisted testing of the involved muscles, weakness usually is not associated with myofascial pain syndromes unless the weakness is the result of pain inhibition.

PALPATION

Patients with myofascial pain syndromes usually present with trigger points in the suboccipitals, upper trapezius, levator scapula, and rhomboids. Palpation of these areas can elicit tenderness and referred pain throughout the upper extremity.

SPECIAL TESTS

A thorough assessment of patients with myofascial pain syndromes is necessary to rule out thoracic outlet syndrome and adverse neural tension as possible sources of symptoms. Therefore, TOS tests and upper limb tension tests should be used to assess these conditions.

Intervention

Myofascial pain responds well to manual therapy techniques used in conjunction with flexibility exercises and strengthening exercises to address postural impairments and poor ergonomics. Stretching exercises should focus on the tight anterior chest and suboccipital musculature, whereas strengthening exercises should focus on the weak interscapular and anterior cervical musculature. A common method of stretching active myofascial trigger points is spray and stretch techniques (Fig. 10–9).

THORACIC OUTLET SYNDROME

Several peripheral entrapment neuropathies can present with symptoms in the shoulder girdle.[21] The thoracic outlet, a triangular area through which nerves and blood vessels of the upper extremity leave the cervical spine and thorax, is a common area of entrapment.[4,6,22,23] Because most neurovascular structures that innervate the upper extremity actually enter *in* to this space, some of the literature refers to the thoracic outlet as the thoracic *inlet*. This chapter refers to the symptoms produced by compression of these neurovascular structures as TOS.

Thoracic outlet syndrome involves neurovascular compression of the subclavian artery, subclavian vein, or the brachial plexus.[4] More than 95% of the time, pressure on the nerves of the brachial plexus is the problem. However, occasionally the artery or vein is involved. Compression can be the result of tight muscles, ligaments, or bony abnormalities in the thoracic outlet area of the body, which lies just behind the clavicle.

Three areas of potential compression of the brachial plexus and related blood vessels in the area of the thoracic outlet exist; they are the scalene triangle, the costoclavicular junction, and the subcoracoid area.[4] The brachial plexus and subclavian artery and vein run through the posterior triangle of the neck between the anterior and medial scalene muscles. Conditions involving shortening or tightening of these muscles might result in compression of the nerves and artery, subsequently

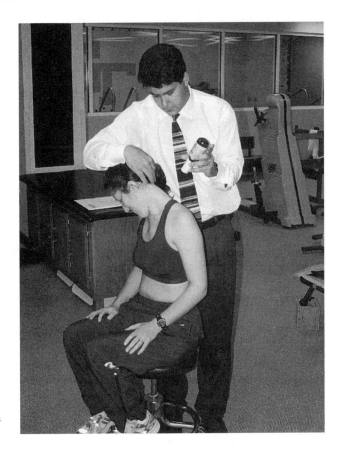

FIGURE 10–9. Spray and stretch to upper trapezius.

causing pain, paraesthesia, or vascular changes in the hand. As the brachial plexus continues its course to the upper extremity, it passes farther distally, between the clavicle and first rib. Finally, the brachial plexus and axillary artery pass underneath the pectoralis minor tendon insertion at the coracoid process. Shortening and tightening of this tendon that occurs with posture changes can result in symptomatic compression neuropathy of the nerves and blood vessels.[23]

Etiology

Entrapment of neurovascular structures can be the result of congenital factors, anatomical factors, or postural impairments. In the past 10 years, adverse neural tension has also been added to the list of causes for TOS. This topic is addressed later in this chapter.

A cervical rib or extended transverse process from the sixth or seventh vertebrae is a congenital anomaly possibly contributing to TOS.[24,25] With cervical rib angulation of the neurovascular bundle, compression might result. With this condition, the inferior portion of the plexus is primarily involved, causing symptoms along the ulnar and median nerve distributions. If the subclavian artery is compressed, symptoms include pain, pallor, coolness, sensitivity to cold, and intermittent claudication.

An anomaly of the first rib is another congenital condition that might compress the lower portion of the brachial plexus. If the rib is unusually broad or angulated, TOS symptoms might be experienced similar to those seen with involvement of a cervical rib.

Many anatomical conditions involving the bone or soft tissues can lead to TOS. Following a fracture, callus formation of the clavicle or first rib can produce neurovascular compression. Hypertrophy or tightness of the anterior and middle scalene, hypomobility of the pectoralis minor, and changes in the costocoracoid ligament might also contribute to the development of TOS. Compression of the neurovascular structures in the thoracic outlet most often occurs in the costoclavicular space.[26] If the arm is elevated with impaired elevation of the clavicle, compression in the underlying neurovascular area might result. Both the brachial plexus and the subclavian artery and vein pass through the space between the clavicle and the first rib. Any deviation in this space can lead to microcirculation problems in the upper extremity.

Impaired posture might be the result of specific lifestyle, body type, or heredity. Common postural impairments associated with TOS include a forward head posture, scapular protraction, and internal rotation of the GH joints. These postural impairments are associated with tight anterior chest musculature (specifically the pectoralis minor) and weak parascapular musculature. The resulting decreased soft tissue mobility in the thoracic outlet can cause compression of the neurovascular bundle.[27] Postural impairments in which the clavicle is maintained in depression can also lead to the compression of these structures under the costoclavicular space. The coracothoracopectoral space is often compressed because of shortening or hypertension of the pectoralis minor. These muscular changes are commonly seen in individuals who lift weights or exhibit impaired posture.

Examination

HISTORY

Patients with TOS usually complain of pain and paresthesia involving the neck, shoulder, forearm, wrist, and hand. Symptoms related to TOS have been documented in 90% of all TOS cases.[28,29] Those symptoms are most often pain, paraesthesia, and paresis of the neck, upper extremity, and hand. Other symptoms include numbness, edema, and muscle weakness. However, symptoms of vascular origin occur in only 5% to 10% of all cases and rarely are the only complaint.[30] The lack of vascular symptoms in a large majority of patients with TOS is significant when considering that many of the clinical tests, such as the Adson's test, the costoclavicular provocative maneuver, or the hyperabduction test, are based on palpating for changes in the radial pulse.

The symptoms typically worsen after activities such as weight lifting or overhead sports. They also might be worse at night. The patient might report a history of overuse or trauma involving the clavicle or first rib.

POSTURE

Patients with TOS usually present with postural impairments, including a forward head and rounded shoulders. Hypertrophy of the anterior chest and cervical musculature, including the pectoralis minor muscle and the anterior and medial scalene muscles, usually accompany this posture. These postural impairments can compromise the space in the scalene triangle, causing compression of the neurovascular structures. For example, the loss of muscle tone and drooping of the shoulders seen in forward head and rounded shoulders can result in depression of the anterior chest wall. The depression of the sternum pulls the anterior thoracic cage downward. This in turn pulls the shoulder girdle down, forward, and close to the chest wall. As a result, the angle between the scaleni muscles is decreased, and the clavicle is pulled closer to the first rib.[31]

RANGE OF MOTION

Because of the increased compression on the neurovascular bundle, end-range shoulder elevation might be limited by pain inhibition in patients with TOS. Active overhead elevation, however, does raise the clavicle. Therefore, patients with compression of the brachial plexus between the clavicle and first rib might experience alleviation of symptoms with overhead elevation. Cervical range of motion might be limited at the end range of rotation to either direction because this movement can narrow the space of the scalene triangle. Scapular retraction might also be restricted because of the soft tissue restriction of the anterior chest musculature.

RESISTED MUSCLE TESTING

Muscle weakness might be detected in patients with TOS if compression of a peripheral nerve causes pathological changes. Some muscles of the shoulder girdle might also test weak in different positions because of pain inhibition.

PALPATION

Tenderness on palpation of the scalene triangle is usually exhibited by patients with TOS. Manual compression in this area might elicit referred symptoms into the upper extremities. Palpation for elevation of the first rib in the scalene triangle is essential (Fig. 10–10). Decreased intervertebral mobility and tenderness might be noted throughout the cervical and thoracic spine.

SPECIAL TESTS

Many provocative tests are used to determine compression of the thoracic outlet. Each of these tests uses different forces to determine if a specific structure is involved. For example, the Adson's maneuver uses compression of the scalenes to determine the effect on the radial pulse, whereas the Allen and Halstead maneuvers use traction of the scalenes. The costoclavicular syndrome test and Roos test are used to determine if narrowing of the costoclavicular space is causing compression of the neurovascular structures. The Wright's maneuver is used to determine if tightness of the pectoralis minor is causing compression of these structures on the first rib or clavicle. The reliability and validity of each of these tests varies depending on which study is referenced. Many studies recognized the problem with the high incidence of false positives and false negatives that occur with these tests.[32] However, a clinician treating a patient with TOS should be less concerned with treating tissue structures and more concerned with resolving the impairments that led to the TOS. Therefore, if TOS is suspected through the history and one or two tests, then performing all these tests might be unnecessary because they will not guide treatment. Treatment focuses on addressing the associated impairments.

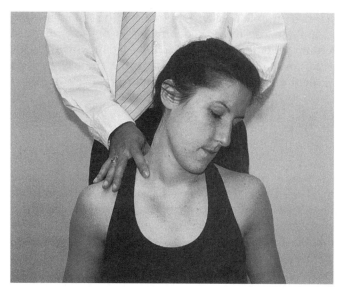

FIGURE 10–10. Palpation of the scalene triangle.

Intervention

After ruling out the cervical and thoracic spine and shoulder area as a source of symptoms, impairments must be identified. Specific treatment involves manual therapy to restore the soft tissue mobility around the anterior chest musculature, emphasizing the pectoralis minor and scalenes (Fig. 10–11). In addition, manual therapy should include joint mobilization of the first rib, sternoclavicular (SC), acromioclavicular (AC), and ST joints. Once soft tissue and joint mobility have been restored and maintained with a home flexibility program, strengthening of the posterior shoulder and interscapular musculature can be initiated. Patient education emphasizing proper posture and sitting ergonomics is also an important part of treatment.

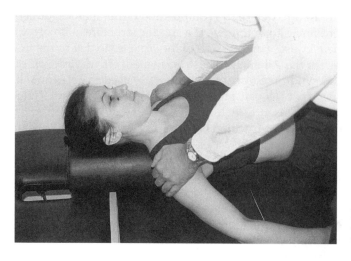

FIGURE 10–11. Stretching of the anterior chest musculature over a foam roll.

OTHER PERIPHERAL ENTRAPMENT NEUROPATHIES

Suprascapular Nerve Entrapment

Suprascapular nerve entrapment (C5 to C6) should be considered for patients with acute shoulder pain and muscle weakness. This nerve, the origin of which is in the C5 or C6 nerve roots, then passes posteriorly through the supraclavicular fossa and the scapular notch to reach the supraspinatus fossa. The transverse scapular ligament holds the nerve within the notch. This area can become stenotic, leading to nerve compression. In addition, if forward head posture and rounded shoulders are present, usually an increase in scapular protraction and downward rotation of the inferior angle of the scapula occurs. This positional change might cause traction in the brachial plexus at the origin of the suprascapular nerve.[21] The suprascapular nerve supplies motor innervation to the supraspinatus and infraspinatus muscles and sensory innervation to the AC joint, and subacromial bursa.

Common causes of suprascapular lesions include fracture of the scapula, acute trauma, overuse, chronic irritation, and ganglion cysts. Sudden scapula motion, such as protraction and abduction, can pull the nerve against the medial wall of the scapula notch or the ligament. The nerve is also stretched with external humeral rotation and shoulder elevation. Individuals working with overhead activities, such as painters, electricians, volleyball players, baseball players, tennis players, and weight lifters are more susceptible to suprascapular nerve pathology.

Any disease process that limits the mobility of the nerve will increase the risk of damage. Various causes of shoulder pain can alter shoulder function and place the suprascapular nerve at risk. Suprascapular neuropathy might be a result of changes in normal scapulohumeral rhythm that occur with conditions such as adhesive capsulitis of the GH joint.

Dorsal Scapular Nerve Entrapment

The dorsal scapular nerve arises from the upper trunk of the brachial plexus, piercing the body of the scalene medius muscle. A forward head position can increase tension in the anterior cervical spine, possibly causing myoligamentous laxity. Hypertrophy and hyperactivity of the medial scalene might result in entrapment of this nerve, causing limited hand and arm movement.[21] Clinical symptoms of dorsal scapular nerve entrapment include scapular pain radiating to the lateral shoulder and arm.

Examination

HISTORY

For patients with peripheral nerve entrapment, symptoms might be experienced in any tissue innervated by that nerve. In the upper quarter, the two nerves discussed above can refer pain to the shoulder if they become entrapped. Neither of these conditions has a specific mechanism of onset. Shoulder pain with suprascapular nerve involvement is usually located along the posterior and lateral aspects of the shoulder and trapezius. Because the suprascapular nerve is a motor nerve, symptoms are experienced as a deep dull ache. If a large traction stress is applied to the nerve, symptoms might radiate into the common wrist extensor group in the forearm.

Symptoms that arise from the dorsal scapular nerve involvement are experienced on the medial border of the scapula on the involved side, with some pain radiating into the lateral aspect of the upper arm and forearm.

POSTURE

Although postural impairments might be observed in patients with peripheral entrapment neuropathies, the most common finding is selective atrophy of the muscles innervated by the entrapped nerve. Patients with suprascapular nerve entrapment might have observable atrophy of the supraspinatus and infraspinatus muscles. These patients might report night pain when in the side-lying position, because this position might increase traction stress on the nerve. A patient with entrapment of the dorsal scapular nerve might have swelling in the supraclavicular region, possibly holding the head in rotation and lateral flexion to the involved side. In addition, atrophy of the rhomboid muscles and scapular winging might be observed.

RANGE OF MOTION

Range of motion for patients with suprascapular nerve entrapment might be limited for any movement that increases the traction stress on the nerve. Movements that might be limited include scapular protraction and elevation. Patients with entrapment of the dorsal scapular nerve might have limited cervical range of motion, particularly for rotation and side-bending away from the involved side.

RESISTED MUSCLE TESTING

Because the suprascapular nerve innervates both the supraspinatus and infraspinatus, patients with injury to this nerve might present with weakness in external rotation and initiating abduction. Patients with injury to the dorsal scapular nerve might have weakness of the rhomboids, often observed as scapular winging.

PALPATION

Tenderness on palpation of the scapular notch is seen in patients with suprascapular nerve entrapment. Conversely, tenderness on palpation of the medial scalene is seen in patients with dorsal scapular nerve entrapment.

SPECIAL TESTS

Patients with suprascapular nerve entrapment might have positive upper limb tension tests (Figs. 10–5 to 10–8). Patients with dorsal scapular nerve entrapment might demonstrate positive results for both thoracic outlet syndrome and upper limb tension tests.

Intervention

Treatment of patients with peripheral neuropathies focuses on the presenting impairments. Resolving postural impairments through flexibility and strengthening exercises, mobilizing restricted joint structures, and neural mobilization are common methods of treatment.

ADVERSE NEURAL TENSION

Unlike peripheral entrapment and compression neuropathies, adverse neural tension is a condition where the nerves are unable to glide freely in the nerve bed.[33] Elvey[34] states that neural tissue can be involved in many upper extremity conditions. The mobility of both the nerve root and peripheral nerve needs to be assessed when determining the source of shoulder symptoms. Decreased mobility of the peripheral nerves could alter the mobility of the GH joint.

Butler[33] has done extensive work examining the mobility of the neuromeningeal tissues in the upper extremity. His work applied some of the concepts of Brieg[35] and Elvey[34] that focused on testing the range of movement of the nerve in the nerve bed and designing treatment strategies based on the results. This approach recognized that all the components of the nerve, including the epineurium, perineurium, and endoneurium, should be considered as potential sources of symptoms because all these structures have sensory and autonomic innervation. Additionally, each structure has to move freely to accommodate changes in position of the upper extremity.[1,33–35] Persistent inflammation or compression leads to the laying down of scar tissue in the intraneural or extraneural space by fibroblasts, inhibiting movement. This hypomobility of the neuromeningeal structures leads to pain.

In the upper limb, three major peripheral nerves, the median, radial, and ulnar nerves, derived from the brachial plexus, are capable of producing shoulder symptoms. The median nerve (lateral and medial cords) has axons from the ventral rami of C5, C6, C7, C8, and T1 spinal nerves. The radial nerve (posterior cord) is comprised of fibers from C6, C7, C8, and T1 with a variable C5 contribution. The ulnar nerve (medial cord) is composed of fibers from the ventral rami of C7, C8, and T1. Various upper limb tension tests have been used to assess the mobility of these peripheral nerves in the upper extremity (Figs. 10–5 to 10–8). These tests are similar to the straight leg raise test of the lower extremity. Because these tests involve end-range passive motion of AC, SC, GH, elbow, wrist, and finger joints, these areas should be cleared prior to examination.

Each nerve has a specific pattern of movement that is used for assessment and treatment.[33] In testing neural tissue, a gentle progressive nerve stretch is used to provoke pain in the upper extremity and to identify the involved nerve. Caution in conjunction with gentle stretching techniques is necessary to prevent overstretching and additional inflammatory reactions. When the mobility of neural structures is impaired, pain and other symptoms are generated through direct stimulation of axons and chemical activity.

Examination

HISTORY

Patients with symptoms related to adverse neural tension can present with a variety of complaints, depending on the specific nerve involved. Typically, symptoms are described as burning, aching, or tingling in the shoulder or upper extremity. The patient might have a history of immobilization resulting from injury or surgery.

POSTURE

No specific postural impairments are associated with patients who have adverse neural tension. A forward head posture might be noted. Also, the patient might seek out positions of the upper extremity that cause the least amount of tension on the nerves. This position is usually scapular protraction, glenohumeral internal rotation and adduction, elbow flexion, forearm pronation, and wrist flexion.

RANGE OF MOTION

Range of motion for patients with adverse neural tension will depend on the level of irritability. In extreme cases, patients might have difficulty moving to the extreme end ranges of shoulder, elbow, and hand motion.

RESISTED MUSCLE TESTING

Resisted testing is usually normal for patients with adverse neural tension. However, if adverse neural tension causes prolonged muscle guarding, disuse atrophy accompanied by muscle weakness might result.

PALPATION

Patients with adverse neural tension might report tenderness on palpation in common entrapment site areas. For example, the ulnar nerve might be tender in the ulnar groove at the elbow, the median nerve might be tender to palpation at the wrist or cubital fossa, and the radial nerve might be tender to palpation in the brachialis region and the dorsum of the forearm.

SPECIAL TESTS

Patients with adverse neural tension will have positive upper limb tension tests (Figs. 10–5 to 10–8).

Intervention

Treatment of patients with adverse neural tension focuses on addressing the impairments. Impaired posture, cervical and thoracic joint/soft tissue hypomobility, and neural hypomobility are common impairments associated with this condition. Therefore, treatment will include joint and soft tissue mobilization of the cervical and thoracic spine, joint mobilization of the shoulder girdle, flexibility exercises for the anterior chest musculature, strengthening of the posterior shoulder and interscapular musculature, and neural mobilization techniques using the upper limb tension test positions. The work of Butler[33] should be consulted for specific neural mobilization techniques.

COMPLEX REGIONAL PAIN SYNDROMES (CRPS)

Complex regional pain syndrome (CRPS), also known as *reflex sympathetic dystrophy* (RSD), *causalgia, Sudeck's atrophy,* or *shoulder-hand syndrome,*[36] is a term used to classify

---

BOX 10–1 Terms Used to Describe Complex Regional Pain Syndrome
- Acute bone atrophy
- Algodystrophy
- Causalgia
- Chronic pain syndrome
- Neurodystrophy
- Osteopenia
- Pain-dysfunction syndrome
- Posttraumatic dystrophy
- Reflex neurovascular dystrophy
- Shoulder/hand syndrome
- Sympathalgia
- Sympathetic overdrive syndrome
- Sympathetic mediated pain syndrome

---

a group of signs and symptoms that might follow injury to bone, soft tissue, or nerve (Box 10–1). The terms *RSD* and *causalgia* were used interchangeably in the literature causing a great deal of confusion.[37] In 1996, the International Association for the Study of Pain (IASP)[36] determined that the terms RSD and causalgia should be replaced by CRPS I and II. CRPS type I is a syndrome that develops after a nonneural noxious event such as a fracture, laceration, or contusion, whereas type II develops after a direct injury to a nerve.[37] This classification of CRPS more accurately represents the signs and symptoms of the disorder. The following terms are used as a name for this condition because each name describes the signs and symptoms.

Complex:	Varied signs and symptoms such as inflammation, autonomic changes in sweating, hair growth, and temperature regulation, motor changes that distinguish this from other pain
Regional:	Wider distribution of symptoms beyond area of original lesion
Pain:	Pain that is disproportionate to the inciting event
Syndrome:	Constellation of signs and symptoms

According to the International Association for the Study of Pain (IASP), the following three components are necessary to meet the criteria for CRPS: (1) sensory abnormalities, including spontaneous burning pain and/or allodynia, (2) vascular and sweating abnormalities, edema and trophic changes in skin, subcutaneous tissue, joint, and bone, and (3) motor abnormalities, including impairment of active/passive function, tremor, and dystonia.[36]

Clinical Course of the Syndrome

CRPS I and II are characterized by a specific sequential progression of symptoms through three stages: hyperemic, ischemic, and atrophic stages. However, no time limits exist for each stage, and a patient might or might not go through all stages.

HYPEREMIC STAGE

The acute (*hyperemic*) stage is characterized by constant burning pain with edema and tenderness, initially localized to the area of injury. Sensory changes, such as allodynia and hyperpathia, in which nonnoxious stimuli elicit pain, are often present. Several researchers have noted that vasomotor instability will cause either increased or decreased temperature changes, without any logical sequence.[38,39] Therefore, the distal part of the extremity might be warm, red, and sweaty or cool, cyanotic, and dry. This stage might last only a week, or might persist for as long as 6 months. Radiographs are often negative, whereas the triple-phase bone scan will show positive results at an earlier date.[40]

ISCHEMIC STAGE

The dystrophic (*ischemic*) stage usually follows the acute stage. This stage includes spreading edema, increased stiffness, and increased muscular wasting. Persistent edema in the hand acts as an internal hand splint that obstructs joint motion, changes the moment arm of joint motion, and decreases tendon gliding. Edema lifts the skin from the joint axis, causing perpendicular orientation of connective tissue. The result is limited longitudinal movement of the skin, further restricting motion.[41] Edema also can lead to compression of nerve endings and tissue anoxia, which increases pain. Because edema fluid is an excellent culture medium for bacteria, persistent edema increases the risk of infection. The protein-rich fluid also contains fibrinogen, which promotes scarring and fibrosis.

During this phase, the pain might radiate from the site of injury, possibly involving the entire extremity. Both hyperpathia and allodynia are usually more pronounced at this stage. The skin might be cool or hot, moist or dry, and cyanotic. Trophic disturbances, such as coarse hair and rigid and brittle nails, are also common findings during this stage. Signs of muscle atrophy become more prominent. Radiographs usually reveal patchy osteoporosis, and the triple-phase bone scan is positive. The patient will usually experience spontaneous pain aggravated by movement. In some cases, movement of the involved limb is accompanied by a tremor.[38,39,42] During this stage, sympathetic blocks might still be effective in reversing the process, although the response to blockage might be short-lived and less pronounced.[38,42]

ATROPHIC STAGE

The third stage (*atrophic*) is characterized by marked trophic changes of the skin and osteopenia that eventually become irreversible. Pain is now less prominent, and the skin becomes glossy and tight. The skin temperature often is lower than normal, with the extremity appearing pale or cyanotic. Muscle atrophy of the hand and forearm is more pronounced. The joints in the hand and wrist become fixed or ankylosed. Both x-ray and bone scan might reveal soft tissue and bony changes. At this stage, the condition might not respond to sympathetic nerve blocks.[38,42]

Examination

HISTORY

CRPS I and II of the shoulder might have a variety of predisposing events including trauma (which might be trivial); inflammatory disorders; immobility of the upper extremity associated with myocardial and cerebral infarction; cervical osteoar-

TABLE 10–1 Causes of Shoulder and Upper Extremity CRPS

Type	Example
TRAUMA	
Accidental injury	1. Sprain, fracture, dislocation of upper extremity including shoulder
	2. Minor cuts or lacerations, contusion
	3. Crushing injury of the upper extremity
	4. Nerve trauma
	5. Brachial plexus injury
Surgical intervention	1. Rotator cuff repair
	2. Nerve decompression
	3. Surgical scar
	4. Injections or irritants
	5. Mastectomy
DISEASES	
Cardiac disorders	Myocardial infarction
Neurological disorders	1. Central vascular accidents
	2. Spinal cord tumors: syringomyelia
	3. Spinal nerve disease: herpes zoster, radiculitis
	4. Carcinoma from the breast, apex of the lung or pelvis
Infections	1. Soft tissue and skin
	2. Periarticular infections
Vascular disease	1. Periarthritis nodules
	2. Diffuse arteritis
	3. Arteriosclerosis
	4. Thrombophlebitis
Musculoskeletal disorders	1. Postural impairments
	2. Myofascial trigger points
Idiopathic disorders	1. Complex regional pain syndrome
	2. Complex mediated pain syndrome

thritis and other degenerative joint diseases; surgery; musculoskeletal strains, sprains, or dislocations; burns; and malignancy (Table 10–1).[38] However, the cause of CRPS is unknown in about 35% of cases. Regardless of the mechanism, most patients will present with similar signs and symptoms, including edema, stiffness, severe burning pain, temperature changes, and trophic changes of the skin in the involved limb.[36] Many patients with CRPS localized at the hand or wrist also have shoulder complaints.[43]

The symptoms might appear immediately or might be delayed by weeks, months, or years. The hallmark sign includes burning pain that is often exceedingly intense and out of proportion to the pain expected from original tissue damage.[39] Although the initial injury might be confined to the shoulder girdle, associated symptoms are commonly seen in the distal region of the involved extremity. In some instances, symptoms occur in the uninvolved side. Although the symptoms vary in intensity, some researchers have noted a similar course of progression.

TESTS AND MEASURES

The diagnosis of CRPS is often made through a clinical examination, based on the symptomology described. Clinical evaluation is critical for determining vasomotor instability, pain out of proportion to the injury, persistent edema, and trophic changes in the involved limb. Diagnostic studies and sympathetic nerve blocks might be used to confirm the diagnosis.[44]

Although radiographs are important early to rule out fractures, triple-phase bone scanning (scintography) is more effective than other tests for detecting early bony changes for patients with CRPS.[45–48] Radiographs might detect patchy demineralization and increased rate of bone turnover if periarticular osteopenia is present.[45] The classic patchy osteopenia on radiographs is seen in approximately 50% of cases. Bone scans can demonstrate local increased bone turnover, believed to reflect increased blood flow from loss of sympathetic vasoconstriction.

A positive response to a sympathetic blockade may also be used to diagnose CRPS.[49] According to Toumey,[49] this response is considered to be the most important diagnostic criterion in the evaluation of CRPS. The results of a positive block would be decreased pain, temperature changes, and the ability to move the limb more comfortably. In more recent literature, blocks have been used to confirm the presence of autonomic hyperactivity.[49]

When the patient with CRPS presents to physical therapy, guarding of the involved upper extremity might be noted (Fig.10–12).[41] Trophic changes of the skin and edema in the hand might also be observed (Fig. 10–13). Range of motion is usually limited in the fingers and wrist because of pain and swelling. If the condition persists, range of motion for the elbow and shoulder might also be limited. Subsequently, the patient might develop adhesive capsulitis. Hypomobility of the cervical and thoracic spine is a common finding for patients with CRPS.[41] Additional findings include positive upper limb tension tests and weakness of the upper extremity muscles secondary to pain inhibition.

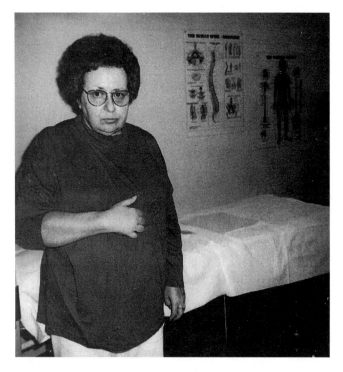

FIGURE 10–12. Muscle guarding of the upper extremity.

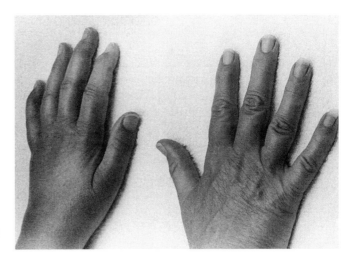

FIGURE 10–13. Trophic changes in the hand.

Intervention

Successful rehabilitation of patients with chronic CRPS I and II requires a knowledgeable team of professionals. For patients with severe involvement, evaluation and treatment by a pain management team of physical therapists, occupational therapists, psychologists, vocational rehabilitation counselors, nutritionists, nurses, physicians, case managers, and social workers might be necessary.

PHYSICAL THERAPY

Successful treatment is predicated on a comprehensive physical therapy program, designed at interrupting the vicious cycle of dysfunction (Fig. 10–14).[41] Prevention and early recognition are the key to successful management of this condition. According to Stralka and Akin,[41] self-imposed or applied immobilization is the benchmark in the development of this syndrome. Early recognition of vasomotor instability, the avoidance of any type of prolonged immobilization, and immediate intervention, can lessen the severity of trophic changes and lead to a more positive outcome.

Any unrecognized and untreated pathology or impairments will result in continuation of the syndrome.[37,39,40,42] Emphasis on only one impairment might temporarily improve symptoms, but the cycle will recur unless all components are treated appropriately.[37,40] Guidelines might be set to develop a treatment protocol including the following:

1. Addressing physical impairments: vasomotor control, pain, edema, joint hypomobility
2. Addressing psychological impairments: stress, depression, anxiety
3. Promoting weight bearing
4. Integrating functional and work-related activities (when possible)

Modalities for Control of Pain and Edema

Because the pathophysiology of CRPS often is associated with hyperactivity of the regional sympathetic nervous system, management focuses on interrupting this

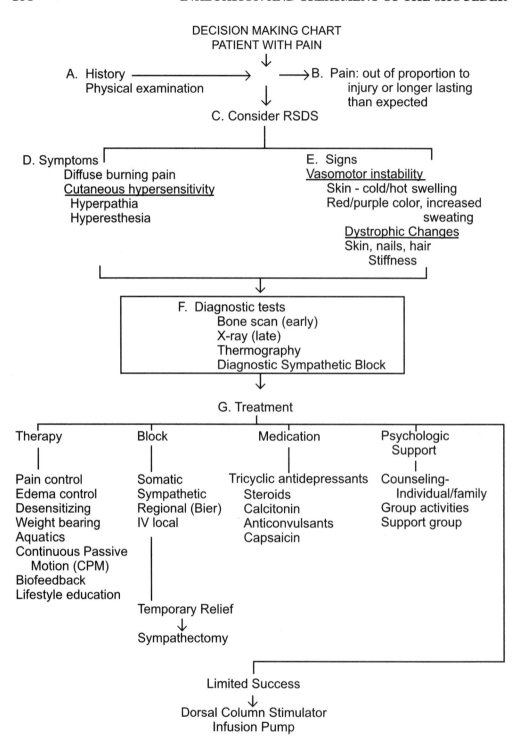

FIGURE 10–14. Decision making chart: patient with pain. (Adapted from Stralka, SW: Reflex sympathetic dystrophy syndrome. Brotzman, SB (ed): Orthopaedic Rehabilitation: A Practical Approach. Mosby Yearbook, St Louis, 1995).

cycle.[39,40] Control of pain and edema with modalities can decrease the hyperactive sympathetic activities and promote movement. Pain control also helps to decrease muscle guarding, allowing for more effective soft tissue mobilization, stretching, joint mobilization, and postural training.[41] Research indicates that transcutaneous electrical neurovascular stimulation (TENS) can be effective in controlling pain for patients with vasomotor instability of the upper extremity.[50–52] High Volt Pulsed Current (HVPC) has been used successfully by this author to decrease both pain and edema in the hand and wrist. The use of a glove and high-volt pulsed current, along with elevation, often is effective in decreasing edema.[41] If joint stiffness is present, ultrasound might be used to increase tissue extensibility.

Range of Motion and Soft Tissue Mobilization

Passive range of motion helps to decrease edema, slow bone demineralization and fibrosis formation, and prevent the development of joint contractures. Continuous passive motion machines can be used, but should not replace active use of the extremity. The individual should be encouraged to use the upper extremity as much as possible. Soft tissue mobilization and elevation of the limb help to decrease arterial hydrostatic pressure, increase lymphatic and venous drainage, and decrease interstitial volume.

Splinting

Static or dynamic splints are worn at night to help decrease joint stiffness and deformity. However, splinting must be fully integrated with an active exercise program throughout the day. Splinting forces should be low enough not to exacerbate the patient's pain or the inflammatory process.

Spinal Mobilization

Some evidence suggests that T4 mobilization can increase skin temperature and decrease pain for patients with CRPS.[53] A recent case study of a 38-year-old woman indicated that after thoracic spinal mobilization was added to treatment, a reduction of dystrophic and allodynic symptoms was noted, accompanied by improved hand functions.[45] Mobilization might be effective because of the physical attachment of the sympathetic nervous system to the somatic nervous system. The anatomical relationship between the sympathetic nervous system and the thoracic spine might indicate that the sympathetic nervous system responds to movement just as the somatic nervous system does.[33] Thus, small-amplitude thoracic joint mobilizations might cause mechanical alteration of the sympathetic trunk.

Slater[54] stated that a direct pathophysiological connection exists so that mechanical alteration might influence physiological functions of the sympathetic nervous system. Spinal mobilization is believed to produce changes in neurophysiologic activity in tissue by activating mechanoreceptors. Improvement in spinal mobility following mobilization might also decrease pain by reducing nociceptor input. Mechanoreceptor discharge is theorized to exert an inhibitory effect on the presynaptic cells of the substantia gelatinosa. In turn, nociceptive activity is depressed.

Local muscle spasm in the thoracic area is common among patients with upper extremity CRPS. Immobilization of the limb and abnormal posturing causes local muscle spasm in the thoracic area. Spinal mobilization might send afferent impulses to the central nervous system to reduce the fusimotor neuron discharge, thus causing muscle relaxation.[55]

Patients with CRPS often have impaired postures of the shoulder girdle because of upper extremity immobilization or guarding. Prolonged upper extremity guarding can result in muscle imbalances around the shoulder girdle. Mobilizing the thoracic spine and preventing guarded movement is another hypothesis for why mobilization might be helpful for patients with CRPS.

Biofeedback and Relaxation Training

Patients are also taught self-management methods to decrease the sympathetic response. Relaxation, either by breathing or visual imagery, can decrease blood pressure, oxygen consumption, heart rate, and ventilation rate. Grunert et al.[56] reported that a combination of biofeedback, relaxation training, and psychological support increased hand temperatures an average of 7° in 20 patients. From this group, 14 of the patients maintained normal temperatures in their limbs a year later. Pain ratings (visual analog scale, 0 to 10) improved from an average of 7.6 before treatment to 4 after treatment. Relaxation techniques that can help patients reduce tension and anxiety also might physiologically decrease the amount of adrenaline released.

PHARMACOLOGICAL INTERVENTION

A variety of medications are used in the management of patients with CRPS.[57] A disturbance of the normal sleep cycle can cause hyperirritability of the musculoskeletal and sympathetic nervous system, which might exacerbate symptoms. Thus, tricyclic antidepressants, which produce a sedative and analgesic effect allowing the individual to sleep, might be helpful. Nonsteroidal anti-inflammatory drugs (NSAIDs) can be effective in reducing pain and inflammation associated with CRPS. Corticosteroids might also help with decreasing pain and inflammation, as well as alleviating or depressing symptoms of redness, tenderness, edema, and loss of function, especially in the hand.

Drugs that prevent further bone demineralization, such as calcitonin (Calcimar) and alendronate (Fosamax), can be used for patients with osteopenia. Often, anticonvulsive medications are used for patients with symptoms of dystonia, such as difficulty in initiated movement or increased tone.[37,38,42] Antianxiety drugs are commonly used to decrease posttraumatic stress symptoms. Transdermal patches of clonidine (Catapres) have been used to control symptoms of hyperpathia, hyperalgesia, or allodynia in patients with CRPS. Other medications such as capsaicin (Zostrix), have been effective in decreasing hypersensitive areas.

McLesky[58] reported moderate improvements in pain, edema, and vasoconstriction after treatment with oral prazosin (Minipress). Other adrenergic blocking agents such as phentolamine (Regitine) have been reported to relieve pain and improve skin temperature.[41,58] Intravenous phentolamine has also been useful in diagnosing and treating CRPS.

NERVE BLOCKS

Sympathetic nerve blocks can be used for diagnostic, prognostic, or therapeutic goals.[38,42] Diagnostic nerve blocks help differentiate the source of the symptoms. Prognostic blocks usually are performed with a local anesthetic substance that allows the patient to feel the effects of the denervation. For therapeutic use, a series of blocks is administered, either peripherally or aimed at the sympathetic nerves, to re-establish a sensitized central pain signal in the neuron. Therapeutic peripheral nerve blocks should be scheduled in conjunction with physical therapy to allow the patient to actively perform exercises such as muscle contraction, tendon gliding, and desensitizing, which have shown improvement in hand circulation. The exercise program after blocking should not elicit pain, especially as the effects of the block diminish.

Sympathetic nerve blocks are used for patients with CRPS to interrupt the abnormal reflex mediated by the dysfunctional sympathetic system.[38,42] Raj[39] noted that sympathetic blockage and physical therapy are the mainstays of current therapeutic management. Most patients respond dramatically to sympathetic blockade, and permanent resolution of symptoms is possible if therapy is instituted before irreversible changes occur.

For CRPS of the upper extremity, stellate ganglion or brachial plexus nerve blocks decrease symptoms in both the head and neck and upper limb. If a stellate ganglion block is not sufficient, selective peripheral nerve blocks can be performed to aid in the diagnosis of complex pain syndromes.[59] A series of peripheral blocks can be performed if success is achieved and the symptoms are decreased. Additional blocks, such as epidural and steroid injections, are indicated for inflammation, especially of the nerve root areas.[59]

PSYCHOLOGICAL INTERVENTION

Evaluation and treatment of any patient with persistent pain must consider psychosocial and behavioral factors that can affect management strategies. In recent years, pain clinics have stressed the importance of controlling psychosocial and behavioral problems along with using comprehensive treatment programs. Psychological intervention should be aimed at developing coping skills for patients with depression, anxiety, or chronic traumatic stress syndrome. Counseling should involve family members and significant others so that the individuals closest to the patient have an understanding of what is expected from the patient and what is expected of them.

Occasionally, rehabilitation must be postponed until some of the psychological disorder is controlled. For example, it might be impossible to effectively treat an individual with posttraumatic stress syndrome in a certain setting because that setting stimulates anxiety. After dealing with the psychological aspect, treatment can be resumed. Continued counseling in the form of support groups might be indicated.

SUPPORT GROUPS

Support groups for patients with CRPS can be an adjunct to physical treatment. The coping skills development group is a time-limited, short-term intensive counseling and education program. Goals of the program are to assist complex pain patients in learning skills to cope better with their pain and health problems.[60] Components of this program include taking control of the pain problem, understanding the purpose and meaning of pain, learning to reduce and manage stress, using the minimum amount of pain medication, understanding how nutrition and pain interact, adopting healthy attitudes about health problems, and using communication skills to help alleviate some of the relationship stresses with significant others.

Initially, patients meet with a health services psychologist to determine the degree of depression, anxiety, and other dysfunction that might interfere with recovery. At this time, a treatment plan also is developed to assist in decreasing depression. Patients should participate in setting realistic and achievable goals and in understanding what they have been experiencing, both physically and emotionally.[60] When a comprehensive pain program is not available, other options should be provided, for example, other health care professionals and patients who work with these patients, clergy support, and on-line communication with the RSD bulletin board.

CRPS Summary

Because both CRPS I and II are ongoing vasomotor instability problems, the patient might be experiencing vasodilation, vasoconstriction, or a combination of both. The therapist treating patients with CRPS should immediately attempt to identify the current vasomotor state, perform baseline skin measurements, and monitor the progress of the skin temperature to ensure clinical effectiveness and an improved functional outcome.[41]

The goal of the treatment program is to interrupt the dysfunctional circle of pain, edema, stiffness, bone loss, and dystonia. This goal is accomplished by addressing the impairments of joint mobility, muscle performance, and endurance. The therapist must remember to empower the patient and to assist with the emotional and psychological aspects of this disorder.

REFERRED PAIN

Although referred pain from visceral structures is not included as part of these practice patterns, an upper quarter examination must include a medical screening of visceral structures to rule out potential sources of shoulder pain.[61] Referred pain, a symptom perceived in a location other than its origin, occurs either segmentally or in a dermatomal distribution specific to the tissue involved. For a comprehensive medical screening examination, see the work of Boissonnault.[61,62]

Cardiac Induced Pain

Angina pectoris, defined as an imbalance of myocardial oxygen supply and demand arising when the available blood supply is inadequate to meet the metabolic requirement of the cardiac muscle, is often noted in the left shoulder, arm, or substernal area.[62] The pain on the inside of the arm is usually in the ulnar distribution. Atypical angina might occur in the face, jaw, teeth, either or both shoulders, and in either or both arms. If shoulder pain is accompanied by the above complaints, the patient should be immediately referred to the physician.

Pulmonary Induced Pain

Shoulder pain associated with pulmonary conditions is usually from overuse of the accessory muscles. Commonly, patients in respiratory distress will use the accessory muscles of respiration (sternocleidomastoid), paraspinal muscles, and the shoulder girdle muscles to breathe. Additionally, respiratory muscle dysfunction might result from weakness secondary to myasthenia gravis, Guillain-Barre syndrome, and other diseases. Referred pain to the shoulder area might occur because of postural abnormalities and overuse of accessory muscles. Examination of the shoulder girdle would rule out shoulder dysfunction versus respiratory problems.

Gastrointestinal System Disease Induced Pain

Pathology of the gastrointestinal system generally leads to low back pain, leg pain or thoracic spine complaints rather than shoulder pain. However, esophageal spasm, a combination of colic and dysphagia of unknown cause, can refer pain to the left shoulder, upper thoracic spine, and anterior rib cage.

Inflammation of the liver and/or the gallbladder are conditions that can present as right shoulder pain and upper quadrant abdominal pain. Gallbladder symptoms develop in the right upper abdominal quadrant or might be referred to the scapula, right shoulder, and anterior chest wall. Pain with pancreatitis often radiates to the lower thoracic area, scapula, and supraspinatus area.

Gastrointestinal pathology refers symptoms to multiple areas, requiring the physical therapist to rule out the musculoskeletal structures as the underlying cause. A thorough history and physical evaluation should raise questions as to the source of the symptoms. A pattern of symptoms that is atypical for a musculoskeletal condition should result in a referral to a physician.

Tumor Induced Pain

Osteogenic sarcoma, which represents 25% of primary malignant tumors, is most commonly found in the metaphysis of long bones such as proximal humerus, lower femur, and upper tibia. Males are twice as likely as females to develop osteosarcoma. The most common clinical finding is pain varying from mild to severe and from intermittent to continuous in the upper humerus and shoulder girdle. Because this tumor is first grade, it might be painful and the pain might increase with shoulder girdle movement because of size.

Chondroblastoma, a rare primary neoplasm of cartilaginous origin, is found in the epiphyseal region of long bones such as the humerus or femur. Clinical symptoms are pain and tenderness of the shoulder area with joint limitations in movement.

CASE STUDY 10–1

EXAMINATION
History

A 35-year-old male weight lifter presents to the physical therapy clinic with a chief complaint of pain and paresthesia radiating from the anterior aspect of the right shoulder to the biceps region and forearm. He states that he has been experiencing these symptoms for 4 weeks, but he is unable to recall any specific incident that led to these symptoms. He reports that he has been an avid weight lifter for 15 years and has never had any problems like this before. He also reports that he has increased his weight training program over the past 3 months in preparation for a competition. The symptoms are aggravated by overhead movements, worsening at the end of the day and when lying in bed with his arms positioned above his head.

Tests and Measures

Physical evaluation reveals numerous postural impairments including a forward head posture, bilateral scapular protraction, bilateral glenohumeral internal rotation, increased thoracic kyphosis, and increased cervical lordosis. Hypertrophy of the upper trapezius, pectoralis, and neck musculature is also noted, resulting in loss of range of motion at the end range of shoulder elevation. Assessment of flexibility reveals tightness in the anterior chest musculature, suboccipital musculature, and biceps. Weakness of the interscapular musculature by one muscle grade is noted with resisted muscle testing.

Range of motion for the cervical spine is limited by 25% for forward bending and left rotation, and limited by 50% in right rotation. The patient reports paresthesia at the end range of right rotation. Decreased intervertebral mobility is noted with unilateral PA pressures applied to the right side of the C5 to T1 spinal segments. Generalized hypomobility is noted when central PA pressures are applied to the mid-thoracic spine.

Upper limb tension testing with a median nerve bias (see Fig. 11–6) on the right side reproduces the patient's symptoms. The patient is able to extend the elbow to 45° before the symptoms are elicited. Any attempt to side-bend the head to the left in this position is met by heavy guarding and increased symptoms. Similar testing on the left side elicits minor symptoms in the cubital fossa, but the clinician is able to extend the patient's elbow to 5° of flexion. Wright's maneuver and the Adson test are both positive.

EVALUATION

The history and tests and measures indicate that this patient has referred symptoms related to spinal impairments and thoracic outlet syndrome. Therefore, this patient is classified into musculoskeletal practice pattern G and neuromuscular practice pattern D, according to the *Guide to Physical Therapist Practice*. Musculoskeletal practice pattern G describes impaired joint mobility, motor function, muscle performance, and range of motion resulting from spinal disorders; whereas neuromuscular practice pattern D describes impaired motor function and sensory integrity associated with peripheral nerve injury.

DIAGNOSIS

This patient presents with impaired posture, joint mobility, range of motion, and motor control associated with thoracic outlet syndrome and adverse neural tension. These symptoms most likely developed as a result of increased intensity of weight training. The increased intensity probably led to increased muscle hypertrophy and impingement of the neurovascular structures around the thoracic outlet. Goals for this patient include increasing flexibility of the anterior chest and cervical musculature, increasing joint mobility of the cervical and thoracic spine and shoulder girdle, increasing neural mobility, and increasing strength of interscapular musculature.

INTERVENTION

Initial treatment sessions consist of flexibility exercises for the anterior chest and scalene musculature, mobilization to the cervical and thoracic spine, mobilization of the first rib, and soft tissue mobilization of the scalenes and surrounding musculature. In addition, the patient is placed on a home exercise program emphasizing flexibility exercises for the anterior chest and cervical musculature. The goal of this program is to provide enough soft tissue and joint mobility to allow this patient to move into scapular retraction without discomfort. This phase of the treatment continues for five sessions.

Neural mobilization is added to the treatment program on the fifth visit to enhance the mobility of the brachial plexus and peripheral nerves. Strengthening of the interscapular and parascapular muscles is also initiated at this time, emphasizing the rhomboids, middle trapezius, and lower trapezius. After 3 weeks of treatment, the patient reports that he only experiences symptoms when lying supine with his hands clasped behind his head. This position is used as a stretch, with the therapist pulling the elbows back into extension using hold-relax techniques. The patient is educated in proper lifting techniques and is discharged at the end of 4 weeks.

CHAPTER SUMMARY

This chapter reviews the practice patterns that include conditions that can be indirect sources of shoulder pain. Although specific tissue pathologies are presented, most of these conditions have common impairments that include muscle imbalances, impaired posture, and impaired muscle performance. Successful treatment is accomplished by addressing these impairments through flexibility exercises, joint and soft tissue mobilization, postural retraining, and strengthening exercises.

REFERENCES

1. Sunderland, S: Nerves and Nerve Injuries, ed 2. Churchill Livingstone, Edinburgh, 1978.
2. Grimsby, O, and Gray, JC: Interrelationship of the spine to the shoulder. In Donatelli, R (ed): Physical Therapy of the Shoulder, ed 3. Churchill Livingstone, New York, 1997.
3. Sunderland, S, Koppel, HP, and Thompson, WAL: Peripheral Entrapment Neuropathies, ed 2. Robert E. Krieger, New York, 1976.
4. Overton, LM: The causes of pain in the upper extremities: A differential diagnosis study. Clin Orthop 51:27, 1967.
5. Kellgren, J: Observations of referred pain arising from muscle. Clin Sci 3:175, 1938.
6. Ridell, DH: Thoracic outlet syndrome: Thoracic and vascular aspects. Clin Orthop 51:53, 1967.
7. Campbell, SM: Referred shoulder pain: An elusive diagnosis. Postgrad Med 73:193, 1983.
8. Leland, JS: Visceral aspects of shoulder pain. Bull Hosp J Dis 14:71, 1953.
9. Hawkins, RJ, et al: Cervical spine and shoulder pain. Clin Orthop Rel Res 258:142, 1990.
10. Wells, P: Cervical dysfunction and shoulder problems. Physiotherapy 68:66, 1982.
11. Guide to Physical Therapist Practice. American Physical Therapy Association, Alexandria, VA, 1998.
12. Hisrch, D, et al: The anatomical basis for low back pain. Acta Orthop Scand 33:1, 1963.

13. Mooney, R, and Robertson, J: The facet syndrome. Clin Orthop Rel Res 115:149, 1976.
14. Kiernan, JA: Barr's, The Human Nervous System, ed 7. Lippincott-Raven, Philadelphia, 1998.
15. Cloward, RB: Cervical discography: A contribution to the etiology and mechanisms of neck, shoulder, and arm pain. Ann Surg 150:1052, 1959.
16. Bogduk, N, and Mauland, A: The cervical zygapophyseal joint as a source of neck pain. Spine 13:610, 1988.
17. Norkin, CC, and Levangie, PK: Joint Structure and Function: A Comprehensive Analysis. FA Davis, Philadelphia, 1983.
18. Yong-Hing, K, and Kirkaldy-Willis, WH: The pathophysiology of degenerative disease of the lumbar spine. Orthop Clinics North Am 14:491, 1983.
19. Janda, V: Muscles, central nervous system regulation and back problems. In Korr, IM (ed): The Neurobiologic Mechanisms in Manipulative Therapy. Plennum Pub. New York, 1978.
20. Travell, JH, and Simons, DG: Myofascial Pain and Dysfunctions: Trigger Point Manual. Williams & Wilkins, Baltimore, 1983.
21. Koppell, HP, and Thompson WAL: Peripheral Entrapment Neuropathies, ed. 2. R E, Kreiger, New York, 1976.
22. Karas, S: Thoracic outlet syndrome. Clin Sports Med 9:297, 1990.
23. Roos, DB: New concepts of thoracic outlet syndrome that explain etiology, symptoms, diagnosis, and treatment. Vasc Surg 13:313, 1979.
24. Coote, H: Pressure on the axillary vessels and nerve by an exostosis from a cervical rib interference with the circulation of the arm. Removal of the rib and exostosis recovery. Med Times Gaz 11:108, 1861.
25. Roos, B: Congenital anomalies associated with thoracic outlet syndrome. Am J Surg 132:771, 1975.
26. Pecina, MM, et al: Tunnel Syndromes. CRC Press, Boca Raton, 1991.
27. Edgelow, PI: Neurovascular consequences of cumulative trauma disorders affecting the thoracic outlet: a patient-centered treatment approach. In Donatelli, R (ed): Physical Therapy of the Shoulder, ed 3. Churchill Livingstone, New York, 1997.
28. McGough, EC, et al: Management of thoracic outlet syndrome. J Thorac Cardiovasc Surg 77:169, 1979.
29. Roos, DB: The place for scalenectomy and first-rib resection in thoracic outlet syndromes. Surg 92:1077, 1982.
30. Pisko-Dubienski, ZA, and Hollingsworth, J: Clinical application of Doppler ultrasonography in thoracic outlet syndrome. Can J Surg 21:145, 1978.
31. Greenfield, BH: Upper Quarter Evaluation: Structural Relationships and Interdependence. In Donatelli RA, and Wooden, M (eds): Orhtopaedic Physcial Therapy. Churchill Livingston, New York, 1989.
32. Winkel, D, et al: Diagnosis and treatment of the upper extremity: Thoracic outlet syndrome. Aspen Publishers, Gaithersburg, MD, 1997.
33. Butler, DS: Mobilization of the Nervous System. Churchill Livingstone, Melbourne, 1993.
34. Elvey, RL: The investigation of arm pain. In Grieve, GP (ed): Modern Manual Therapy and the Vertebral Column. Churchill Livingstone, Edinburgh, 1986.
35. Brieg, A: Adverse Mechanical Tension in the Nervous System. John Wiley & Sons, New York, 1978.
36. Merskey, H, and Bogduk, N: Classification of Chronic Pain: Descriptions of Chronic Pain Syndromes, ed 2. IASP Press, Seattle, 1994.
37. Boas, RA: Symptoms, signs and differential diagnoses. In Janig, WS, and Stanton-Hicks, M (eds): Reflex Sympathetic Dystrophy: A Reappraisal. IASP Press, Seattle, 1996.
38. Janig, WS: The sympathetic nervous system in pain. In Stanton-Hicks, M (ed): Physiology and Pathology. Kluwer Academic Publishers, Boston, 1990.
39. Raj, PP: Multidisciplinary management of reflex sympathetic dystrophy. In Stanton-Hicks, M (ed): Current Management of Pain, Kluwer Academic Press, Boston, 1990.
40. Raj, PP: Taxonomy of pain syndromes. In Raj, PP (ed): A Comprehensive Review of Pain Medicine. Mosby, St. Louis, 1996.
41. Stralka, SW, and Akin, K: Reflex sympathetic dystrophy. In Brotzman, SB (ed): Orthopaedic Rehabilitation: A Practical Approach. Mosby, St. Louis, 1995.
42. Raj, PP: Reflex sympathetic dystrophy. In Raj, PP (ed): A Comprehensive Review of Pain Medicine. Mosby, St. Louis, 1996.
43. Steimbrocker, O, and Friedman, H: The shoulder: Reflex sympathetic dystrophy of the upper extremity. Ann Int Med 29:22, 1948.
44. Baron, R, et al: Clinical characteristics of patients with complex regional pain syndrome in Germany with special emphasis on vasomotor function: Reflex sympathetic dystrophy–A reappraisal. In Janig, W, and Stanton-Hicks, M (eds): Progress in Pain Presentation, IASP Press, Seattle, 1996.
45. Genant, HK, et al: The reflex sympathetic dystrophy syndrome. Radiology 117, 1975.
46. Greyson, ND, and Tepperman, PS: Three-phase bone studies in hemiplegia with Reflex SD and the effect of disuse. J Nucl Med 25:425, 1984.
47. Kozin, F, et al: Bone scintography in reflex sympathetic dystrophy syndrome. Radiology, 138:437, 1981.
48. MacKinnon, SE, and Holder, E: The use of three-phase bone scan in the progression of RSDS. J Hand Surg 9A(4):556, 1984.
49. Toumey, PF: Reflex sympathetic dystrophy and surgery. Gynecol and Obstet 100:97, 1955.

50. Finney, J, et al: Low frequency transcutaneous nerve stimulation in reflex sympathetic dystrophy. J Neurol Orthop Med Surg 12:270, 1991.
51. Omer, G: Symposium on pain evaluation and treatment of painful upper extremity. Gen Hand Surg 9B:20, 1984.
52. Kaada, B. Vasodilatation induced by TENS in peripheral ischemia (Raynaud phenomenon and diabetic neuropathy). Eur Heart J 3:303, 1982.
53. Menck, J, et al: Mobilization of the thoracic spine. Management of a patient with CRPS in the upper extremity. A case report. Poster presentation at the APTA Combined Sections Meeting. Seattle, WA, 1999.
54. Slater, H, et al: Sympathetic slump: The effects of a novel manual therapy technique on peripheral sympathetic nervous system function. J of Man and Manip Ther 1;2(4):156, 1994.
55. Maitland, GD: Vertebral Manipulation, ed 4. Butterworth, London, 1997.
56. Grunert, BK, et al: Thermal self-regulation for pain control in reflex sympathetic dystrophy syndrome. J Hand Surg 15A:615, 1990.
57. Hooshmand, H: Chronic Pain: Reflex Sympathetic Dystrophy Prevention and Management. CRC Press, Boca Raton, 1993.
58. McLeskey, CH: Use of cold-stress test and intravenous reserpine block to diagnose and treat reflex sympathetic dystrophy. Anesthesiol 59A:199, 1993.
59. Yarnitsky, D, and Ochoa, J: Differential effect of compression: Ischemic block in warm sensation and heat-induced pain. Brain 114:907, 1991.
60. Caudill, MA: Managing Pain Before it Manages You. Guilford Press, New York, 1994.
61. Boissonnault, WG: Examination in Physical Therapy Practice. Churchill Livingstone, New York, 1991.
62. Michel, TH, and Downing, J: Screening for cardiovascular system disease. In Boissonault, WG (ed): Examination in Physical Therapy Practice: Screening for Medical Disease. Churchill Livingstone, New York, 1991.

CHAPTER 11

Musculoskeletal Pattern I: Impaired Joint Mobility, Motor Function, Muscle Performance, and Range of Motion Associated with Joint Arthroplasty

Susan W. Stralka, MS, PT
Penny L. Head, PT, SCS, ATC

INTRODUCTION

Conditions such as bone tumor, rheumatoid arthritis, osteoarthritis, Paget's disease, and avascular necrosis of the humeral head often result in *total shoulder arthroplasty* (TSA) to improve function and relieve pain.[1] During the last several years, the number of TSAs performed has been on the rise. This increase can be traced to improved prosthetic designs and surgical techniques.[2,3] However, successful functional outcome is based primarily on rehabilitation offered by the physical therapist, who must recognize the impairments and functional limitations commonly associated with TSA.

According to the *Guide to Physical Therapist Practice* (the *Guide*),[4] the practice pattern for patients who have undergone TSA is pattern I. Pattern I includes patients who present with functional limitations resulting from the following impairments: impaired joint mobility, motor function, muscle performance, and range of motion. Patients excluded from this pattern are those with failed surgical procedures and unrelated postoperative complications during recovery and rehabilitation (e.g., fall with fracture). Physical therapists working in clinical settings with a large postoperative orthopaedic population can expect to manage patients with TSA. Therefore, they should have a working knowledge of the surgical determinants of surgery, as well as patterns of practice delineated by the *Guide*.[4]

This chapter provides the content and process information needed to assist the practicing physical therapist to competently examine, diagnose, and treat patients who have undergone TSA. Specifically, this chapter reviews the historical development of TSA, including the evolution of prosthetic designs, surgical approaches, and soft tissue morbidity related to TSA, postoperative examination and complications, and rehabilitation. Case studies presented at the end of the chapter describe the examination and treatment of patients following TSA, using the elements of the preferred practice pattern (examination, evaluation, prognosis, diagnosis, and intervention).

HISTORICAL DEVELOPMENT OF TOTAL SHOULDER ARTHROPLASTY

The earliest report of shoulder arthroplasty was recorded in 1893 when Pean, a French surgeon, implanted a platinum and rubber device for a glenohumeral (GH) joint destroyed by tuberculosis.[1] This prosthesis remained in place for approximately 2 years but then was removed due to uncontrollable infection. In 1953, Neer successfully replaced the humeral head with a Vitallium prosthesis and reported on his results in 1955.[5] This prosthesis was used to treat patients with irregular (degenerated) articular surfaces resulting from fracture or osteonecrosis and those with traumatic degenerative and arthritic conditions of the shoulder.[5]

In 1974, Neer developed the Neer II humeral prosthesis that successfully combined prosthetic humeral head replacement and glenoid resurfacing with a polyethylene unit for chronically painful incongruities involving both the humeral head and the glenoid cavity.[6] The criteria developed by Neer for successful TSA are listed in Box 11–1. In 1974, Kenmore et al.[7] reported on the development of a polyethylene glenoid liner for use with a Neer humeral head replacement. Shortly after, implant fixation to bone by polymethylmethacrylate was begun (Figs. 11–1 and 11–2).[7]

Currently, either press fit fixation with or without porous coating, or cement fixation using polymethylmethacrylate is used to fixate the humeral component. Indications for cemented fixation included the following: (1) failure to achieve adequate press fit fixation; (2) poor bone stock secondary to the underlying disease process such as rheumatoid arthritis; (3) previous arthroplasty; (4) fractures of the proximal humerus in which the tuberosities no longer provide rotational stability; and (5) degenerative cysts of the humerus. Noncemented humeral components are indicated in younger patients with good bone stock. They also have been found to

---

BOX 11–1 Neer Criteria for Successful Total Shoulder Replacement
1. Restoration of anatomic shape of the glenoid and humeral head for maximum ROM
2. Minimum bone removal for insertion of prosthesis
3. Avoidance of mechanical locking of prosthetic component
4. Repair and rehabilitation of all soft tissue

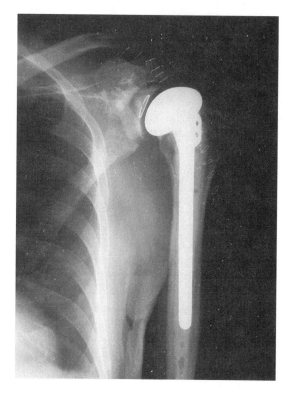

FIGURE 11–1. Postoperative anterior-posterior view of shoulder showing Neer II type of cemented humeral prosthesis and a nonmetal backed polyethylene glenoid.

work well in older patients with few complications. Cement should not be used for revision surgery for component loosening, especially if extensive bone loss has occurred.

Modular components are currently designed to allow precise tensioning of soft tissue, including the rotator cuff tendons, and, if necessary, the ease of revision. The

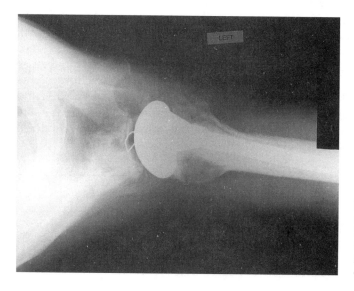

FIGURE 11–2. Axillary lateral x-ray showing cemented humeral and glenoid Neer II components. Small metallic marker shown in base of polyethylene glenoid component.

complications of the modular component designs are glenoid loosening and metal on metal wear. Nonconforming designs, in which the curvature of the glenoid diameter is larger than that of the humeral diameter, have recently come on the market. These allow for improved humeral head translation and reduced glenoid rim loading and polyethylene wear.[1] TSA using a constrained unit (see the following section) in patients with loss of rotator cuff, but with a functional deltoid muscle, was popular in the 1970s but had limited success.

PROSTHETIC DESIGN OF THE TOTAL SHOULDER COMPONENT

Prostheses are classified into constrained (ball and socket), semiconstrained, and unconstrained anatomic devices.[8] The type of the prosthesis used is an important factor in rehabilitation prognosis and treatment planning. The primary goal of surgery with a constrained prosthesis is elimination of pain, with functional elevation of the upper extremity as a secondary concern. In the presence of either a semiconstrained or unconstrained prosthesis, the goal of surgery is the restoration of functional (overhead) elevation of the upper extremity. The constrained prosthesis has a linked ball and socket joint allowing for rotation but preventing translation. The constrained prosthesis has a high failure rate because of the lack of humeral translation that increases stresses along the bone/cement interface.[4–13] Therefore use of a constrained prosthesis is uncommon, except in cases of tumor resection with significant loss of the humeral head or glenoid fossa. With a rotator tendon cuff deficiency, a semiconstrained prosthesis restricts superior migration of the humeral prosthesis.

The unconstrained prosthesis is the most commonly used prosthesis variety. The unconstrained prosthesis has similar radii for the humeral and glenoid components, allowing for greater range of motion. The prosthesis also has different links to allow for better fitting into the humeral shaft. The humeral heads are often modular and can be interfixed on the humeral stem.

Several design modifications of the unconstrained prosthesis have been made. The glenoid component, made of polyethylene, comes in different sizes. Because a small percentage of polyethylene glenoid components have shown wear (deformation), metal backing has been added as an option. Biomechanical testing has shown that loosening and breakage of the polyethylene glenoid component can occur under excessive loads, but the metal backing improves the fixation strength.[8–12] The metal backing might also slightly improve stress transfer to cortical bone underneath the glenoid fossa.

The primary indications for a Neer II type of unconstrained total shoulder replacement include pain caused by incongruency of the glenoid and humeral head, loss of function, and diminished shoulder range of motion (ROM). The pathologies in which the glenoid is intact, such as acute fractures, avascular necrosis, neoplasm of the proximal humerus, and some old injuries in young patients, are best treated by replacement of the humeral head.

Total shoulder arthroplasty is an especially difficult procedure because optimal function after surgery requires reconstruction of the rotator cuff and the deltoid muscles and the orientation of the implant. The stability of the unconstrained implant also depends on preservation of the humeral bone length and the proper orientation of the articular surfaces of the implant. Pain relief following surgery is reported to be quite good.[1,13–15] However, the restoration of ROM has been shown to vary, depending on the presurgical shoulder dysfunction, patient motivation, and the skill of the surgeon. Patients with osteoarthritis generally achieve the best outcomes because the rotator cuff is usually intact and the bone stock is good.[1] In patients with rheumatoid arthritis, the quality of the musculotendinous tissue is often compromised, directly influencing the functional result. In the presence of damaged rotator cuff tendon, or with significant bone stock loss, a hemiarthroplasty is recommended.[1,16] Recently, high incidents of glenoid component loosening, deformation, and wear have been reported in patients with a deficient rotator cuff.[1,16] However, the overall durability of TSA over time is as good as that for any other joint.

SHOULDER ARTHROPLASTY

In certain situations, *hemiarthroplasty*, or the implantation of the humeral component alone, is indicated. The rationale for performing a hemiarthroplasty is that the surface of the glenoid is judged to be in good condition with minimal deformity or incongruity.[17] Indications for a humeral head replacement alone include the following: (1) osteonecrosis of the humeral head; (2) recent four-part and head-splitting fractures of the proximal humerus; (3) recent three-part fractures of the proximal humerus in the elderly; (4) some proximal humeral neoplasms; (5) malunions and nonunions of old proximal humerus fractures; and (6) insufficient glenoid bone stock to support a glenoid component.[18]

Total shoulder arthroplasty (replacement of the humeral head and glenoid articular surface with prosthetic components) is indicated primarily in individuals with pain resulting from glenohumeral arthritis, including loss of function that has not responded to conservative treatment.[1] Surgical factors influencing outcome of TSA can be found in Box 11–2.

Certain diagnostic groups often result in pain and destruction that require arthroplasty. Patients with rheumatoid arthritis, primary or secondary osteoarthritis, and arthritis associated with old trauma such as fractures, fracture dislocation, or recurrent dislocations are primary candidates for arthroplasty. Other indications include rotator cuff arthropathy, failed previous surgery, and osteonecrosis.[3] Other less common diagnoses include septic arthritis, ankylosing spondylitis, lupus erythematosus, hemophilia, and other synovial diseases.[3] Sisk and Wright[1] report that stiffness in the absence of pain rarely is an indication for shoulder arthroplasty.

Contraindications to shoulder arthroplasty include a neuropathic joint, infection, and paralysis with loss of the deltoid, or the rotator cuff. If the deltoid or the rotator cuff musculature is involved, shoulder arthroplasty can be performed with muscle transfer or other soft tissue procedures. Individuals considered to be candidates for

---

BOX 11–2 Surgical Factors Influencing Outcome of Total Shoulder Arthroplasty
- Preservation of deltoid origin
- Reconstruction of rotator cuff musculature
- Release of capsular and musculotendinous contractures
- Balancing of all soft tissue

TSA should not have any medical contraindications to the surgery and should be well motivated and informed about the anticipated results.

Specific Indications for TSA

The following are specific pathologies and rehabilitation concerns commonly associated with TSA. For additional reference, pathologies associated with humeral head replacement and TSA performed at the Mayo clinic from 1975 to 1992 are listed in Table 11–1.

OSTEOARTHRITIS

Patients with osteoarthritis often have flattening posterior erosion of the glenoid and an enlarged or deformed humeral head.[7,11] Finding osteophytes located inferiorly is common. In the general osteoarthritic population, those individuals with shoulder complex problems usually have an intact rotator cuff, whereas the subscapularis muscle often is shortened and limits external rotation. Typically, the acromioclavicular (AC) joint is arthritic, thus requiring excision of the distal clavicle.[1,5,7]

SOFT TISSUE LESIONS

Proper management of shoulder soft tissue is extremely important because it affects final ROM after surgery. The resultant ROM is directly proportional to the soft tissue tension.[11] The deltoid is the key muscle in functional shoulder recovery. In the postoperative rehabilitation program, the surgeon should inform the therapist of the expected postoperative external rotation motion that will be possible.

RHEUMATOID ARTHRITIS

In patients with rheumatoid arthritis, changes are often noted with the rotator cuff.[7,11] The bone is often osteopenic (porous bone or inadequate calcified bone) with erosion and cysts. Attenuation of the glenohumeral capsule and the rotator cuff can lead to a functionally insufficient cuff that simulates a full thickness rotator cuff tear. In these patients, the coracoacromial ligament should be kept intact to act as a restraint to superior migration of the humeral head.[7,11]

TABLE 11–1 Diagnosis of Patients Requiring Joint Arthroplasty
at the Mayo Clinic from 1979 to 1992

Diagnosis	Humeral Head #	Total Shoulder #
Osteoarthritis	67	354
Rheumatoid arthritis	109	206
Traumatic arthritis	126	109
Osteonecrosis	33	40
Cuff tear arthropathy	36	22
Failed surgery	16	134
Other	7	6
Total	394	871

ROTATOR CUFF DEFICIT OF THE SHOULDER

Problems such as arthritic changes, previous musculoskeletal injury, synovial crystals and enzymes can cause rotator cuff disuse. The pathologic sequelae of cartilage loss, bone loss, and extensive rotator cuff tearing is called a "Milwaukee shoulder," leading to progressive degenerative changes. Neer[6] discusses the same progression and bone resorption along with the previously noted symptoms. TSA for this type of shoulder with multiple tissue destruction might be unsuccessful due to the multiple tissue problems.

With rotator cuff tears, superior migration of the humerus articulating with the undersurface of the acromion and considerable weakness in external rotation occurs. With rotator cuff damage, the inferior insertions from the subscapularis and infraspinatus should be preserved. Any salvageable tendon from the internal or external rotator muscles can be reinserted to bone. Preserving the coracoacromial ligament in the rotator cuff-deficient patient is important because this ligament becomes a major anterior-superior constraint as well as a fulcrum for motion instead of the glenoid. Additional stability can be achieved by the use of a large prosthesis having a congruous articulation with the coracoacromial arch.

POSTTRAUMATIC DEGENERATIVE DISEASE

Operations performed after old trauma are difficult, demonstrating high complication rates along with special rehabilitation concerns.[2,5,7] These concerns are related to several factors such as scarring of the rotator cuff and capsule from previous surgery, bony deformities, or erosion from trauma. Muscle contractures, atrophy, and peripheral nerve deficits also complicate this procedure. Thus, rehabilitation must address all of these problems.[1,2,5,7]

AVASCULAR NECROSIS

Patients with avascular necrosis usually have good results with TSA.[3,6] Avascular necrosis results in destruction of articular cartilage and underlying cortical bone because of interruption of blood supply and nutrition to these tissues. At the shoulder, the pathology usually involves only the humeral head. The rotator cuff tendons and GH joint capsule are often intact. The indications for replacing only the humeral head include acute fractures and painful chronic glenohumeral incongruities. Pain is often the primary consideration in the decision to perform TSA.

Preoperative Planning and Evaluation

Prior to arthroplasty, the shoulder should be carefully evaluated for bony deficiency as evidenced by radiographs or diagnostic imaging. The patient who presents with osteoarthritis requiring TSA usually has a history of progressive shoulder pain along with stiffness and loss of motion. The patient commonly complains of grinding or grating in the shoulder that is often disturbing and painful. Evaluating the glenoid for loss of joint space and erosion of bone stock is important. Patients with osteoarthritis often have posterior glenoid wear, osteophyte formation, and humeral head flattening, and possible subluxation of the humeral head.

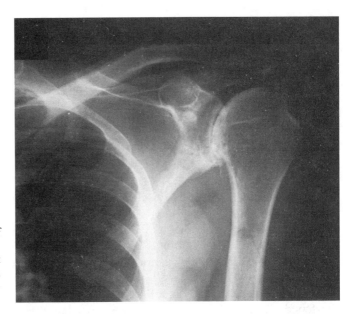

FIGURE 11–3. AP x-ray of GH joint with typical osteoarthritic changes of the joint space narrowing subchondral cyst and hypertrophic osteophytes.

In patients with rheumatoid arthritis, there is usually erosion in the base of the coracoid process. Examination of the shoulder should be documented prior to arthroplasty with consideration of bony deficiency, the presence and amount of glenohumeral instability, or tightness, especially with internal rotation. Stability of the GH joint is affected by bony deficiency. If the GH joint is stable, minimal bone deficiency does not require treatment. However, if the GH joint is unstable, the bony deficiencies must be corrected to prevent failure of the arthroplasty.

Anterior-posterior, axillary lateral, and scapular-Y views are the standard roentgenograms (Figs. 11–3 and 11–4). These particular views provide information

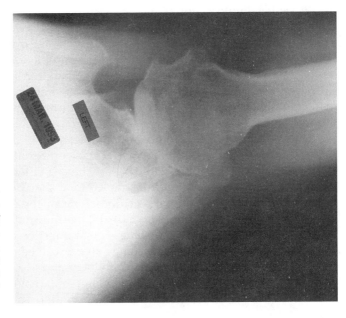

FIGURE 11–4. Axillary lateral-shoulder-best view for demonstrating the total loss of articular cartilage with bone-on-bone involvement between humeral head and glenoid. This view is crucial in preoperative planning to assess the adequacy of the glenoid.

about degenerative changes of the GH joint, humeral head elevation, tuberosity position, glenohumeral wear, subluxation, and osteophyte formation.[1] Electromyography and nerve conduction studies should be obtained preoperatively in patients with suspected peripheral or nerve root defects.[3] If a patient has a history of infection, surgery, or aspiration, then nuclear medicine studies are often necessary to determine the status of that area. Evaluation of the AC joint before surgery is important because unrecognized AC joint pathology can compromise the TSA results.

Surgery

Total shoulder arthroplasty is an especially difficult procedure, because optimal function after surgery requires a great deal of skill in the reconstruction and rehabilitation of the rotator cuff and deltoid muscles and in the orientation of the implants.[1,2,5,7,14,19] The stability of the unconstrained implant also depends on preserving the humeral and glenoid length and the direction of the articular surfaces of the implants. The soft tissue repair around the implant is as important to the functional result as is the orientation of the components. If the subscapularis muscle is shortened, it should be dissected free and lengthened enough by coronal plane z-plasty. If a tear of the rotator cuff requires repair, the tendons should be moved so that they can be reattached without tension with the arm at the side.[20,21] Surgical techniques vary. Refer to Campbell's *Operative Orthopedics,* 9th Edition, Volume I[22] for more information.

Complications of Total Shoulder Replacement Arthroplasty

Total shoulder arthroplasty is associated with numerous complications including prosthetic loosening, glenohumeral instability, tears of the rotator cuff, periprosthetic fracture, infection, neural injury, and deltoid dysfunction.[23] Constrained total shoulder prosthesis has limited clinical success and has been associated with more complications than the unconstrained implants. Reoperation is common after constrained total shoulder arthroplasty, with rates reportedly ranging from 4% to 54%. Complications with the constrained prosthesis include mechanical loosening, instability, failure of the implant secondary to plastic deformation fracture, or loosening of the components.[3] Currently, most orthopaedic surgeons use constrained TSA as a salvage operation following tumor resection or in the presence of irreparable rotator cuff tears and failed unconstrained TSA.

Unconstrained total shoulder arthroplasty has been shown to be a highly successful procedure with good and excellent results reported for most of the shoulders evaluated at the time of early and midterm follow up.[23–26] The most common complications with unconstrained total shoulder arthroplasty, in descending frequency, include the following: (1) loosening of the component, (2) glenohumeral instability, (3) tear of the rotator cuff, (4) periprosthetic fracture, (5) infection, (6) failure of the implant, and (7) weakness or dysfunction of the deltoid.[27–32] Most cases of clinical and radiographic loosening have involved failure of the fixation of the glenoid component. Although rare following a TSA, infection has potentially devastating complications. As with other joint replacements, treatment depends on the isolation of the pathogen from the tissue or fluid samples. If a patient has been diagnosed with infection, the treatment options include antibiotic suppression, irrigation and debridement, removal of the prosthesis, reimplantation, resection arthroplasty, arthrodesis, and in severe instances, amputation.

Failure of shoulder replacement might be the result of the following: disassociation or loosening of the polyethylene glenoid from its metal tray, fracture of the keel or metal glenoid backing, fracture of the fixation screws, subluxation, or dislocation of polyethylene spacers.[18] Occasionally, weakness of the deltoid muscle occurs because of failed operative repair or injury to the axillary nerve. Optimum operative exposure is important. This can be done when surgery is performed through an extended deltoid pectoral approach without detaching the origin or insertion of the deltoid muscle.[31] In a report on 40 revision arthroplasties by Neer and Watson[13] the cause of failure resulting from arthroplasty was assigned to one of the following three groups: (1) preoperative conditions, (2) operative or prosthetic complications, or (3) postoperative problems. The most common causes of failure among all three groups include scarring and detachment of the deltoid muscle, loss of external rotation resulting from contracture of the subscapularis muscle, prominence or retraction of the greater tuberosity, loss of glenoid bone, and inadequate postoperative rehabilitation.[13]

TOTAL SHOULDER ARTHROPLASTY REHABILITATION

Total shoulder arthroplasty has been successful in relieving pain for many patients with disabling shoulder problems. However, successful restoration of shoulder function following TSA is highly dependent on a well-designed rehabilitation program. The TSA has been called the "most challenging and least forgiving of joint arthroplasties," and full recovery is more therapy-dependent than with other total joint procedures.[19]

The primary goals of rehabilitation following joint replacement include preventing adhesions through early ROM, maximizing joint mobility, protecting rotator cuff repair if applicable, and maximizing muscle strength. Critical factors that might affect the rehabilitation process include the integrity of the soft tissue and bony structures, the stability of the prosthesis, the fixation technique used, and any concomitant injuries or specific disease states. Another factor that might affect the rehabilitation process is patient selection, in terms of motivation, compliance, and expectations. Patients must be made aware of their responsibilities in the rehabilitation programs. Educating the patient regarding the nature and scope of therapy will improve compliance with rehabilitation and thus improve the outcome.

Examination and Evaluation

The initial examination process gathers data by means of the patient history, relevant systems review, and pertinent tests and measures. These data allow the physical therapist to diagnose the nature and extent of the problem (impairments and functional limitations). Selection of examination procedures and the depth of the examination following TSA will vary based on the patient's age, stage of recovery (acute, subacute, chronic), phase of rehabilitation (early, intermediate, late, return to activity), and home, community, or work situation.[4]

Common examination methods following TSA include a history and systems review to determine factors such as age, health status, past medical history, family and/or caregiver resources, prior functional status and activity level, and initial integumentary status. Determining whether or not the patient has tissue deficiencies or specific disease states that might affect the rehabilitation process, for example, rotator cuff arthropathy or rheumatoid arthritis, is crucial. During this process, the patient should also be questioned regarding his or her goals on the completion of the rehabilitation program. The examination continues with common tests and measures employed by the therapist to assess pain, edema, status of wound healing, posture, joint mobility, range of motion, soft tissue restrictions, muscle performance, and functional capacity with regard to self-care and home management (see Chap. 5 for a review of clinical examination techniques).

Evaluation and interpretation of the data gathered during the examination process reveal the patient's functional impairments and allow the therapist to establish the diagnosis and prognosis. Common postoperative impairments following TSA include pain, hypomobility of the GH, sternoclavicular (SC), and AC joints and the scapulothoracic articulation, loss of ROM, decreased muscle performance, postural abnormalities, and decreased capacity to perform self-care, and home management activities involving the upper extremity.

Prognosis

Once the impairments and functional limitations have been determined, the plan of care (prognosis) should be developed. The plan of care should specify goals and outcomes, treatment interventions to be used, the frequency and duration of treatment required for attaining the stated goals, and criteria for discharge.

Interventions

Many different rehabilitation programs have been described following TSA (Table 11–2). The most complete rehabilitation program has been described by Neer[6] and has been modified over time. Neer suggested dividing patients into the following two groups: (1) those who could undergo a reasonably "normal" rehabilitation program, and (2) those with tissue deficiencies, usually involving the muscles and/or bone, who must be placed in a "limited-goals" rehabilitation program.

Rehabilitation programs for patients demonstrating joint hypomobility, decreased ROM, and decreased muscle performance, with no concomitant rotator cuff repair or tissue deficiency, should address early ROM and early muscle strengthening. Early ROM is initiated to prevent the formation of adhesions that would limit mobility and function. Early muscle strengthening is initiated to retard muscle atrophy and to improve functional use of the upper extremity.

For patients with concomitant rotator cuff repair or tissue deficiency, rehabilitation is aimed at maintaining joint stability and obtaining lesser range of motion with reasonable muscle control in this limited range. Range of motion is slowed to allow better scar formation, thus enhancing joint stability (Table 11–3).

As a general rule, patients with osteoarthritis or avascular necrosis fit into the "normal" rehabilitation category, and can progress with a vigorous early active ROM program. Patients with rheumatoid arthritis, old trauma, or rotator cuff arthropathy

TABLE 11–2 Rehabilitation Program for Shoulder Arthroplasty
With No Tissue Deficiency

Phase	Goals	Treatment Interventions
Phase I. Immediate Motion Phase	Increase passive ROM Prevent adhesions Decrease pain Prevent rotator cuff shutdown	Sling immobilization except with exercise CPM use if requested by physician Modalities as necessary to minimize pain/swelling Elbow, wrist, and hand ROM/gripping exercises Pendulum exercises Passive ROM for forward flexion, scapular plane elevation, ER (neutral to 30° abduction) to 45°, and IR (neutral to 30° abduction) Basic scapular stabilization exercises Progressive PROM exercises Active-assisted ROM (AAROM) exercises with cane and/or pulley for forward flexion, scapular plane elevation, ER, and IR Isometrics for IR, ER, and abduction in neutral
Phase 2. Early Strengthening Phase	Improve ROM Increase functional strength	Progressive PROM exercises Progressive AAROM exercises Joint mobilization as necessary to restore arthrokinetics AROM exercises for forward flexion, scapular plane elevation, and abduction (progress supine to seated short arm ranges) Tubing exercises for ER and IR in neutral Progressive scapular stabilization program Upper body ergometer Biceps/triceps and forearm strengthening
Phase 3. Maximum Strengthening Phase	Improve shoulder strength/endurance Improve functional capacity	Continued PROM, AAROM, and joint mobilization to restore functional ROM Continued progression of strength program for deltoid, rotator cuff, and scapular muscles Functional retraining as necessary

Adapted from Campbell Clinic Physical Therapy Department and Foundation, Memphis, Tennessee.

typically fit into the "limited-goals" category and must focus on a passive range of motion program and delay active range of motion for several weeks, depending on the status of the rotator cuff repair.[19]

Progression of the rehabilitation program will depend on the patient's responses to the treatment interventions and requires periodic re-evaluation by the physical therapist. Treatment interventions vary depending on the impairments discovered in the examination process and the presence or absence of tissue deficiencies or pre-existing systemic disease. The rehabilitation process should begin as soon after surgery as the physician will allow. Good communication between the surgeon and physical therapist is essential, because only the surgeon knows the extent of soft tissue damage and repair. The therapist must be made aware of any deviations from the normal postoperative progression to modify the rehabilitation program for the individual.

RANGE OF MOTION

Joint hypomobility following total joint arthroplasty can lead to debilitating functional impairment. Initiating ROM exercises early in the rehabilitation process is

TABLE 11–3 Rehabilitation Program for Shoulder Arthroplasty with Tissue Deficiency

Phase	Goals	Treatment Interventions
Phase 1. Immediate Motion Phase	Increase passive ROM Decrease pain Retard muscle atrophy	Sling immobilization except with exercise CPM use if requested by physician Modalities as necessary to minimize pain/swelling Elbow, wrist, and hand ROM/gripping exercises Pendulum exercises Basic scapular stabilization exercises Passive ROM for forward flexion and scapular elevation to 90°, ER and IR in neutral to 30°
Phase 2. Early Strengthening Phase	Improve ROM Increase functional strength	Progressive PROM exercises AAROM exercises with cane and/or pulley for forward flexion, scapular elevation, ER, and IR Isometrics for IR, ER, and abduction in neutral Progressive scapular stabilization program Progressive PROM and AAROM exercises Joint mobilization as necessary to restore arthrokinematics AROM exercises for forward flexion, scapular plane elevation, and abduction (progress supine to seated short arc ranges) Tubing exercises for ER and IR in neutral Upper body ergometer Biceps/triceps forearm strengthening
Phase 3. Maximum Strengthening Phase	Restore functional ROM Improve shoulder strength/endurance Improve functional capacity	Continued PROM, AAROM, and joint mobilization to restore functional ROM Continued progression of strength program for deltoid, rotator cuff, and scapular muscles as tolerated Functional retraining as necessary

Adapted from Campbell Clinic Physical Therapy Department and Foundation, Memphis, Tennessee.

the key to restoring functional mobility. Early ROM minimizes the formation of adhesions. Passive and/or gentle active-assistive ROM exercises generally can be initiated within the first 24 to 48 hours postoperatively for forward flexion and for external rotation with elbow at the side. Passive and/or active-assistive motion for internal rotation and abduction can be initiated within 2 to 4 weeks postoperatively. The status of the rotator cuff is the primary factor in determining the type of motion (passive versus active) and the ranges of motion allowed in the early postoperative period.

The ROM portion of the rehabilitation program is designed to progressively increase mobility of the shoulder complex. The therapist must consider motion not only at the GH joint, but the ST, AC, and SC joints as well. Specific treatment interventions to improve joint mobility and ROM might include passive, active, and active-assistive stretching; joint mobilization; soft tissue mobilization; and the use of a continuous passive motion machine (Figs. 11–5 to 11–8). Physical agents and electrotherapeutic modalities such as hot/cold packs, ultrasound, and electrical stimulation might also be used for the purpose of decreasing pain, reducing soft tissue swelling, and/or facilitating improved joint range of motion.

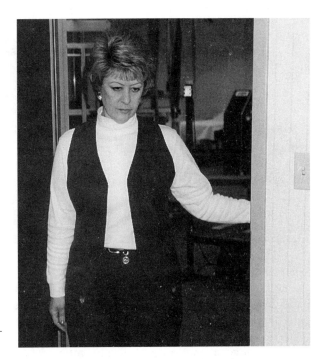

FIGURE 11–5. Passive external rotation.

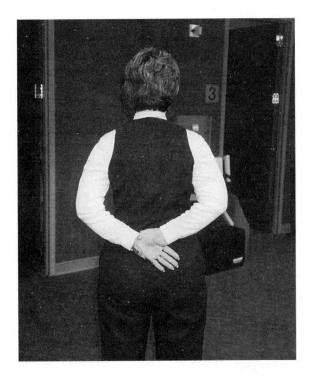

FIGURE 11–6. Passive internal rotation.

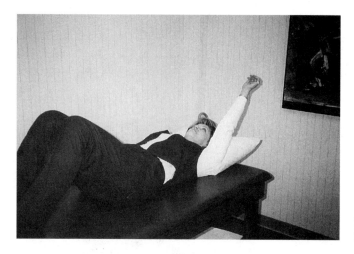

FIGURE 11–7. Active flexion in the supine position.

Initially, passive ROM (PROM) is performed manually by the therapist. The patient can also perform passive and active-assistive ROM exercises, including pendulum swings, pulley exercises, and/or wand exercises (Figs. 11–9 to 11–12).

The cautious use of joint mobilization, by a therapist skilled in mobilization, to improve range of motion is typically initiated between the fourth and eighth week postoperatively, depending on the integrity of the rotator cuff tendons. Joint mobilization is used to restore normal arthrokinematics of the shoulder complex. It is

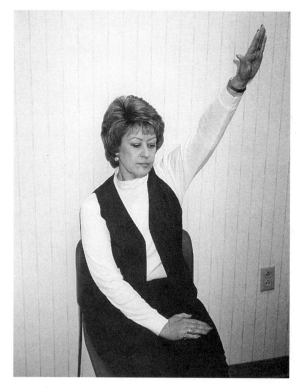

FIGURE 11–8. Active flexion in the sitting position.

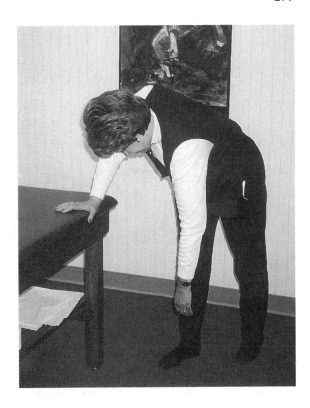

FIGURE 11–9. Pendulum exercises.

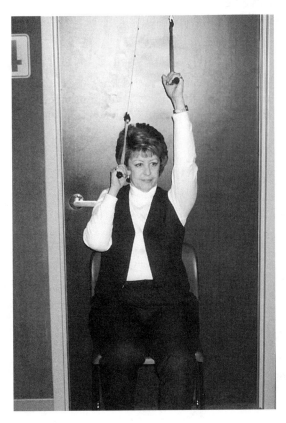

FIGURE 11–10. Pulley exercises for forward flexion.

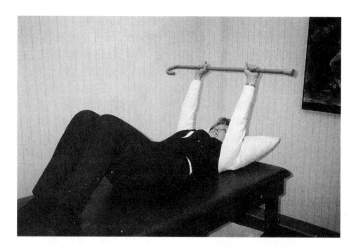

FIGURE 11–11. Wand exercise for flexion.

indicated when the lack of extensibility of the periarticular tissues limits the arthrokinematic movement of the joint surfaces.

Continuous passive motion (CPM) might be used as an adjunct to rehabilitation following TSA. The reported value of this modality varies in the literature. Craig[33] and Neer[34] reported that use of CPM resulted in earlier recovery of motion, diminished pain, and a shorter hospital stay. Brems et al.[35] suggested that patients become dependent on the use of CPM for rehabilitation. Certain situations might be potentially more appropriate for the use of CPM, for example, patients having bilateral shoulder problems precluding the use of the uninvolved extremity for assisted ROM. However, donning the apparatus is difficult and usually requires assistance.

STRENGTH TRAINING

Decreased muscle performance (strength, power, and endurance) is another common impairment following TSA. Neuromuscular shutdown of key muscle groups, including the scapular stabilizers and the rotator cuff, can occur with prolonged immobilization following surgery.

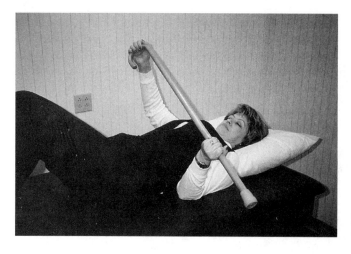

FIGURE 11–12. Wand exercise for external rotation.

Early initiation of strengthening exercises will help to prevent neuromuscular shutdown, to retard muscle atrophy, and to improve functional mobility; however, the strengthening program should be graded to prevent damaging the surgical repair. Once again, the status of the rotator cuff will be the primary factor in determining the progression of the strengthening program.

The strengthening portion of the rehabilitation program is designed to progressively improve muscle performance and functional joint mobility, ultimately leading to improved ability to perform self-care and home management activities. Specific treatment interventions to improve muscle performance might include aquatic exercises; active, active-assistive, and resistive exercises; and neuromuscular facilitation techniques. Electrotherapeutic modalities such as biofeedback and electrical stimulation might also be used to facilitate neuromuscular re-education.

As ROM progresses during the course of total shoulder rehabilitation, strengthening programs may begin. Early emphasis should be placed on scapular stabilization exercises, such as shoulder shrugs, shoulder retractions, and scapular PNF patterns, to prevent neuromuscular shutdown of this key muscle group. These exercises can be initiated very early in the rehabilitation program without risk to a tissue-deficient patient. Resistive exercises include isometric and isotonic strengthening (Figs. 11–13 to 11–15). Isometric exercises for the rotator cuff and middle deltoid are generally initiated within the first 2 to 4 weeks of rehabilitation, with progression to gentle isotonic strengthening within the fourth to sixth week. Resistance can be applied manually or with weights, pulleys, and elastic bands. Resistive exercises can also be performed in a water environment. The properties of water allow buoyancy of the upper extremity to assist with ROM and resistance to allow strengthening capabilities (see Chap. 16).

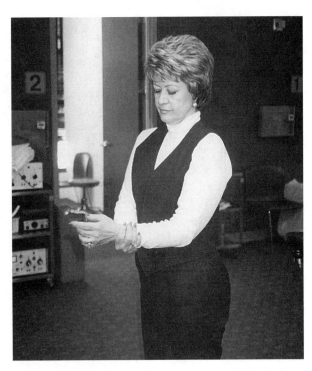

FIGURE 11–13. Isometric external rotation in neutral.

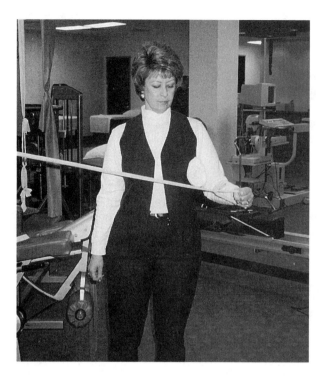

FIGURE 11–14. Resisted external rotation with Thera-Band.

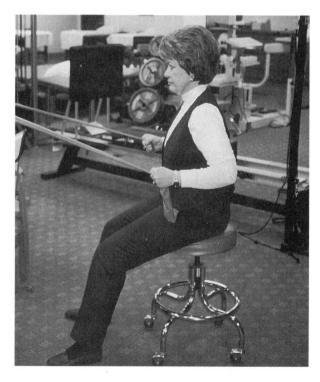

FIGURE 11–15. Seated rows with Thera-Band.

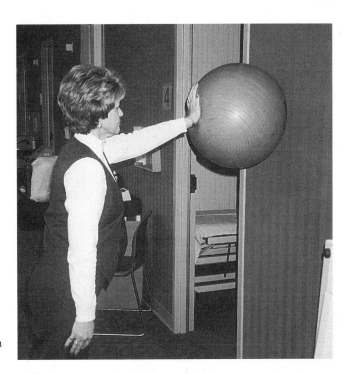

FIGURE 11–16. Closed chain scapular stabilization.

The strength program is emphasized, becoming the central focus of rehabilitation, 10 to 12 weeks after surgery. Proprioceptive and closed chain exercises are also progressed at this time (Fig. 11–16). Resisted exercises for both the glenohumeral and scapulothoracic muscles are performed with increasing amounts of intensity, repetitions, and frequency. Delaying muscle strengthening 10 to 12 weeks from surgery allows sufficient time for tissue healing following the surgical procedure. Muscle strengthening is a slow process. Therefore, the patient must be encouraged to be persistent with the exercise program.

Reexamination should be performed often in the course of total shoulder rehabilitation. The process of reexamination allows the therapist to evaluate the patient's progress and to modify treatment interventions appropriately. For example, through the process of reassessing ROM and joint mobility, the therapist can define the appropriate time to begin using joint mobilization techniques.

As joint mobility and muscle performance improve, rehabilitation should focus on functional retraining. Treatment interventions should include techniques to improve the patient's ability to perform physical tasks related to self-care, home management, work, and leisure activities. Re-examination allows the therapist to determine when these treatment interventions can take place.

CASE STUDY 11–1: HEMIARTHROPLASTY

INITIAL EXAMINATION

This patient is a 58-year-old neurosurgeon who fell while jogging and suffered a three-part comminuted fracture of the proximal humerus on the nondominant left side involving the greater tuberosity, humeral head, and humeral shaft. The patient also sustained a nondisplaced fracture of the lesser tuberosity. He was initially treated in the emergency room and immobilized with a sling and swathe. Two days after injury, the patient underwent hemiarthroplasty to replace the humeral head. Physical therapy (PT) was initiated on the second postoperative day.

EXAMINATION

The patient presented to PT with significant hematoma formation throughout the entire upper extremity as a result of the trauma. He reported only minimal pain in the area of the incision and in his elbow. An avid runner, he stated that he would like to return to this activity. His primary goal was to resume operating within 3 months.

Active ROM of the shoulder was not assessed during the initial evaluation because of the patient's postoperative status. Passive forward flexion and abduction were limited to 110° and 85°, respectively. External and internal rotation were not assessed at the orthopaedist's request because of the tuberosity fractures. The patient complained of mild discomfort with passive movement. Motion was limited by a muscular end-feel. Moderate swelling was noted in the forearm, wrist, and hand. Atrophy of the biceps, triceps, and forearm musculature was noted, as well as the deltoid, pectoralis, supraspinatus, infraspinatus, and parascapular muscles. A manual muscle test of the shoulder musculature was not performed at this time. The patient demonstrated full ROM of the cervical spine, elbow, forearm, wrist, and fingers. Gross weakness was noted for biceps, triceps, wrist flexors and extensors, and grip.

EVALUATION AND PROGNOSIS

The patient presents with limited shoulder motion secondary to the trauma and subsequent surgery. Postsurgical active movement of the shoulder is avoided. Passive movement is limited to forward flexion and abduction only. The patient's chief complaint is decreased biceps and grip strength and the inability to resume his duties as a neurosurgeon. A moderate amount of swelling is noted in the forearm, wrist, and hand. However, pain is minimal.

Goals established for this patient include decrease in pain and swelling, increase in joint mobility and ROM, increase in muscle performance, increase in independence with self-care and home management activities, and full return to function as a neurosurgeon. The initial treatment plan focuses on increasing shoulder ROM in flexion and abduction and improving capsular extensibility by passively applying tensile stress to the GH joint. Passive and active-assisted ROM exercises and joint mobilizations are used to achieve the goals for improved joint mobility and range of motion. The strategy also includes maintaining scapular mobility and restoring neuromuscular control of the scapula through the use of stabilization exercises.

Treatment is performed at a frequency of three times per week. Prognosis for reaching the stated goals is 4 months.

INTERVENTION

Two days following surgery, gentle PROM for forward flexion and abduction of the shoulder, as well as active ROM for the elbow, forearm, wrist, and hand is initiated. Scar mobilization and soft tissue mobilization of the pectoralis and latissimus dorsi muscles are also performed. The patient receives ice to the shoulder following treatment to control pain and inflammation. His wife is instructed in a home program consisting of PROM for flexion and abduction and retrograde massage of the hand and forearm to decrease swelling.

Scapular stabilization exercises in neutral and scapular mobilization techniques to maintain scapular mobility are initiated on the second visit. The patient attends physical therapy three times per week for the first 3 weeks, for PROM, scapular stabilization exercises, and soft tissue mobilization. Passive motion for rotation is not initiated to allow adequate healing of the tuberosity fractures.

RE-EXAMINATION AND INTERVENTION

At 3 weeks following surgery, the patient demonstrates 130° of passive flexion and 125° of passive abduction with no reports of pain. At this time, the frequency of visits is decreased to two times per week, with continuation of the home program three times per day. Emphasis continues on PROM for flexion and abduction and scapular stabilization exercises.

At 4 weeks after surgery, low grade (grades 1 and 2) joint mobilization for inferior glide is initiated to facilitate progression of ROM. Tightness of the inferior GH joint capsule is noted during reassessment. Patient rapidly progresses to 145° of passive flexion and 150° of passive abduction with initiation of joint mobilizations.

At 5 weeks after surgery, PROM for external and internal rotation with the humerus in neutral is initiated. Active ROM exercises, including supine flexion, isometrics for external and internal rotation, supine serratus punches, and tubing exercises for shoulder extension and seated rows, are initiated for strengthening. Use of the sling is discontinued. The patient is able to resume seeing patients in his office at this time.

At 6 weeks, he demonstrates 165° of passive flexion, 160° of passive abduction, 45° of external rotation in neutral, 60° of external rotation with the humerus in 90° of abduction, and 55° of internal rotation in 90° of abduction. Active ROM is limited to 110° of flexion and 95° of abduction in the sitting position. Substitution of the upper trapezius occurs as a result of deltoid and rotator cuff weakness. At this time the rehabilitation program progresses to include strengthening exercises against gravity for the deltoid, use of the upper body ergometer, and tubing exercises for the rotator cuff. Scapular exercises are advanced to include closed chain exercises. Higher grade joint mobilizations (grades 3 and 4) for inferior glide are initiated to facilitate progression of end ROM.

At 8 weeks, the patient demonstrates full PROM for flexion and abduction, 60° of passive external rotation in neutral, 80° of passive external rotation in 90° abduction, and 70° of passive internal rotation in 90° abduction. Active ROM had also improved to 160° of flexion, 155° of abduction, 45° of external rotation in neutral, and 70° of external rotation in 90° abduction. The patient also demonstrates a significant improvement in functional strength. He is able to return to full duty as a neurosurgeon. Frequency of treatment is decreased to one time per week to monitor his progress. This is continued until 12 weeks after surgery, at which time the patient is discharged from physical therapy. The patient continues with daily stretching exercises as well as progression of his strengthening program for 9 months postoperative.

CASE SUMMARY

It is worth noting that this patient's rapid progress in rehabilitation and ability to resume full function so quickly are a result of several factors. Although his age could have worked against him, his high level of fitness prior to the trauma benefited him. This patient was also highly motivated, both personally and professionally, which increased his compliance with physical therapy and his home program. The patient's spouse was extremely supportive, attending every rehabilitation session and also working diligently with him at home. And, finally, because of lack of trauma to other tissues, for example, the rotator cuff, rehabilitation was initiated very early following surgery, allowing scar tissue modeling as the healing process took place, thus preventing excessive adhesions. Early initiation of physical therapy is extremely important for a good outcome following shoulder arthroplasty.

CASE STUDY 11–2: TOTAL SHOULDER ARTHROPLASTY

INITIAL EXAMINATION

This patient is a 70-year-old retired schoolteacher with a history of significant degenerative joint disease of the right GH joint. The decision was made to perform a TSA based on her pain level and loss of function of the upper extremity. She was no longer responding to conservative measures of treatment, such as nonsteroidal anti-inflammatory drugs (NSAIDs) physical therapy, and cortisone injections.

Prior to surgery, the patient demonstrated the following active ROM of the right shoulder:

Flexion	118°
Abduction	105°
Ext. rot.	56°
Int. rot.	40°

She reported pain at rest and with activity and a decrease in functional use of her arm with activities of daily living (ADLs) such as brushing her hair, tucking in her shirt, fastening her seatbelt, and fastening her bra.

During surgery, significant tears of the supraspinatus and infraspinatus tendons were noted. A repair of the rotator cuff was performed in conjunction with the TSA. Following surgery, the patient began using a continuous passive motion machine (CPM) on the first postoperative day for forward flexion in a limited range from 0° to 90°.

EXAMINATION

The patient presents to physical therapy 4 weeks after surgery, immobilized with a sling and abduction pillow in neutral rotation and 30° abduction. She reports a lack of compliance with use of her CPM at home because of pain with passive movement of the shoulder. Her chief complaint is decreased functional use of her dominant right shoulder. Her primary goal is to restore normal functional use of her shoulder to allow independence with ADLs. She is not involved in recreational activities other than playing cards or board games.

Active ROM of the shoulder is not assessed at this time because of the rotator cuff repair. Passive forward flexion is limited to 76° and passive external rotation in neutral is limited to 7°. Pain and a muscular end-feel were noted with passive ROM. Generalized atrophy of the entire upper extremity and parascapular musculature are noted. The patient demonstrates full ROM of the elbow, forearm, wrist, and fingers, and limited but functional ROM in the cervical spine. No gross weakness is noted for these areas with the exception of grip.

EVALUATION AND PROGNOSIS

The patient presents with limited shoulder motion as a result of the surgery; however, her motion was also limited prior to surgery. The surgical report does not indicate the amount of motion obtained following surgery. Postsurgical protocol does not allow for active movement of the shoulder because of the repair of the rotator cuff. Passive motion is limited to forward flexion and external rotation 0° to 20° in neutral. The patient's chief complaint is pain with passive movement.

Goals for this patient include decreased pain, increased joint mobility and range of motion, increased muscle performance, and increased independence with self-care and home management activities. The initial treatment plan is to gradually progress PROM of shoulder flexion and external rotation by passively applying tensile stress to the GH joint, while protecting the rotator cuff repair. Strategies also include decreasing pain to allow progression of ROM, maintaining scapular mobility, and restoring neuromuscular control of the scapula through the use of stabilization exercises. Treatment is performed at a frequency of three times per week. Prognosis for reaching stated goals is 6 months.

INTERVENTION

Gentle PROM for forward flexion and external-internal rotation in neutral, active ROM for the elbow, forearm, and wrist, and gripping exercises are initiated. Scar mobilization and soft tissue mobilization of the pectoralis major, upper trapezius, and latissimus dorsi are performed. Interferential current is used during PROM to decrease pain with this activity, thus allowing increased gains in motion. The patient receives ice to decrease pain and inflammation following treatment. The patient is encouraged to be compliant with use of the home CPM unit and is instructed in a home program consisting of pendulum exercises, PROM for forward flexion and external rotation in neutral (not to exceed 20), and scapular stabilization including shoulder shrugs and retraction.

The patient attends PT three times per week for PROM, scapular stabilization, and soft tissue mobilization.

RE-EXAMINATION AND INTERVENTION

At 2 weeks following surgery, the patient demonstrates only minimal gains in passive motion (80° of flexion, 10° of external rotation in neutral, and 14° internal rotation in neutral). She continues to report lack of compliance with the home CPM unit, and also reports noncompliance with her home exercise program because of pain. Pulley exercises for flexion ROM and submaximal isometrics for shoulder abductors and extensors are initiated.

At 4 weeks after surgery, the patient demonstrates 86° passive flexion, 14° passive external rotation in neutral, and 20° passive internal rotation in slight humeral abduction. She reports better compliance with her home program. The CPM unit is discontinued at this time. Active-assisted ROM exercises using a cane are initiated for flexion, scaption (elevation in the scapular plane), and external rotation in neutral and 30° abduction. Submaximal isometrics for internal and external rotators in neutral are also instituted. Scapular stabilization exercises are advanced to include tubing exercises for shoulder extension and seated rows. She continues PT three times per week, with emphasis on passive motion, soft tissue mobilization, and scapular mobilization and stabilization. Moist heat is used prior to PROM to help facilitate motion. Use of interferential current is discontinued, because it no longer has an effect on her pain during ROM activities. The sling is also discontinued at this time.

At 6 weeks postoperative status, the patient demonstrates moderate gains in PROM. She is able to achieve 105° flexion, 94° of elevation in scaption, 20° external rotation in neutral, and 24° internal rotation in slight abduction. At this time, active ROM (in supine) is assessed, and the patient demonstrates 84° flexion, 75° of elevation in the scapular plane, and 10° of external rotation in neutral. Active internal rotation is limited to the ability to place the back of her hand on her right sacroiliac joint. Passive motion for flexion, elevation in scaption, internal-external rotation (neutral, 45°, and 90° abduction), and scapular mobilization are continued. At this time, low-grade joint mobilizations for anterior, inferior, and posterior glides are started to increase capsular extensibility. Active ROM for strengthening, including supine flexion, seated short arc flexion, and scaption (45° to 90°), and tubing exercises for internal-external rotation in available ROM also are initiated. Aquatic exercises are started to promote both ROM and strength. The patient has access to a pool and is instructed in an independent exercise program for both ROM and strength progression. The patient is advised to begin using her right upper extremity for light functional activities below shoulder level.

At 8 weeks postoperative status, the patient continues to demonstrate consistent gains in both active and passive ROM. She reports compliance with her pool program and her land-based home program. The treatment routine continues three times per week through 12 weeks after surgery, with progression to high-grade (grade 4) joint mobilizations as needed. Low load progressive stretching using exercise bands is instituted for flexion and external rotation. At 12 weeks postoperative, the patient reports increased functional use of her right upper extremity, for example, she is now able to tuck in her shirt, put on her seatbelt, fasten her bra, and do light household chores. Her PROM has progressed to 148° flexion, 140° of elevation in scaption, and 63° of external rotation in abduction. Actively she is able to perform 140° flexion, 136° of elevation in scaption, 58° external rotation, and internal rotation to the level of T8. The patient is less compliant with attending physical therapy beginning at 10 weeks postoperative status. Therefore, the frequency of treatment is decreased to one time per week to monitor her strength and ROM and to increase and modify her home program.

At 20 weeks postoperative status, the patient demonstrates functional active ROM and strength. Passively she is able obtain 156° flexion, 148° of elevation in scaption, and 68° of external rotation in abduction. Actively, she can perform 150° of flexion, 144° of elevation in scaption, and 61° external rotation in 90° abduction. Internal rotation has not changed. The patient reports that she is generally noncompliant with her home exercise program, but appears to be satisfied with her present functional level. She reports minimal pain with activity and no pain at rest. At this time, the patient is discharged from physical therapy but encouraged to resume her home program to make additional ROM and strength gains.

CASE SUMMARY

This patient would be considered a part of the tissue-deficient rehabilitation group. Her rehabilitation was successful because the functional use of her right upper extremity was restored and pain was decreased. Although she did not achieve full ROM capability, her stability and function were considered more important. Several factors affected the outcome of this particular case, including age and general deconditioned state prior to surgery, lack of ROM prior to surgery, motivational level and noncompliance early in the rehabilitation process, lack of family help with the home program, and tissue deficiency with subsequent repair of the rotator cuff. Although progression of both active and passive motion is delayed to allow healing of the rotator cuff repair, rehabilitation should still be initiated early with the tissue deficient patient.

CHAPTER SUMMARY

Although the widespread use of unconstrained total shoulder prostheses has resulted in a marked decrease in complications, difficulties necessitating reoperation have been reported by many investigators.[36–41] However, analysis of prosthetic survivorship in TSA involving long-term clinical studies is limited. Current emphasis of orthopaedic clinic studies should be directed toward outcome research and the effects of treatment on the health of patients and their subsequent quality of life.[42] Cofield[43] performed an estimated 176 unconstrained total shoulder prostheses and predicted a 9.6% cumulative probability of failure at 5 years. The criterion for failure was defined as a need for major reoperation, which was performed on eight shoulders (5%). The indications for reoperation included early dislocation of three shoulders, loosening of the glenoid component in three shoulders, muscle transfer for paralysis of the axillary nerve in one shoulder, and resection arthroplasty and infection in one shoulder.[43]

Both proper exposure and surgical technique are necessary for proper component placement and soft tissue reconstruction. The postoperative rehabilitation program should be individualized according to the surgical indications, with the initial early goal of return of shoulder motion with gradual progression dictated by the patient's shoulder pathology and motivation. TSA requires much attention to detail not only in the choosing of the individual candidate and the surgical technique, but also in the rehabilitation program.

The goals of total shoulder rehabilitation include maximizing joint mobility through early ROM, protecting rotator cuff repair if applicable, and maximizing strength through a progressive exercise program. Optimal outcomes following TSA include improving the patient's health-related quality of life, returning the patient to his or her maximal level of independence with self-care and home management activities, and optimizing the patient's return to his or her role function (e.g., worker, spouse, grandparent).

A well-designed rehabilitation program is essential for achieving a successful outcome following TSA. Optimal recovery of function requires coordinated involvement of the patient, surgeon, and physical therapist in the rehabilitation process. The rehabilitation program itself needs to be a well-defined, logical sequence that respects tissue healing as well as joint mobility and stability, muscle strength, and function.

REFERENCES

1. Sisk, TD, and Wright, PE: Arthroplasty of the shoulder and elbow. In Crenshaw, AH (ed): Campbell's Operative Orthopaedics, ed 8. Mosby, St. Louis, 1992.
2. Massey, BF, and Ank, N: Biomechanics of the shoulder. In Rockwood, C, and Master, R (eds): The Shoulder. WB Saunders, Philadelphia, 1990.
3. Bergmann, G: Biomechanics and pathomechanics of the shoulder joint with reference to prosthetic joint replacement. In Koelbel, R, et al (eds): Shoulder Replacement. Spring-Verlag, Berlin, 1987, p 33.
4. Guide to Physical Therapist Practice. American Physical Therapy Association, Alexandria, VA, 1997.
5. Neer, CS: Articular replacement of the humeral head. J Bone Jt Surg [Am] 37A:215, 1955.
6. Neer, CS, et al: Cuff tear arthropathy. J Bone Jt Surg [Am] 65A:1233, 1983.
7. Cofield, RH: Degenerative and arthritic problems of the glenohumeral joint. In Rockwood, C, and Master, R (eds): The Shoulder, WB Saunders, Philadelphia, 1990.
8. Radosky, MW, and Bigliani, LU: Surgical treatment of nonconstrained glenoid component failure. Oper Tech in Orth 4:4 226, 1994.
9. Coughlin, MJ, et al: The semiconstrained total shoulder arthroplasty. J Bone Jt Surg [Am] 61A:574, 1979.
10. Engelbrecht, E, and Stelbrink, G: Totale schulterendoprosthese modell. St. Georg Chirurg 47:525, 1976.
11. Fenlin, JM Jr: Total glenohumeral joint replacement. Orthop Clin North Am 6:525, 1975.
12. Gristina, AG, and Webb, LX: The monospherical shoulder prosthesis (abst). Orthop Trans 8:88, 1984.
13. Neer, CS, et al: Recent experiences in total shoulder arthroplasty. J Bone Jt Surg [Am] 64:319, 1982.
14. Norris, TR, and Iannotti, JP: Prospective outcome study comparing humeral head replacement (HHR) vs. total shoulder replacement (TSR) for primary osteoarthritis. J Shoulder Elbow Surg [Am](Abstract) March/April, 1997.
15. Gartsman, GM, et al: Modular shoulder arthroplasty. J Shoulder Elbow Surgery July/Aug 1997, p 333.
16. Freeman, BG, and Allaryce, TV: Hemiarthroplasty in rotator cuff tear arthroplasty. Oper Tech in Orth 4:4 253, 1994.
17. Gristina, AG, et al: Total shoulder replacement. Orthop Clin North Am 18:445, 1987.
18. Competo, CA, et al: Arthroplasty and acute shoulder trauma: reasons for success and failure. Clin Orth and Rel Res, 7:27, 1956.

19. McGlynn, FJ: Total Shoulder Arthroplasty. In Andrews, JR, and Wilk, KE (eds): The Athletic Shoulder, Churchill Livingstone, Edinburgh, 1994.
20. Garaners, JC, et al: Milwaukee shoulder. Arthritis Rheum 24:484, 1981.
21. Halverson, DB, et al: Milwaukee shoulder-synovial fluid studies. Arthritis Rheum 24:474, 1981.
22. Azar, FS, and Wright, PE: Total Shoulder Arthroplasty. In Canale, ST (ed): Campbell's Operative Orthopaedics, ed 9. Mosby, Philadelphia, 1998, p 473.
23. Wirth, MA, and Rockwood, CA: Complications of total shoulder-replacement arthroplasty. J Bone Jt Surg, Current Concept Review, Vol 78A, No 4, 1996.
24. Barrett, WP, et al: Nonconstrained total shoulder arthroplasty in patients with polyarticular rheumatoid arthritis. Orthop Trans 11:466, 1987.
25. Barrett, WP, et al: Total shoulder arthroplasty. J Bone Jt Surg [Am] 69-A:865, 1987.
26. Frich, LH, et al: Shoulder arthroplasty with the Neer Mark-II prosthesis. Arch Orthop and Trauma Surg 107:110, 1988.
27. McCoy, SR, et al: Total shoulder arthroplasty in rheumatoid arthritis. J Arthroplasty 4:105, 1989.
28. Matsen, FA III, et al: Glenohumeral instability. In Rockwood, CA, and Matsen, FA III (eds): The Shoulder, Vol 1. WB Saunders, Philadelphia, 1990, p 534.
29. Martin, SD, et al: Total shoulder arthroplasty with an uncemented glenoid component. Read at the Annual Meeting of the American Shoulder and Elbow Surgeons, Orlando, Florida, February 1995.
30. Mazas, F, and de la Caffiniere, JY: Total arthroplasty of the shoulder: Experience with 38 cases. Orthop Trans 5:57, 1981.
31. Pollock, RG, et al: Prosthetic replacement in rotator cuff-deficient shoulders. J Shoulder and Elbow Surg [Am] 1:173, 1992.
32. Wainwright, D: Glenoidectomy. J Bone Jt Surg [Am] 58-B:377, 1986.
33. Craig, EV: Continuous passive motion in the rehabilitation of the surgically reconstructed shoulder: A preliminary report. Orthop Trans 10:219, 1986.
34. Neer, CS, et al: Earlier passive motion following shoulder arthroplasty and rotator cuff repair: A prospective study. Orthop Trans 10:219, 1986.
35. Brems, JJ, et al: Interscalene block anesthesia and shoulder surgery. Orthop Trans 14:250, 1990.
36. Boyd, AD Jr, et al: Total shoulder arthroplasty versus hemiarthroplasty: Indications for glenoid resurfacing. J Arthroplasty 5:329, 1990.
37. Brenner, BC, et al: Survivorship of unconstrained total shoulder arthroplasty. J Bone Jt Surg [Am] 71-A:1289, 1989.
38. Brostrom, LA, et al: Should the glenoid be replaced in shoulder arthroplasty with an unconstrained Dana or St. Georg prosthesis? Ann Chir Gynaecol 81:54, 1992.
39. Cofield, RH, and Daly, PJ: Total shoulder arthroplasty with a tissue-ingrowth glenoid component. J Shoulder and Elbow Surg 1:77, 1992.
40. Cruess, RL: Shoulder resurfacing according to the method of Neer. In Proceedings of the British Orthopaedic Association. J Bone Jt Surg [Br] 62-B(1):116, 1980.
41. Hawkins, RJ, et al: Total shoulder arthroplasty. Clin Orthop 242:188, 1989.
42. Gartland, JJ: Orthopaedic clinical research: Deficiencies in experimental design and determinations of outcome. J Bone Joint Surg [Am] 70-A:1357, 1988.
43. Cofield, RH: Unconstrained total shoulder prosthesis. Clin Orthop 173:97, 1983.

CHAPTER 12

Musculoskeletal Pattern J: Impaired Joint Mobility, Motor Function, Muscle Performance, and Range of Motion Associated With Bony or Soft Tissue Surgical Procedures

Lori Thein Brody, MS, PT, SCS, ATC

INTRODUCTION

Although impaired joint mobility develops at the shoulder for a variety of reasons, most operative procedures are followed by a period of decreased mobility. Postoperative hypomobility might result from pain, swelling, and muscle impairment. Mobility can also be decreased by actual biomechanical alterations made during surgery. For example, a procedure that tightens the joint capsule might alter the previous relative glenoid and humeral positions. Previous stabilization procedures such as the Bristow involve the insertion of actual mechanical barriers to movement. The clinician has many tools available to improve range of motion. However, deciding which tools to use and when to use them postoperatively can be challenging.

This chapter reviews common shoulder surgical procedures and discusses postoperative management of impaired joint mobility. Understanding the intent of the surgical procedure provides the clinician with the necessary guidelines and framework for appropriate treatment decision making, even though each surgeon might have individual adaptations of these procedures, necessitating rehabilitation modifications. (The specific details of therapeutic exercise are covered elsewhere in this book; see Chaps. 16 to 17). The chapter concludes with a case study that reviews clinical decision making, evaluating a patient, and implementing a treatment program to prevent impaired joint mobility following surgery.

SOFT TISSUE HEALING

Understanding the soft tissue healing process provides the basis for choosing the right intervention at the right time. Hypomobility might result from too little activity in the early phases, whereas hypermobility might result from too much activity in some cases. The intervention must be matched to the impairment or functional limitation at the correct time. The phases of healing provide guidance for these choices.

A surgical procedure is like any other acute injury. The tissues progress through a series of healing phases beginning with the inflammatory response.

Phase I: Inflammatory Response

Healing of acute injuries passes through three major phases, beginning with the acute vascular-inflammatory response. When soft tissues are damaged, injured cells in the area release chemical substances that initiate the inflammatory response. Local bleeding occurring during surgery acts as a strong chemotactic stimulus, attracting white blood cells that help rid the site of bacteria and cellular debris via phagocytosis. Vasodilation increases local blood flow, whereas altered capillary permeability allows greater exudation of plasma proteins and white blood cells. In this phase, the damaged tissues and microorganisms are removed, fibroblasts are recruited, and some wound strength is provided by immature collagen fibers.[1] This phase is initiated at the time of surgery and lasts 3 to 5 days.[1]

Clinical signs and symptoms characteristic of the inflammatory phase include pain, warmth, palpable tenderness, and swelling. Joint or muscle range of motion are generally limited because of pain or direct tissue damage.

Phase II: Repair-Regeneration

The repair-regenerative phase, which follows the inflammatory phase, lasts from 48 hours to 8 weeks. The hallmark of this phase is the presence of the tissue macrophage, which directs the cascade of events of this phase. Fibroblasts actively resorb old collagen and synthesize new collagen, characterized by small fibrils, disorganized in orientation, and deficient in cross-linking.[1] This tissue is easily damaged by overly aggressive activity. As this phase progresses, tissue macrophage and fibroblast activity gradually decreases. During this phase, the warmth and edema resolve, and the palpable tenderness decreases. Tissues will now tolerate gentle loading, which will help align the healing collagen fibrils.

Phase III: Remodeling-Maturation

The maturation-remodeling phase is characterized by increased organization of extracellular matrices. Although some synthesis still occurs, the main activity is the organization and strengthening of randomly placed fibrils to form new collagen. This new collagen must orient and align along the lines of stress to accommodate the shoulder's functional loads. Tension, in the form of stretching, active contraction, resistive loads, or electrical stimulation guides this process. The exact end point for tissue remodeling is unknown. However, months to years are believed to be necessary for completion of remodeling.

STABILIZATION PROCEDURES

The glenohumeral (GH) joint sacrifices inherent structural stability to enhance its functional mobility (see Chap. 1). As such, this joint is susceptible to hypermobility problems. Surgical stabilization is indicated when hypermobility results in functional limitations or disability that are unresolved with conservative treatment. Individuals who experience instability with routine daily activities (reaching into the back seat of a car, working overhead, rolling over in sleep) are candidates for stabilization procedures. These symptoms can be disabling if the individual is unable to fulfill expected roles (e.g., worker, student, spouse, parent) because of the instability. Many procedures are available, and the treatment choice depends on factors such as the direction(s) of instability, age of the patient, physical demands on the shoulder, and the history of instability.[2–4] Additionally, some of the same procedures are performed openly via arthrotomy (creation of a full incision in the joint through which surgery is performed) in some cases and arthroscopically (small porthole incisions are made into the joint to view inside the joint with a scope) in others.

Stabilization procedures are generally classified into capsular repairs, subscapularis muscle procedures, bone blocks, coracoid transfers, and miscellaneous procedures (fascia lata slings, osteotomies).[3] Some procedures use bioabsorbable materials, whereas others use sutures or hardware left in place. Most procedures are performed for chronic instability, although procedures for acute stabilization also are being performed.[2] The most common stabilization procedures and the postoperative treatment guidelines are discussed in this chapter. Capsular repair procedures, which address the primary pathology in anterior instability and maintain full or nearly full mobility postoperatively, are most widely accepted by orthopaedic surgeons.[3]

Anterior Instability: The Bankart Repair

The Bankart repair, one of the most common stabilization procedures performed because of its common indications, is performed to address the "essential lesion" or *Bankart lesion* occurring in approximately 80% to 97% of acute traumatic anterior dislocations.[3–6] The Bankart lesion is an avulsion of the ligaments, capsule, and labrum from the anteroinferior glenoid rim.[3,7,8] The Hill Sachs lesion, which often accompanies a dislocation, is a compression fracture of the posterior humeral head resulting from impaction of the humeral head, on the glenoid rim (Fig. 12–1). The surgeon's goal is to repair the Bankart avulsion back to the glenoid through an open incision or arthroscopy.

Whereas the Bankart lesion is termed the *essential lesion*, no single lesion is common to all cases.[9] Variable disruption is possible with injury primarily to the inferior glenohumeral ligament, or the ligament and capsulolabral structures. The inferior glenohumeral ligament might be stretched or torn, alone or in combination

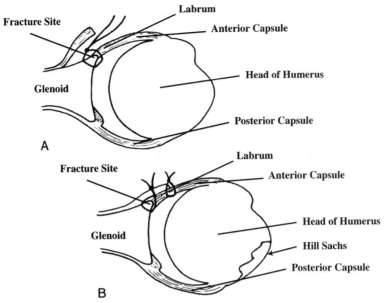

FIGURE 12–1. *(A)* Bankart lesion is a fracture of the anterior rim of the glenoid fossa with the attached labrum where the labrum is pulled away from the anterior glenoid, along with a small piece of glenoid. *(B)* The Hill Sachs lesion is compression fracture of the postero-lateral humeral head after a traumatic anterior dislocation of the GH joint.

with other injuries. The adjacent joint capsule and the attachments at the glenoid labrum might be disrupted. Detachments of the capsulolabral complex are common. Additionally, avulsion of ligaments from the humerus and glenoid fractures can occur.[10,11]

The function of surgery is to restore *normal anatomy.* Thus, all injured structures must be identified either preoperatively or at the time of surgery to ensure all contributors to instability are addressed. The Bankart lesion by itself is generally insufficient to allow complete glenohumeral dislocation.[5]

Indications for a Bankart repair include an individual with a history of a traumatic anterior dislocation and a discrete Bankart lesion without rotator cuff pathology or arthritis.[9] Voluntary instability (the ability to voluntarily dislocate one's own shoulder) is an absolute contraindication for any stabilization procedure. In this situation, the patient has learned a neuromuscular pattern of dislocation that will not be corrected with surgery. Neuromuscular retraining is necessary prior to considering surgical stabilization.

The Bankart procedure may be performed via an arthrotomy or arthroscopy. If performed arthroscopically, the shoulder joint and subacromial space are examined arthroscopically as part of the repair procedure. Visualization of these two spaces is difficult with an open repair. As a result, some surgeons examine the shoulder arthroscopically prior to the open Bankart repair. Swenson and Warner[9] noted a 20% conversion rate of arthroscopic to open procedures based on their examination under anesthesia (EUA) and arthroscopic findings. Benefits of the open repair included potentially greater stability postoperatively, whereas benefits of the arthroscopic repair included improved cosmesis and increased external rotation motion. As with any surgical procedure, these benefits vary by surgeon and patient.

Typically, the surgical procedure begins with an EUA similar to the clinical examination. Translation in each direction is checked, asymmetries noted, and the presence of any clicking or grinding and the direction that produces these findings is acknowledged.[12] Following the EUA, arthroscopy of both the GH joint and the subacromial space is performed.[4,7] This procedure provides the surgeon with the additional benefit of looking inside the shoulder joint to verify the clinical findings.

The Bankart repair is accomplished with staple fixation, transosseous suture repair, or absorbable polyglyconate "tacking" devices.[13–16] However, the absorbable tacking devices lose their holding strength and might resorb over a 4- to 6-week period following implantation.[13] In some cases, resorption might take as long as 6 months.[9] Biodegradable tacking device materials are preferred because of the increased risk of complications associated with loosening, migration, and breakage of metallic implants.[17] These tacking devices also eliminate the need for transglenoid drilling or suture tying.

The arthroscopic Bankart repair has been criticized for a higher number of failures as compared to when the open procedure is used.[13,18–20] A weaker repair resulting from less concomitant capsular scarring combined with the low pull-out strength (resistant to tensile forces) of all these procedures might impact the success rate of the arthroscopic procedure. Failure of arthroscopic Bankart repairs might also be affected by the population treated. Individuals younger than 30 years old and who participate in collision sports might be at greater risk for failure.[21]

The most common complication following surgical stabilization is impaired mobility. Other complications includes loosening of surgical hardware such as staples or tacks, osteoarthritis, infection, pain, and inability to return to the previous level of activity.[22] Recognition of both ends of the impaired mobility continuum (hyper- and hypomobility) ensures appropriate treatment modification. Recurrent instability and motion loss contribute to dissatisfaction following surgery. A study that reviewed failed arthroscopic Bankart procedures found 60% of the Bankart lesions to be healed at the time of revision (usually done as an open procedure).[23] Redundant anterior capsules were present in 75% of these patients. Although capsular laxity is difficult to quantify arthroscopically, and might be underestimated in many patients, many individuals with acute dislocations also have significant capsular laxity.[17] Failure to successfully treat the Bankart lesion results in dislocations, whereas failure to address the capsular laxity produces subluxations.[23]

At the other end of the continuum, hypomobility can be a significant problem. A biomechanical study of Bankart reconstruction procedures found the shoulder capsule to be very sensitive to anterior capsular shortening.[24] Patients who were evaluated nearly 12 years post-Bankart procedure were found to have a mean loss of 12° of external rotation.[25] A 2- to 8-year follow-up of arthroscopic Bankart and/or capsulorrhaphy procedures found a mean loss of 3° of external rotation.[15]

Anterior or Multidirectional Instability: Capsulorrhaphy Procedures

Capsular tightening procedures are performed alone or in combination with Bankart procedures. Capsulorrhaphy is performed alone when instability without a Bankart lesion exists. When a Bankart lesion is also present, the procedure is sometimes called a *modified Bankart procedure,* which combines a Bankart repair with various techniques of reefing or plicating a redundant capsule.[26,27] Many different versions of capsulorrhaphy exist, and postoperative rehabilitation will vary depending on the surgeon's findings and preferred procedures.

Surgery is indicated in those individuals who have failed conservative management and who continue to have severe pain, disabling instability with activities of daily living, or persistent paresthesias.[28] Capsular shift procedures are indicated when the inferior capsule and glenohumeral ligaments are lax. This situation occurs following acute anterior dislocations when the ligaments are stretched with or without sustaining a Bankart lesion.[15] The capsular laxity occurring after traumatic dislocations can be overlooked in the presence of a Bankart lesion.[11,16,17] The goal of the inferior capsular shift is to reduce the volume of the joint capsule anteriorly, posteriorly, and inferiorly, providing balance around the humeral head.[29]

Several types of capsular tightening procedures are performed, either openly or using arthroscopically-assisted techniques. An anterior or posterior approach can be used. A T-plasty is combined with repair of a Bankart lesion (if present) to decrease the inferior axillary recess. The inferior and lateral capsule is advanced medially and superiorly via a transverse capsular incision, with a vertical incision made either medially along the glenoid or laterally along the humeral head.[26,27] If two vertical incisions are made, it is considered an H-plasty (Fig. 12–2).[4] A variable amount of capsule is resected, depending on the amount of redundancy in the capsule.[15] The free edge of the capsule is then repaired to the glenoid margin adjacent to the labrum. This procedure tightens the capsule and also provides an additional anterior soft tissue block.

Capsular tightening procedures are also performed in individuals with multidirectional instability. The inferior capsular shift is a final course of treatment once conservative measures have failed. Thus, the surgical decision making in this population is more difficult than that involving the individual with traumatic instability. The inferior capsular shift is performed to reduce capsular redundancy and to provide symmetric tightening of the capsule. Additionally, this procedure may be modified as determined by the direction of greatest laxity. An anterior approach advances the inferior and posterior capsule anteriorly on the humeral neck. The posterior approach advances the redundant capsule posteriorly.

Some surgeons use other tools such as the holmium: yttrium-aluminum-garnet (Ho-YAG) laser or radiofrequency devices to shrink redundant capsule arthroscopically.[30–32] This procedure addresses the capsular laxity seen in traumatic (with or without a Bankart lesion) and atraumatic instability. These tools provide shrinkage and tightening of the capsule, with results simulating a capsulorrhaphy. Long-term results and their resultant rehabilitation implications are yet to be determined. Currently, rehabilitation follows the guidelines for traditional capsulorrhaphy.

Rehabilitation Considerations for Anterior Stabilization

Although postoperative expectations vary by surgeon and surgical technique, an understanding of general range of motion (ROM) expectations guides the intervention choices. Some surgeons prefer restricted motion in the early postoperative phase to protect the stabilization.[3] Because this is primarily a soft tissue procedure, adequate time is allowed for healing to occur at the surgical site. The shoulder is placed in an immobilizer for 2 to 3 weeks, with removal for elbow, wrist, and hand motion. Although passive external rotation is avoided for the first 6 weeks, pendulum

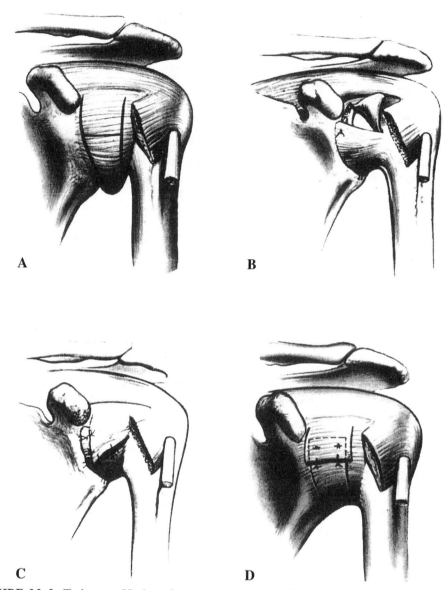

FIGURE 12–2. T-plasty or H-plasty for capsular laxity. *(A)* Capsular incisions for performing a T-plasty or H-plasty. *(B)* The inferior portion of the T-plasty advanced superiorly and medially to decrease the inferior redundancy. *(C)* The superior portion of the T-plasty advanced inferiorly to reinforce the repair. *(D)* The completed H-plasty, performed for marked inferior laxity. (From Nicholas, JA, and Hershman, EB: The Upper Extremity in Sports Medicine. CV Mosby, St. Louis, 1990.)

exercises and active range of motion activities are started by the third week. Despite these early motion restrictions, full motion is expected by 10 to 12 weeks in most individuals and by 6 to 8 weeks in throwing athletes.[22] External rotation is at greatest risk of restriction, and loss of motion at the shoulder is associated with degenerative joint disease.[33] As such, restoration of normal range of motion without placing the repair at risk is imperative.

Posterior Stabilization

Posterior instability is often overlooked in the clinic because nearly 95% of shoulder instability occurs in an anterior direction.[3,4,34] However, posterior instability can be problematic for many individuals. Posterior subluxation is a more common problem than posterior dislocation. Functional activities such as pushing doors open, pushing carts, or weightbearing on the hands are painful in individuals with posterior instability. Acute traumatic posterior instability also occurs and is often associated with a posterior Bankart lesion.[35] Hawkins and Janda have categorized patients with posterior instability into four groups (Box 12–1).

Treatment considerations for posterior instability are the same as those for anterior instability. A trial of conservative care may precede any surgical intervention. Like anterior stabilization procedures, posterior procedures are generally categorized as repair of the posterior soft tissues, posterior bone blocks, glenoid osteotomy, or a combination of procedures.[27,36,37] In most situations, the posterio-inferior capsular shift corrects the problem. Augmentation with a posterior bone block is reserved for unusual cases.[38] Historically, failure rates following surgical repair for posterior instability have been high.[34,37,39]

Like anterior or multidirectional instability, surgery, performed via arthrotomy or arthroscopy, begins with an examination under anesthesia. Arthroscopic examination of the GH joint and subacromial space can confirm clinical findings. Common findings at surgery include redundancy in the posterior and inferior capsular pouches, partial or complete detachment of the posterior labrum, and labral wear and chip fractures of the posterior glenoid.[36] The same biodegradable tacks used anteriorly can be used posteriorly to reattach detached capsule and labrum (posterior Bankart) (Fig. 12–3). A capsular stabilization procedure (T-plasty, H-plasty) is performed if capsular redundancy is contributing to posterior instability.

REHABILITATION CONSIDERATIONS

Postoperative rehabilitation recommendations following posterior capsulorrhaphy include 4 to 6 weeks of immobilization followed by passive ROM for 2 weeks, active ROM and stretching for an additional 4 weeks, and subsequent strengthening.[37] Early passive motion into external rotation may be initiated for throwers. Internal rotation and elevation in the sagittal plane are avoided for the first 6 weeks to prevent excessive forces on the posterior capsule. Following posterior stabilization, internal rotation motion loss is the major impaired joint mobility problem. Gentle strengthening exercises are initiated approximately 2 weeks after immobilization is discontinued, with return to light throwing at 4 months.[34]

BOX 12–1 Classification of Posterior Shoulder Instability

1. Acute posterior dislocation, with and without impression defect
2. Chronic posterior dislocation, locked with impression defect
3. Voluntary recurrent posterior subluxation, habitual and muscular control
4. Involuntary recurrent posterior subluxation, positional and nonpositional

---

Adapted from Hawkins, RJ, and Janda, DH: Posterior instability of the glenohumeral joint: a technique of repair. Am J Sports Med 24(3):275, 1996.

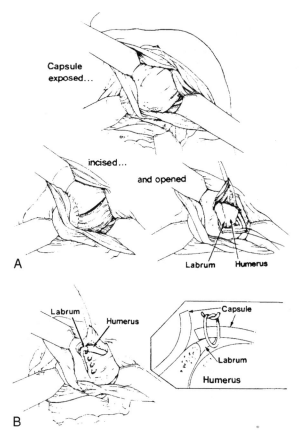

Capsule
exposed...

incised...

and opened

Labrum   Humerus

A

Labrum

Humerus

Capsule

Labrum

Humerus

B

FIGURE 12–3. Posterior stabilization procedure. *(A)* The capsule is exposed and a transverse incision is made. Two capsular flaps are developing by "T-ing" the capsule parallel to the glenoid and adjacent to the labrum. *(B)* The inferior capsular flap is advanced superiorly and medially and attached to the labrum. (From Rockwood, CA, and Matsen, FA:The Shoulder. WB Saunders, Philadelphia, 1990, p 985, with permission.)

Management of Impaired Joint Mobility Following Stabilization Procedures

Tests and measures used in this situation include patient history and measures of impairments (loss of motion, decreased joint accessory motion, pain) and functional limitations (inability to comb hair, hook bra). These test results provide the guide for rehabilitation. These examination findings must be considered in light of the surgical procedure, presurgical impairments and functional limitations, any comorbidities, and the time from surgery. An understanding of the expected mobility following different surgical procedures guides the implementation of different mobilization techniques.

If hypomobility persists beyond expectations following shoulder stabilization, the number of physical therapy visits might fall outside the expected range for this pattern. Greater supervision and manual treatment might be necessary to ensure the expected outcome. Additionally, the reason for falling outside the normal mobility expectations should be determined. Range of motion examination, joint accessory testing, and scar examination should clarify the hypomobility source. A capsular pattern of limitation versus a unidirectional loss of motion (such as external rotation in anterior stabilization or internal rotation in posterior stabilization) will guide interventions chosen. Any scar tissue adhesions around the surgical site might be an additional source of noncapsular hypomobility. Impaired muscle performance or pain might contribute to hypomobility because of an inability to move through expected ranges postoperatively. If hardware was used in the procedure, failure of that hardware, for example, migration, should be considered as a potential cause of hypomobility. Nonadherence with the home exercise program, reinjury, or other comorbidities can contribute to persistent hypomobility.

Interventions chosen for the hypomobile shoulder are directed at the cause of the motion limitation. Motion loss resulting from true capsulitis might fall into musculoskeletal pattern D: impaired joint mobility, motor function muscle performance, and range of motion associated with capsular restriction. Direct interventions include therapeutic exercise, functional training, manual therapy, and modalities. Therapeutic exercise and manual therapy include stretching, mobilization, and strengthening activities performed on land or in the pool. Techniques include connective tissues massage, passive range of motion, and joint or soft tissue mobilization. Aggressive mobilization to lengthen a shortened capsule can be used after 4 months if motion restrictions remain. If an inferior capsular shift was performed, the normal glenohumeral biomechanics during elevation should be considered. As the arm is elevated, the humeral head must drop inferiorly, putting stress on the inferior capsule. If the patient is getting primary impingement symptoms during elevation, limited inferior mobility might be the cause. Conversely, this movement is approached cautiously in individuals with hypermobility to avoid any stretching of the inferior capsular pouch.

If motion loss is the result of isolated loss of external or internal rotation exceeding the postsurgical expectations, manual therapy and range of motion techniques should focus on restoring this motion. Close communication with the surgeon will alert the clinician to any anomalies that might be contributing to this hypomobility. Additional pathology, such as labral lesions and degenerative changes, might compromise postoperative motion gains. In the absence of these factors, intervention to restore unidirectional loss of motion should be instituted when the patient begins to fall outside the usual postoperative range norms.

The skin is examined to determine if restrictions around the surgical site are contributing to hypomobility. After the surgical incisions close, massage over the wounds is instituted to maintain mobility of the skin and underlying fascial layers. This mobilization is continued until the soft tissue mobility around the incisions is similar to the surrounding area.

As new range of motion develops, muscle control in the new range is necessary to maintain that motion. Individuals with significant weakness might develop hypomobility because of an inability to move the shoulder into expected ranges. If the primary problem is impaired muscle performance, the patient might fall into musculoskeletal pattern C: impaired muscle performance (see Chap. 4). In this case, a combination of range of motion and mobilization exercises coupled with progressive resistive exercise should be instituted. For example, if the external rotator muscles are weak, a combination of resistive exercises for this muscle group along with mobilization into external rotation can be used. Increasing the range into external rotation simultaneously decreases the amount of torque necessary to attain the same degree of rotation.

If pain is the chief cause of hypomobility, the cause of pain must be determined and treated. Electrotherapeutic, mechanical, or thermal modalities may accompany other techniques to decrease pain.

Despite the risk of development of instability, aggressive mobility exercises should be instituted if significant motion loss still exists beyond typical postoperative expectations. The clinician must consider *how much* motion is lost and whether this loss impairs *function* or could lead to the development of osteoarthritis. Any loss of function at the shoulder will be accommodated for by adjacent joints or the other shoulder, placing these structures at risk. The development of osteoarthritis has significant disability implications. Thus, restoration of motion following these procedures can provide tertiary care and prevent secondary residual disability.

SUBACROMIAL DECOMPRESSION

Primary impingement syndrome is a common problem treated in the clinic. Most cases of impingement syndrome resolve with conservative management, including physical therapy interventions and medical management using oral and injectable medications. However, some cases do not resolve despite appropriate conservative measures. In these cases, subacromial decompression or acromioplasty may be performed. An acromioplasty presumes the cause of symptoms to be related to an expansion of the contents of the subacromial space, a decrease in the size of the subacromial space, abnormal biomechanics, or abnormal anatomy.[40] These conditions produce pain in the shoulder, particularly pain with overhead movement. Decompression is performed primarily to relieve the patient's pain.[41] Additionally, if a rotator cuff repair is performed, a simultaneous decompression provides extra room for the repair. Like other shoulder surgical procedures, the outcome is the result of appropriate patient selection, good surgical technique, and appropriate postoperative rehabilitation.

Decompression consists of several different procedures, some or all of which might be performed on any given patient. These procedures might include resection of the coracoacromial ligament, the anterolateral undersurface of the acromion, the lateral portion of the clavicle, and any osteophytes (Fig. 12–4). The acromioclavicular joint is not routinely removed as part of this procedure, although resection might be indicated when this joint is painful.[42] The subacromial decompression can be performed either openly or arthroscopically. Early reports of arthroscopic decompression were less satisfactory when compared to the open procedure, but as experience with the arthroscope at the shoulder progressed, outcomes have improved.[43]

Arthroscopy offers the advantage of better intraarticular visualization and the lower likelihood of overlooking rotator cuff pathology and labral tears. Additionally, less trauma to the deltoid muscle and less scarring enhance immediate postoperative function.[42–44] A 1-year follow-up of open versus arthroscopic decompression results showed that the arthroscopic groups had earlier gains that are matched by the open group at 1 year.[45]

Complications following open acromioplasty include persistent pain, acromial fracture, glenohumeral hypomobility, weakness, infection, and detachment of the deltoid.[42,46] Many of these complications can be attributed to problems with the following three keys to successful intervention: appropriate diagnosis, surgical technique, and adequate postoperative rehabilitation. Diagnostic errors include overlooking underlying instability or the early signs of degenerative joint disease. Surgical errors include removing too little or too much bone.[43] Complications following arthroscopic acromioplasty are fewer, and are primarily related to inadequate tissue removal necessitating additional surgery.[42] Patients generally have difficulty returning to high demand sports following acromioplasty procedures.[43]

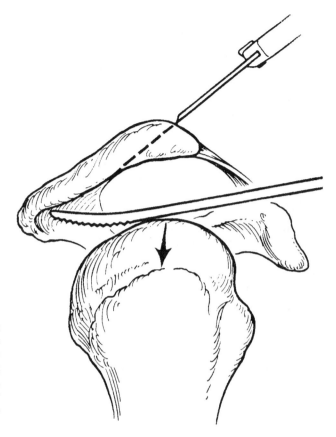

FIGURE 12–4. One component of the decompression procedure includes resecting the anterioinferior surface of the acromion using an osteotome. (From Rockwood, CA, and Matsen, FA: The Shoulder. WB Saunders, Philadelphia, 1990, p 641, with permission.)

Rehabilitation Considerations and Management of Impaired Joint Mobility

Continued pain postoperatively is one of the primary treatment considerations. However, restoration of motion is critical to the long-term outcome of the procedure. Gentle range of motion exercises, including pendulum and elbow, wrist, and hand mobility activities, are initiated immediately after surgery. Passive range of motion into flexion is allowed within pain tolerance. After the first week, active range of motion and gentle progressive resistive exercises are added. The patient should have full motion by 4 to 6 weeks postoperatively.

If hypomobility persists postoperatively, the history will play an important role. Those patients with hypomobility prior to and at surgery might not achieve full motion postoperatively. A study of 40 patients found three to require manipulation after decompression.[47] Although only three underwent manipulation, ten patients had forward elevation less than 120°. Limited motion before surgery might persist after surgery, and the prognosis might need to be modified.

Examination for impairments and functional limitations should consider the altered biomechanics that often result from long-standing impingement syndrome. Hypomobility might be the result of a true capsulitis with capsular pattern motion loss, or elevation might be the primary direction lost because of impingement pain with movement in this direction. Loss of mobility in the joint capsule can produce an impingement by preventing humeral head depression during humeral elevation. Restoration of the normal arthrokinematics (whether unidirectional or multidirectional) is essential to returning the patient to a pain-free state. Interventions for hypomobility resulting from capsular or extraarticular restrictions focus on range of motion activities and manual techniques. Soft tissue massage might be necessary when postoperative scarring contributes to hypomobility. If hypomobility is the result of pain or impaired muscle performance, these impairments must also be addressed.

Postural examination might reveal habitual postures such as excessive scapular protraction contributing to impingement. The patient might fall into musculoskeletal pattern B: impaired posture. Long-standing impingement might also produce faulty movement patterns and substitution patterns that minimize pain. For example, the patient might elevate the arm with abnormal scapulohumeral rhythm using primarily scapular elevators. This faulty movement pattern results in poor motor programming and a subsequent loss of mobility in the inferior capsule. This pattern will further compound hypomobility resulting from impingement. Interventions will include therapeutic exercise to stretch shortened soft tissues, muscle reeducation and subsequent strengthening, coupled with joint and soft tissue mobilization.

ROTATOR CUFF REPAIR

The rotator cuff can be a source of pain for many individuals. Rotator cuff pathology can occur as a result of tensile failure, compressive impingement, instability, traumatic tears, and calcific rotator cuff tendonitis. These injuries can occur interstitially, on the bursal side, or on the articular side, and can give rise to some of the classification systems for rotator cuff pathology. Treatment depends on several factors including the cause of the pathology, the age of the patient, size and location of the tear, and the duration of symptoms.[48] Other pathology such as long head of the biceps rupture might accompany rotator cuff tears. Many individuals with rotator cuff tears do well without surgical intervention.[49,50] Pain following a rotator cuff tear often comes from sources other than the tear. These sources might be mechanical (impingement, edge instability) or biological (synovitis, intraarticular pathology, adhesive capsulitis).[49,50] Rehabilitation to restore motion and function can return individuals to function without pain in activities of daily living and in some light sports. However, others in heavy labor or vigorous sports often require surgical intervention to debride, repair, and decompress the rotator cuff. Repair might include tendon-to-tendon repair and tendon advancement to bone.[51] Fixation involves the use of sutures through bone tunnels or suture anchors. The suture anchors have been found to be as strong as or stronger than suture repair to bone.[50]

The goals of rotator cuff surgery are to relieve pain and to restore function, achieved by simple debridement or rotator cuff repair.[52] Simply relieving the pain ultimately restores function in some individuals who have disabling pain. In others, pain relief allows full participation in a rehabilitation program that restores function, or the surgical procedure itself restores muscle function. Because long-standing pain or dysfunction often leads to disuse of the limb, hypomobility might compound the problem. Operative intervention in the presence of significant hypomobility is contraindicated because of the likelihood of further hypomobility.[53]

Surgical procedures for the rotator cuff vary depending on several factors. As with other surgical procedures, rotator cuff repair is performed arthroscopically, openly, or as a combination procedure, called a *miniopen*.[48] A distinct advantage of arthroscopic procedures is lack of disruption to the deltoid muscle. If the rotator cuff tear is the result of compressive impingement, decompression with arthroscopic or open rotator cuff repair is performed. Repair generally includes creating a trough into the vascularized bone, followed by drilling holes for the sutures. The rotator cuff is then pulled through the trough and stabilized with sutures (Fig. 12–5). If the tear has occurred secondary to instability, the shoulder is stabilized before any other procedure is performed. Traumatic tears in young or other high demand individuals are generally repaired through open procedures. However, partial tears in young athletes are being repaired by arthroscopy with good results in some subgroups.[54] A study of 43 athletes found 64% of those with acute traumatic injuries returned to sports following debridement and decompression. Athletes involved in overhead sports were less likely to return to their sports. The nontraumatic subgroups showed only 25% to 50% returned to sports.[54]

Preoperative patient selection is key is critical to postoperative outcome. Careful examination can identify coexisting injuries or clarify the primary diagnosis. For example, a traumatic dislocation in individuals over 40 years of age is more likely to produce a rotator cuff tear than recurrent instability.[55]

Long-standing rotator cuff tears that have been asymptomatic might become symptomatic with increased activity or a subsequent injury. Radiographs demonstrating superior humeral head migration are evidence of an old rotator cuff tear. This

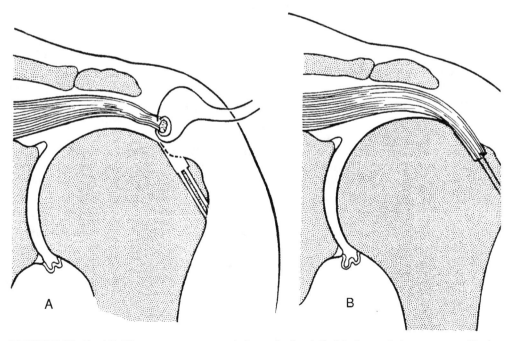

FIGURE 12–5. *(A)* The sutures are passed through the drilled holes and the rotator cuff edge drawn deep into the trough. *(B)* The sutures are tied through the drill holes. (From Rockwood, CA, and Matsen, FA. The Shoulder. WB Saunders, Philadelphia, 1990, p 670, with permission.)

migration might eventually produce subacromial symptoms that are relieved with debridement and decompression.

Surgical failures generally result from the pulling out of sutures from the tendon, suture breakage, postoperative adhesions, inadequate decompression, and deltoid reattachment failure (if done openly).

Rehabilitation Considerations

Rehabilitation following rotator cuff repair depends on factors such as the size of the tear, the quality of the tissue, and any associated pathology. Preoperative range of motion might be decreased, contributing to hypomobility postoperatively. Two years following a miniopen rotator cuff repair, one group of patients had a mean of 49° external rotation, 159° abduction, and 161° flexion. These values were slightly better than the open repair group.[48]

Postoperative rehabilitation for small rotator cuff repairs includes 2 weeks of immobilization with active range of motion of the elbow, wrist, and hand and shoulder shrugs. No active abduction is allowed for the first 3 weeks. Active and passive range of motion and isometric exercises are started at 2 weeks with progressive mobility and strength up until return to activity at 5 to 6 months postoperatively.

Patients with large rotator cuff repairs are immobilized for 4 weeks. Rehabilitation is then progressed in the same manner as that for small tears. Full functional range of motion is expected postoperatively.

Hypomobility following rotator cuff repair can be the result of true capsulitis, pain and secondary disuse, or of poor muscle function. Additionally, because a decompression is generally performed simultaneously, any of the contributors to hypomobility can also occur following rotator cuff repair. As with other surgical procedures, pain or scar restrictions can contribute to hypomobility and should be treated when found.

The examination is the same as for those with hypomobility following other shoulder surgical procedures. History is again important, because decreased mobility prior to surgery often persists postoperatively. Prognosis and the expected range and number of visits might have to be modified.

Intervention for hypomobility focuses on the findings contributing to the hypomobility and functional loss. The key interventions include range of motion and manual techniques. While postoperative motion restrictions might be in place following stabilization procedures, postoperative resistive exercises are often restricted following rotator cuff repair. As such, muscle function might be the greatest contributor to hypomobility. Communication with the surgeon will ensure progression to resistive exercises in a time frame appropriate for each individual patient, given the size and location of the tear and the quality of the tissue. Passive, active-assisted, and active exercise can maintain mobility until more vigorous resistance can be initiated.

OTHER LABRAL PROCEDURES

Although the Bankart procedure is the most common labral repair performed, other labral pathologies can be symptomatic. Labral problems result from acute injuries or chronic wear and tear. The SLAP (superior labrum anterior and posterior) lesion is a common symptom-producing labral injury. This injury is associated with falls on an outstretched arm, sudden deceleration or traction forces such as catching a falling, heavy object, and anterior and posterior instability. Posterior labral tears and rotator cuff tears can be found in cases of chronic instability.[56,57] Cyst formation resulting from fluid leakage under a detached labrum can also produce symptoms.[22] These individuals generally complain of nonspecific posterior pain, increased with overhead activity, instability, and popping.[58,59,60] Some have loss of external rotation motion.[60]

SLAP lesions are classified using a I to IV or I to VII grading system.[60,61] According to the Snyder classification, a type I lesion refers to fraying or tearing of the superior labrum without any instability of the biceps complex, whereas a type II lesion includes instability of the biceps and its labral attachment. Type III lesions are bucket-handled tears without extension into the biceps, and type IV lesions extend into the biceps.[61] Others have found lesions that did not fit into the I to IV classification system and added the following additional classifications: type V, an anteroinferior Bankart lesion continuing superiorly to include separation of the biceps tendon; type VI, an unstable flap tear of the labrum in addition to biceps tendon separation; and type VII, extension of the superior labrum-biceps complex beneath the middle glenohumeral ligament.[60]

Conservative management of these tears often fails, and patients usually require surgery after approximately 10 months from symptom onset.[62] Surgery to treat labral lesions must include an EUA and an arthroscopic examination. Other pathologies such as rotator cuff tears, instability, and acromioclavicular arthritis can accompany labral lesions.[61] Failure to acknowledge and address this associated pathology can lead to postoperative failures. Repair of the labral lesion includes debridement and reattachment of the labrum using techniques similar to Bankart repairs.[62] Specific procedures vary by classification of tear and surgeon preference.

Rehabilitation Considerations

Following surgery, a sling is used for comfort for the first 2 weeks, accompanied by gentle elbow, wrist, and hand motion, and shoulder pendulum exercises. Active and passive range of motion proceeds with pain as a guide. Special attention is given to elevation and avoidance of impingement in the superior aspect of the shoulder. Joint mobilization may be performed in cases in which hypomobility persists. However, the location of injury and surgery and the type of surgical repair must be considered. Overly aggressive mobilization could potentially disrupt the healing labral attachment.

Loss of motion can occur in any direction or in multiple directions, depending on the location of the labral tear. True capsulitis can develop with loss of motion in a capsular pattern. Hypomobility might be unidirectional, depending on the location of the repair. Regardless of capsular or noncapsular patterns of limitation, range of motion and manual techniques will be necessary to restore motion. Restoration of normal arthrokinematics is of particular importance following labral repair to prevent impingement of the humeral head on the repair. Passive and active mobility must be restored to ensure that muscle imbalances do not create an imbalance and impingement despite normal arthrokinematic mobility.

CASE STUDY 12–1

EXAMINATION

JM is a 17-year-old right-handed high school football and baseball player. While playing football near the end of the season, he sustained a left shoulder anterior-inferior dislocation during a pile-up. He was taken to the emergency room where his dislocation was confirmed, then reduced. JM was placed in a sling and instructed to follow up with an orthopaedic surgeon 2 days later. When reevaluated at that time, JM demonstrated apprehension with abduction and external rotation and limited range of motion throughout his shoulder. Radiographs showed a small Hill Sachs lesion (fracture along the posterior and lateral aspects of the humeral head, often the result of a traumatic anterior dislocation, resulting in the posterior lateral humeral head impacting along the anterior rim of the glenoid fossa). No other deformities were noted. The shoulder remained reduced. Shoulder strength was limited by pain, but was normal throughout the distal left arm. Pulses and sensation were intact throughout the extremity.

The prognosis following an acute anterior-inferior dislocation in his age group was explained to JM and his parents. Because it was his nondominant shoulder, they elected conservative management with a surgery option in 2 months if he sustained a reinjury. This plan would allow enough time to rehabilitate in time for summer baseball. Although he had no reinjuries with activities of daily living, JM dislocated his shoulder again playing basketball in physical education classes 9 weeks later. He then opted for surgical reconstruction.

Examination at the time of surgery revealed a Bankart lesion with no other labral damage. He underwent a Bankart procedure using tack fixation. No excessive capsule redundancy was noted, and this, plus the fact that it was the nondominant shoulder, negated the need for a capsular tightening procedure. He was placed in a sling following surgery. He is seen in physical therapy 2 days after his surgery.

JM's passive range of motion ranges from 0° to 58° of flexion, 0° to 50° extension, 0° to 62° abduction, and 0° to 30° internal rotation. External rotation is not tested, because it is prohibited immediately postoperatively. Resisted movements in neutral demonstrate strong contractions throughout all shoulder girdle muscles, with some limitations because of postoperative pain. Neurologic testing is negative.

EVALUATION

JM's history, systems review, and test and measures suggest musculoskeletal pattern J: impaired joint mobility, motor function, muscle performance, and range of motion associated with bony or soft tissue surgical procedures.

DIAGNOSIS

JM demonstrates decreased active and passive range of motion and impaired joint mobility and muscle performance resulting from a Bankart procedure. The patient's underlying problem had been excessive mobility following his dislocations, but he has limited mobility following his surgical procedure.

PROGNOSIS

It is expected that JM will return to his previous level of function over the course of 5 to 7 months.

INTERVENTION

Weeks One to Four

Passive mobility exercises are initiated to prevent further loss of mobility. The sling is removed four to five times daily to perform passive abduction and flexion exercises, as well as gentle pendulum exercises. This passive range of motion can be performed using the other arm, a pulley, or the assistance of another person. Active range of motion for the elbow, forearm, and wrist are performed at the same time. The sling is discontinued and used only for comfort by the third week. At this time, active range of motion into external rotation begins. However, passive force into external rotation is prohibited for the first 6 weeks.

Isometric strengthening of all shoulder girdle muscles begins immediately postoperatively. Strengthening exercises include all the rotator cuff muscles and the scapular stabilizers. The isometric exercise intensity is low enough to prevent increases in shoulder pain. The isometric exercises are performed every hour while awake. Gentle weightbearing exercises are initiated to elicit isometric contraction around the joint. JM places his left hand on a counter and places his body weight on that hand, holding this position for 5 to 10 seconds several times per day. Ice is used after exercise sessions to decrease any postexercise soreness.

Weeks Four to Eight

Passive range of motion in flexion and abduction is progressing well past 90° elevation. Internal rotation is at least 50% of the uninvolved side. Passive range of motion exercises are continued and active and resistive range of motion exercises progress. At the sixth week postoperatively, passive range of motion into external rotation begins. Because this is JM's nondominant side, the need for external rotation range of motion for throwing is less than his dominant side. Our goal is to restore the full 0° to 90° motion but not to gain as much motion as the contralateral side. If this had been JM's dominant shoulder, the external rotation demands would have been greater. Full range of motion is expected by 8 to 12 weeks postoperatively, and JM's range of motion is nearly full by the eighth postoperative week.

Strengthening exercises are progressed at this point. A full complement of exercises to increase muscle performance is initiated. Studies by Townsend[63] and Moseley[64] provide the basis for many of the strengthening exercises chosen. Strengthening for the external rotator, scapular stabilizer, and shoulder elevator muscles are progressed from isometric to isotonic. These are performed through his comfortable, available range of motion using resistive bands and free weights. He also progresses his weightbearing exercises to include wall push-ups, finally progressing to full push-ups from the floor. The goals in this rehabilitation phase are to provide a base of strength on which a functional program will be built. Resistance and repetitions are increased as JM tolerates them.

Weeks Eight to Twelve

During this phase, JM continues his stretching exercises to ensure full glenohumeral mobility. By week 10, his range of motion is full in all directions. His manual muscle test scores are 5/5 without pain. At this point, he is ready for more aggressive exercises to improve his muscle performance. His weightbearing exercises are further progressed to more difficult stairstepping and gymnastic ball activities. JM performs the gymnastic ball exercises at home, and his stairstepping activities in his local gym.

Many of the resistive exercises are progressed to elevations of 90°. Resisted internal and external rotation are performed at 90° elevation using a resistive band at high speeds. These exercises are complemented with plyometric ball activities in overhead and throwing positions. Exercises are performed daily and also include cardiovascular training on land and lap swimming.

Weeks Twelve to Twenty

The muscle performance exercises are continuously progressed to more challenging positions. A full overhead position is used for high speed flexion, extension, internal rotation, and external rotation exercises. Because this is JM's nondominant arm, he is allowed to begin throwing with his dominant side with the rest of the baseball team. He also performs routine baseball drills with his teammates, although he is not allowed to dive or slide yet. He is allowed to begin batting practice at 50% speed.

Weeks Twenty to Twenty-Four

JM is put through a functional progression of baseball activity that includes extended reaching to catch a ball and catching and throwing a ball off-balance. His batting practice is gradually increased to 100% speed. It is recommended that he avoid head-first sliding or diving to protect his shoulder from further injury. JM's home program is modified to reflect a maintenance strength program for his shoulder. He is discharged at week 24.

OUTCOME

JM returned to full sports activity at 24 weeks postoperatively. He had no residual signs of instability and had regained full motion, strength, and function of the left shoulder.

CHAPTER SUMMARY

As surgical procedures change, the therapist must remain current with changes in postoperative rehabilitation. Improvements in surgical techniques have allowed for earlier mobilization with less decreased hypomobility. However, patients might still develop impaired joint mobility for a number of reasons. Hypomobility might be caused by pain, capsular restriction, skin immobility, or impaired muscle performance. Hypomobility that existed prior to the surgical procedure is likely to persist postoperatively. The therapist must recognize hypomobility, differentiating it from normal postoperative range of motion expectations. When hypomobility persists beyond these expectations, intervention is directed at the specific source of hypomobility. For example, pain may be treated with modalities, specific therapeutic exercise, or mobilization techniques, whereas impaired mobility resulting from skin adhesions is treated with mobilization of the skin and scar. Although hypomobility is an impairment, intervention is aimed at both the impairment and the resultant functional limitations. Restoration of full mobility can enhance functional use of the upper extremity and prevent development of secondary problems at the shoulder or adjacent joints.

REFERENCES

1. Leadbetter, WB: An introduction to sports-induced soft-tissue inflammation. In Leadbetter, WB, et al (eds): Sports-Induced Inflammation. American Academy of Orthopaedic Surgeons, Park Ridge, IL, 1990, p 3.
2. Salmon, JM, and Bell, SN: Arthroscopic stabilization of the shoulder for acute primary dislocations using a transglenoid suture technique. Arthroscopy 14(2):143, 1998.
3. Matsen, FA, et al: Anterior glenohumeral instability. In Rockwood, CA, and Matsen, FA (eds): The Shoulder. WB Saunders, Philadelphia, 1990.
4. Skyhar, MJ, et al: Instability of the shoulder. In Nicholas, JA, and Hershman, EB (eds): The Upper Extremity in Sports Medicine. CV Mosby, St. Louis, 1990.
5. Speer, KP, et al: Biomechanical evaluation of a simulated Bankart lesion. J Bone Jt Surg 76A:1819, 1994.
6. Taylor, DC, and Arciero, RA: Pathologic changes associated with shoulder dislocations: Arthroscopic and physical examination findings in first-time, traumatic anterior dislocations. Am J Sports Med 25(3):306, 1997.
7. Caspari, RB, and Geissler, WB: Arthroscopic manifestations of shoulder subluxation and dislocation. Clin Ortho Rel Res 291:54, 1993.
8. Bankart, ASB, and Cantab, MC: Recurrent or habitual dislocation of the shoulder-joint. Br Med J 2:1132, 1923.
9. Swenson, TM, and Warner, JJP: Arthroscopic shoulder stabilization: Overview of indications, technique and efficacy. Clin Sports Med 14(4):841, 1995.
10. Wolf, EM, et al: Humeral avulsion of glenohumeral ligaments as a cause of anterior shoulder instability. Arthroscopy (11)5:600, 1995.
11. Bigliani, LU, et al: Glenoid rim lesions associated with recurrent anterior dislocation of the shoulder. Am J Sports Med 26(1):41, 1998.
12. Wall, MS, and O'Brien, SJ: Arthroscopic evaluation of the unstable shoulder. Clin Sports Med 14(4):817, 1995.
13. Warner, JJP, et al: Arthroscopic Bankart repair with the Suretac device. Part I: Clinical observations. Arthroscopy 11(1):2, 1995.
14. Warner, JJP, et al: Arthroscopic Bankart repair with the Suretac device. Part II: Experimental observations. Arthroscopy 11(1):14, 1995.
15. Torchia, ME, et al: Arthroscopic transglenoid multiple suture repair: 2 to 8 year results in 150 shoulders. Arthroscopy 13(5):609, 1997.
16. Speer, KP, and Warren, RF: Arthroscopic shoulder stabilization: A role for biodegradable materials. Clin Ortho Rel Res 291:67, 1993.
17. Speer, KP, et al: An arthroscopic technique for anterior stabilization of the shoulder with a bioabsorbable tack. J Bone Jt Surg 78A(12):1801, 1996.

18. Lane, JG, et al: Arthroscopic stable capsulorrhaphy: A long-term follow-up. Arthroscopy 9:190, 1993.
19. Grana, WA, et al: Arthroscopic Bankart suture repair. Am J Sports Med 21:348, 1993.
20. Steinbeck, J, and Jerosch, J: Arthroscopic transglenoid stabilization versus open anchor suturing in traumatic anterior instability of the shoulder. Am J Sports Med 26(3):373, 1998.
21. Youssef, JA, et al: Arthroscopic Bankart suture repair for recurrent traumatic unidirectional anterior shoulder dislocations. Arthroscopy 11(5):561, 1995.
22. Wall, MS, and Warren, RF: Complications of shoulder instability surgery. Clin Sports Med 14(4):973, 1995.
23. Mologne, TS, et al: Assessment of failed arthroscopic anterior labral repairs: Findings at open surgery. Am J Sports Med 25(6):813, 1997.
24. Black, KP, et al: In vitro evaluation of shoulder external rotation after a Bankart-reconstruction. Am J Sports Med 25(4):449, 1997.
25. Gill, TJ, et al: Bankart repair for anterior instability of the shoulder: Long-term outcomes. J Bone Jt Surg 79A(6):850, 1997.
26. Altcheck, DW, and Warren, R: T-Plasty modification of the Bankart procedure for multidirectional instability of the anterior inferior type. J Bone Jt Surg 73A:105, 1991.
27. Friedman, RJ: Glenohumeral capsulorrhaphy. In Matsen, FA, et al (eds): The Shoulder: A Balance of Mobility and Stability. American Academy of Orthopaedic Surgeons, Rosemont, IL, 1993.
28. Cooper, RA, and Brems, JJ: The inferior capsular-shift procedure for multidirectional instability of the shoulder. J Bone Jt Surg 74A(10):1516, 1992.
29. Yamagichi, K, and Flatow, EL; Management of multidirectional instability. Clin Sports Med 14(4):885, 1995.
30. Obrzut, SL, et al: The effect of radiofrequency energy on the length and temperature properties of the glenohumeral joint capsule. Arthroscopy 14(4):395, 1998.
31. Pullin, JG, et al: YAG laser-assisted capsular shift in a canine model: Intraarticular pressure and histologic observations. J Shoulder Elbow Surg 6(3):272, 1997.
32. Tibone, JE, et al: Glenohumeral joint translation after arthroscopic, nonablative, thermal capsuloplasty with a laser. Am J Sports Med 26(4):495, 1998.
33. Hawkins, RJ, and Angelo, RL: Glenohumeral osteoarthritis: A late complication of the Putti-Platt procedure. J Bone Jt Surg 72A:1193, 1990.
34. Murrell, GAC, and Warren, RF: The surgical treatment of posterior shoulder instability. Clin Sports Med 14(4):903, 1995.
35. McIntyre, LF, et al: The arthroscopic treatment of posterior shoulder instability: Two-year results of a multiple suture technique. Arthroscopy 13(4):426, 1997.
36. Bigliani, LU, et al: Shift of the posteroinferior aspect of the capsule for recurrent posterior glenohumeral instability. J Bone Jt Surg 77A(7):1011, 1995.
37. Hawkins, RJ, and Janda, DH: Posterior instability of the glenohumeral joint: A technique of repair. Am J Sports Med 24(3):275, 1996.
38. Pollock, RG, and Bigliani, LU: Recurrent posterior shoulder instability: Diagnosis and treatment. Clin Ortho Rel Res 291:85, 1993.
39. Hawkins, RJ, et al: Recurrent posterior instability (subluxation) of the shoulder. J Bone Jt Surg 66A:101, 1988.
40. Gartsman, GM: Acromioplasty: What is it good for and how good is it? In Matsen, FA, et al (eds): The Shoulder: A Balance of Mobility and Stability. American Academy of Orthopaedic Surgeons, Rosemont, IL, 1993.
41. Tibone, JE, et al: Shoulder impingement syndrome in athletes treated by an anterior acromioplasty. Clin Ortho Rel Res 198:134, 1985.
42. Bigliani, LU, and Levine, WN: Subacromial impingement syndrome: Current concepts review. J Bone Jt Surg 79A:1854, 1997.
43. Stephens, SR, et al: Arthroscopic acromioplasty: A 6- to 10-year follow-up. Arthroscopy 14(4):382, 1998.
44. Lazarus, MD, et al: Comparison of open and arthroscopic subacromial decompression. J Shoulder and Elbow Surg 3:1, 1994.
45. T'Jonck, L, et al: Open versus arthroscopic subacromial decompression: Analysis of one-year results. Physiotherapy Research International 2(2):46, 1997.
46. Sachs, RA, et al: Open vs. arthroscopic acromioplasty: Prospective, randomized study. Arthroscopy 10:248, 1994.
47. Nielsen, KD, et al: The shoulder impingement syndrome: The results of surgical decompression. J Shoulder Elbow Surg 3:12, 1994.
48. Baker, CL, and Liu, SH: Comparison of open and arthroscopically assisted rotator cuff repairs. Am J Sports Med 23(14):99, 1995.
49. Burkhart, SS: Reconciling the paradox of rotator cuff repair versus debridement: A unified biomechanical rationale for the treatment of rotator cuff tears. Arthroscopy 10(1):4, 1994.
50. Burkhart, SS, et al: Cyclic loading of anchor-based rotator cuff repairs: Confirmation of the tension overload phenomenon and comparison of suture anchor fixation with transosseous fixation. Arthroscopy 13(6):720, 1997.

51. Matsen, FA, and Arntz, CT: Rotator cuff tendon failure. In Rockwood, CA, and Matsen, FA (eds): The Shoulder. WB Saunders, Philadelphia, 1990.
52. Ellman, H: Rotator cuff surgery: What is it good for and how good is it? In Matsen, FA, et al (eds): The Shoulder: A Balance of Mobility and Stability. American Academy of Orthopaedic Surgeons, Rosemont, IL, 1993.
53. Gazielly, DF, et al: Functional and anatomical results after rotator cuff tear. Clin Ortho Rel Res 304:43, 1994.
54. Payne, LZ, et al: Arthroscopic treatment of partial rotator cuff tears in young athletes. Am J Sports Med 25(3):299, 1997.
55. Neviaser, RF, et al: Anterior dislocation of the shoulder and rotator cuff rupture. Clin Orthop Rel Res 291:103, 1993.
56. Liu, SH, and Boynton, E: Posterior superior impingement of the rotator cuff on the glenoid rim as a cause of shoulder pain in the overhead athletes. Arthroscopy 9:697, 1993.
57. Rodosky, MW, et al: The role of the long head of the biceps muscle and superior glenoid labrum in anterior stability of the shoulder. Am J Sports Med 22(1):121, 1994.
58. Cordasco, FA, et al: Arthroscopic treatment of glenoid labral tears. Am J Sports Med 21(3):425, 1993.
59. Field, LD, and Savoie, FJ: Arthroscopic suture repair of superior labral detachment lesions of the shoulder. Am J Sports Med 21(6):783, 1993.
60. Maffet, MW, et al: Superio labrum-biceps tendon complex lesions of the shoulder. Am J Sports Med 23(1):93, 1995.
61. Snyder, SJ, et al: SLAP lesions of the shoulder. Arthroscopy 6:274, 1990.
62. Mileski, RA, and Snyder, SJ: Superior labral lesions in the shoulder: Pathoanatomy and surgical management. J Am Acad Orthop Surg 6:121, 1998.
63. Townsend, H, et al: Electromyographic analysis of the glenohumeral muscle during a baseball rehabilitation program. Am J Sports Med 19:264, 1991.
64. Moseley, JB, et al: EMG analysis of the scapular muscle during a shoulder rehabilitation program. Am J Sports Med 20:128, 1992.

Treatment Strategies

Clinical Reasoning in the Use of Manual Therapy Techniques for the Shoulder Girdle

Mark A. Jones, BS, PT, MAppSci
Mary E. Magarey, PhD, Grad Dip Man Ther

INTRODUCTION

Although advances in shoulder diagnosis, particularly via arthroscopy and shoulder imaging, have significantly advanced our understanding of common shoulder complex pathologies, clinical diagnosis by physical therapists and orthopaedic surgeons remains largely inexact. For example, a recent investigation compared the diagnostic accuracy of clinical examination by a physical therapist to that of two orthopaedic surgeons. These findings were then compared to the findings at arthroscopic examination.[1] Whereas levels of accuracy varied depending on the condition analyzed, physical evaluation by the orthopaedic or physiotherapy investigators could not achieve 100% agreement with the arthroscopic diagnosis in any case. These results are not surprising given the overlap of presentations of many shoulder disorders. However, this research does highlight the limitation echoed throughout this book that physical therapy management focusing solely on tissue pathology is inadequate. Not only do physical therapists (and orthopaedic surgeons) have limited accuracy in their ability to identify symptomatic structures within the glenohumeral (GH) joint and subacromial space based on clinical examination alone, the multitude of presentations demonstrated by different stages of the same pathology prohibits anything except broad guidelines for management.[1]

Impairment-based management requires treatment options based on the clinical presentation of each patient with consideration of the underlying pathology. For example, a patient with a diagnosis of frozen shoulder might present with an acutely painful shoulder that keeps him or her awake at night. The pain becomes unbearable with any movement, particularly unguarded movement. The joint has relatively normal passive range of movement. Equally, frozen shoulder can present with minimal pain but severe restriction of range of motion (ROM) as a result of capsular tightness. Obviously, treatment administered for "frozen shoulder" in the same manner for both patients will be ineffective for at least one of these two patients.

Manual therapy has different meanings amongst therapists. Clinical concepts of manual therapy range from joint mobilization and manipulation to any hands-on treatment including joint, soft-tissue, and neural mobilizing techniques, to a broader inclusion of all therapeutic procedures, including exercise and education. Clinical judgments regarding appropriate manual therapy techniques and their dosage can only be determined through skilled clinical reasoning and assessment. This chapter briefly reviews the clinical reasoning process, providing a brief overview of this collaborative process, including explanation of the hypothesis categories used to assist the therapist in organizing the process of thinking through the patient's problems. The chapter also discusses the factors influencing the choice of passive treatment used and those influencing the execution and success of passive treatment.

Whereas a broader view of manual therapy is often adopted, this chapter restricts the discussion predominantly to that of clinical reasoning associated with the selection and progression of passive mobilization techniques. The other equally and sometimes more important aspects of management, such as neuromuscular reeducation and therapeutic exercise, are covered in Chapter 14.

Clinical reasoning, or the thinking and decision making associated with a therapist's examination and management of a patient, is the foundation of clinical practice.[2] A good theoretical understanding of clinical reasoning is important to ensure skilled execution and reasoning error reduction. A comprehensive examination of this topic is beyond the scope of this chapter. The reader is referred to the text *Clinical Reasoning in the Health Professions* by Higgs and Jones[3] for a broad review of clinical reasoning across the health professions and to Chapter 12 of that textbook for a specific discussion of clinical reasoning in physical therapy.[2] Figure 13–1 presents a model of the collaborative clinical reasoning process between physical therapists and patients.[2] The therapist's reasoning is portrayed on the left, whereas the patient's thinking is depicted on the right. Central to both the therapist's and the patient's thinking is the understanding by both parties that the problem evolves through the course of the examination and ongoing management. Even in the opening moments of receiving a referral, reviewing case notes, or meeting a patient, the therapist will begin to formulate impressions or hypotheses about the problem and the person, including the context in which the problem exists. Initially these working hypotheses are quite broad, but as further information is revealed through the patient interview, physical examination, and ongoing management, these hypotheses are gradually refined into a more definitive physical therapy diagnosis and plan for management.

The cognitive operations at the core of the reasoning process include hypothesis generation and testing and pattern recognition. Patient cues, including type, area, behavior, and history of symptoms and any psychological, social, cultural, and environmental influences or consequences, can be obtained from the interview. This information, when combined with physical examination findings, generates a range of hypotheses about the patient's problem and its effect on the patient's life. This reasoning process requires pattern recognition based on the therapist's previous academic and clinical experience to weight and combine the cues, forming an

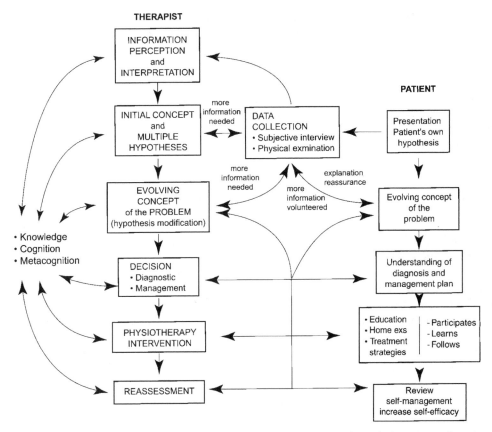

FIGURE 13–1. Collaborative clinical reasoning process between physical therapist and patient. (From Jones, MA: Clinical reasoning and pain. Man Ther 1:17, 1995, with permission.)

interpretation. These patterns include those related to diagnosis, such as impaired ROM due to adhesive capsulitis and others, such as management strategies appropriate for different presentations of impairment. In skilled clinical reasoning, these hypotheses are continually tested through examination and ongoing management, with attention to both supporting and negating evidence.

The nature of the hypotheses is important to the physical therapist's depth of understanding of the problem itself, the management decisions considered, and the ability to predict and inform the patient on a likely outcome. The specific clinical decisions regarding use of passive movement in the treatment of shoulder problems, as discussed later, must be made in the broader context of understanding the patient's functional problems, the dominant pain mechanisms, the source of the symptoms, factors contributing to the development and/or maintenance of the problem, and precautions to physiotherapy examination and management.

Hypothesis Categories

The concept of hypothesis categories, initially introduced by Jones,[4] has since been modified to reflect contemporary thinking and practice within manual therapy and pain management,[2,5–7] The following hypothesis categories represent common areas of clinical decisions that manual therapists should consider:

- Dysfunction/disability (physical or psychological and the associated social consequences)
- Pathobiological mechanisms
- Source of symptoms or dysfunction (often equated with diagnosis or impairment)
- Contributing factors
- Management
- Prognosis

DYSFUNCTION

Dysfunction, possibly physical or psychological, can lead to disability.[8] Examples of physical dysfunction include difficulty dressing, washing hair, making beds or carrying out a sport or a work-related task. The reader is referred to Chapters 3 and 4 for a complete review of the disablement model. Psychological dysfunction relates to patients' understanding of and feelings about their problems. Whereas an incorrect understanding or feeling might be quite natural in the context of a patient's problem and management to date, an understanding or feeling that becomes counterproductive to the patient's health and recovery should be considered dysfunctional. Excessive fear of pain and movement and the belief that complete avoidance of movement will resolve the problem are examples of dysfunctional feelings and understanding. These two dysfunctional feelings are well recognized in the context of chronic low back pain that can also occur with long-standing shoulder problems.

PATHOBIOLOGY

Patients' dysfunction is an expression of their pathobiology. Pathobiological mechanisms include the local tissue mechanisms involved in injury and healing (e.g., inflammation and repair) and the different input, processing, and output mechanisms underlying the patient's impairments and dysfunction.[6] Although management cannot be prescriptively directed by pathology, attention to known pathology and clinical patterns of pathobiological mechanisms will significantly assist therapists' management decisions and prognostic reasoning.

Input Mechanisms

Input mechanisms include the sensory and circulatory systems that inform the body about the environment, both internally and externally.[6,9] For example, two input pain mechanisms are nociceptive and peripheral neurogenic pain. Most clinicians are familiar with the basic mechanism operating when a high intensity stimulus, such as a pinprick, activates high threshold primary afferent nociceptors, resulting in pain. The same mechanism is in operation with acute injuries. Here, injury to target tissues such as ligaments, muscles, and even the connective tissue surrounding nerves will result in mechanical and/or chemical stimulation of nociceptors in what has been called "nociceptive pain."[9,10] The term "peripherally evoked neurogenic symptoms" refers to symptoms that originate from neural tissue outside the dorsal horn or spinal trigeminal nucleus, such as nerve root compression or peripheral nerve entrapment.[9,11] Both nociceptive pain and peripherally evoked neurogenic symptoms have a familiar pattern of presentation to most therapists, with a predictable stimulus-response relationship enabling aggravating and easing factors to be quickly identified by patient and therapist.

Processing

Processing of input occurs in the central nervous system. Therapists should be aware of the clinical features indicative of abnormal CNS processing. For example, abnormal processing can occur in what has been called *Centrally Evoked Symptoms,* where the pathology lies within the central nervous system.[12–14] In this model, the symptoms provoked from a past target tissue injury can be maintained even after the original injury has healed and the symptoms no longer behave with stimulus-response predictability. Another example of the clinical relevance of the processing mechanisms is evident when considering that pain and dysfunction have more than just physical and sensory dimensions. Pain and dysfunction also have affective (i.e., emotional impact such as fear, anxiety, and anger) and cognitive (i.e., thoughts about the pain or dysfunction) dimensions. Patients' feelings and thoughts about their pain and dysfunction can contribute significantly to the maintenance of their problems and the speed of their recovery.

Output Mechanisms

Output mechanisms, influenced through input and central processing mechanisms, operate through the somatic motor, autonomic, neuroendocrine, neuroimmune, and descending pain control systems.[15] Traditionally, therapists are most familiar with assessing and treating the motor system. However, they need to acquire a similar recognition of dysfunction in all of the output systems to understand the complex array of presentations exhibited by patients.[16,17]

SOURCE OF SYMPTOMS

The source of the symptoms refers to the actual structure or target tissue from which the symptoms are emanating. Joints, muscles, soft tissues, and nerves are examples of target tissues that can be injured and thus give rise to pain. The ability of physical therapists to accurately diagnose the tissue at fault and the precise nature of the injury (e.g., tendonitis versus tear) in the shoulder area is limited.[1] However, skilled examination and reasoning allow clinicians to identify the gross structure involved (i.e., local shoulder tissues versus somatic spinal referral) and the associated causal mechanisms (e.g., impingement or dynamic instability). Although being able to discriminate between specific tissue involvement is important, physical therapists' skill in assessing, treating, and monitoring patients' impairments as they relate to their dysfunctions and disabilities is more important.

CONTRIBUTING FACTORS

Contributing factors are any predisposing or associated factors involved in the development or maintenance of the patient's problem. These factors include environmental, psychosocial, and physical-biomechanical components. For example, an inflamed subacromial bursa might be the nociceptive source of the patient's symptoms, with either a tight posterior glenohumeral capsule or "weak" scapular rotator force couples contributing to the altered kinematics that predisposed the bursal irritation. Hypotheses regarding precautions and contraindications to physical examination and treatment serve to determine the extent of physical examination that may safely be undertaken and whether physical treatment is indicated. If treatment is indicated, the clinician must decide whether any constraints to physical treatment (e.g., pain provoking versus nonprovocative treatment techniques) exist.

MANAGEMENT AND PROGNOSIS

Management relates to hypotheses for the overall health of the patient while considering specific physical therapy measures and techniques. Prognosis should be considered with regard to the patient's broader prospects for recovery and return to function.

Patient and Therapist Roles

The boxes on the right in Figure 13–1 represent the patient's thinking in the collaborative reasoning process. Patients develop their own understanding of their problems, shaped by personal experiences and advice from other health practitioners, family, and friends. This understanding, or the meaning patients give to their problems, has been shown to impact on their levels of pain tolerance, disability, and eventual outcome.[18–20] Through a process of evaluating patients' understanding of and feelings about their problems, explanation, reassurance, and shared decision making, the patient and the therapist will develop an evolving understanding of the problem and its management. Responsibility is shared between patient and therapist with the patient taking a more active role in management.

The box on the left in Figure 13–1 emphasizes the importance of the therapist's knowledge, cognition (e.g., data analysis and synthesis), and metacognition (i.e., reflective monitoring of one's own cognitive processes and knowledge organization) to skilled clinical reasoning. For further discussion of these and other external factors influencing therapists' reasoning, refer to Higgs and Jones.[3]

FACTORS ASSISTING IN THE CHOICE OF TREATMENT BY PASSIVE MOVEMENT

Numerous factors involving the problem and the patient require consideration when reasoning about the choice of treatment by passive movement. A broad understanding of the patient's disorder and its effect on his or her life, as gleaned through consideration of the hypothesis categories, will enable the therapist to judge whether passive treatment is appropriate and how it can be used.

Clinicians must consider current and past pharmacological history. Analgesics and anti-inflammatory agents might mask pain and tissue sensitivity, steroids might have weakened tissues, and anticoagulants can increase a patient's susceptibility to bleeding and bruising. Similarly, known or suspected pathology and general health status such as frank instability, rheumatoid arthritis, osteoporosis, and cardiac stability, are also relevant. Although systemic disorders such as rheumatoid arthritis and osteoporosis require extra caution in the use of stronger techniques, suspected pathology within the glenohumeral complex itself must also be factored into specific treatment and broader management decisions. For example, labral injuries, particularly in the athletic population, are likely to be less amenable to manual therapy (including attention to neuromuscular control) because the labrum's poor vascularity suggests that healing is unlikely to occur.[21] No amount of manual therapy can alter the underlying pathology with its potential to disrupt normal function. When the clinical presentation implicates a labral injury, thought should be given to further diagnostic investigation and the possibility of surgery. Additionally, knowledge of structural faults contributing to a primary impingement, such as bony spurs, a calcified coracoacromial ligament, or a type III acromial arch, will assist therapists' recognition of when manual therapy alone is insufficient and when surgical intervention might be required.[22] Clearly, postsurgical management requires similar consideration, with good communication between surgeon, therapist, and patient, to ensure repairs are not compromised.

Pathobiological mechanisms (e.g., pain mechanisms and tissue healing as discussed previously) must also be considered to avoid exacerbation of symptoms, disruption to normal healing, and therapy-induced maintenance of pain.[6,23-25] The precise pain mechanisms dominating a patient's presentation cannot be confirmed. However, clinical patterns of these pain mechanisms and psychosocial (yellow flags) and physical (red flags) risk factors possibly increasing the likelihood of patients developing, or perpetuating, long-term disability and work loss have been proposed.[9,13,14,26] Continued use of passive movement techniques, particularly provocative techniques, when a centrally evoked pain state is suspected will fail to bring any lasting improvement. In fact, it might directly contribute to maintenance of the patient's impairments and disabilities.[24,25] Here, hands-off physical therapy and medical and psychological management are indicated. Clearly, overlapping pain mechanisms frequently occur, in which case, combinations of manual therapy and other services should be utilized.

A knowledge of the normal tissue healing process, including specific healing rates for different structures, will also assist the therapist's assessment of the patient's rate of recovery and appropriate dosage of manual treatment.[23,27,28] For example, overly aggressive treatment in the early stage of an inflammatory process might worsen the impairments and also possibly disrupt the normal healing process, thus prolonging the acute inflammatory stage.[23] In contrast, at the other extreme of the healing process, when dealing with chronically stiff or fibrosed structures, repeated movement and stretching is needed to effect a change. However, such biomedical knowledge alone is insufficient to guide the precise choice and dosage of manual therapy techniques for the many presentations that fall between these extremes. In these cases, therapists need strategies for selecting and applying manual therapy techniques linked to the specific clinical presentations of the impairments unique to each patient.

Many patients will have no general health concerns or other overt medical or psychosocial risk factors. An orthopaedic diagnosis might be available, but two patients with different diagnoses might present with very similar symptoms and signs, depending on the stage of the pathology. For example, symptoms associated with an acute subacromial bursitis might include slight limitation of passive movement and severe pain in the joint with any attempt to move the arm. These symptoms could also be present in the early stages of an acute frozen shoulder. The pathological process and the diagnosis are different, but the same set of treatment techniques might be equally appropriate for both patients. Lack of a definite diagnosis does not necessarily restrict the use of passive movement in treatment.

Once general health and pathobiological considerations have been made, a useful strategy for selection and application of passive movement treatment techniques in a nociceptive dominant presentation is to base treatment on the following:

- The severity and irritability of the disorder
- The relationship between the patient's pain (or any symptoms) to the quality of passive movement (e.g., resistance)
- The symptom response during and immediately following application of the technique
- The physical response and functional capacity following application of the technique

The concept of *irritability* relates to the ease of exacerbation of symptoms, the severity of the symptoms provoked, and the length of time before they subside. Irritability represents a continuum of symptoms. A very irritable condition is aggravated by minimal movement, involves severe pain, and takes hours to settle. Conversely, a nonirritable condition involves minor discomfort, only following extended strenuous activity. This discomfort goes away immediately after the provoking activity is stopped. Irritability is a reflection of the local tissue inflammation and associated primary hyperalgesia. It also can be a manifestation of centrally induced secondary hyperalgesia.[9,13] Understanding the concept of *irritability* helps the physical therapist gauge the depth and amount of mobilization that can be used in treatment without exacerbation of symptoms.

The relationship between the patient's symptoms to the resistance to passive movement can broadly be categorized as dominated by pain or stiffness, or these two impairments can coexist in various combinations.

Pain

When considering selection of treatment techniques for a pain-dominant presentation, such as the patient with an inflamed, irritable disorder in which the symptoms are constant and readily flare with little activity, attention to the kinematics of the shoulder complex is not particularly helpful. Passive treatment is guided by assessment of the movement that can be performed through the largest range with the least pain, regardless of whether the movement is one that occurs as part of normal kinematics. Attention to finding a pain-relieving position in which to treat and a pain-relieving movement to use as a treatment technique is the priority. Frequently, the optimal movement is an accessory one, with the joint resting in a neutral (midrange) position. The application of this passive treatment principle is illustrated in the first case study presented in this chapter.

Stiffness

When addressing a problem dominated by stiffness with little pain or inflammatory features, attention is focused on kinematics. Recent research results have demonstrated that end range GH joint movement is influenced by tension in the passive restraints, such that physiological movements are accompanied by coupled translations, in most instances opposite to the translations occurring in midrange. For example, normal glenohumeral flexion is accompanied by superior and anterior translation and lateral rotation by posterior translation.[29,30] An understanding of the normal kinematics allows physical therapists to recognize when these movements are disturbed. Kinematics might be exaggerated in patients with capsular tightness and might be lost in patients with capsular laxity. Tightness in the capsule, identified by recognition of loss of normal translation, can be effectively addressed by stretching to restore the specific movement lost. However, whereas techniques that follow kinematic principles are clearly effective, therapists should not be bound by these rules, because considerable variation exists in normal range. Other strategies can be equally effective. Whereas stretching into the restricted direction is frequently effective, it might not be the optimal direction for improving overall function. When consideration is given to both the clinical findings of impairment and contemporary understanding of kinematics, a broader range of treatment options is available.

Pain and Stiffness

Most musculoskeletal problems have components of both pain and stiffness. Choice of treatment technique then depends predominantly on the relationship between these two impairments. In general, the greater the presentation is dominated by one of these impairments, the more the selection of passive treatment mirrors the guidelines outlined previously. An example of a presentation in which pain dominates is the patient with a stage 2 frozen shoulder.[31] For this patient, pain, the worst complaint, limits passive movement, but resistance to movement can also be felt. A mobilization technique directed at altering the pain would be the ideal treatment for this patient. In contrast, a patient with a stage 3 frozen shoulder would have stiffness as the dominant component, with slight pain only provoked at the end range of movement. In this case, the choice of treatment is more likely to be a technique aimed at altering the tissue stiffness. The strength of the stretching technique would be strongly influenced by the amount of pain provoked during the technique and the response on reassessment of active movement.

There are many more examples of how pain and stiffness often present in shoulder problems, but it is beyond the scope of this chapter to present these cases and the associated implications to selection and progression of passive treatment. A more thorough discussion of selection of passive treatment can be found elsewhere.[32–34]

MOVEMENT DIAGRAMS

To assist therapists' communication regarding their assessments of the relationships between patient symptoms and quality of passive movement and their choice of treatment techniques and their applications, the concept of movement diagrams and grades of movement will be briefly reviewed. A movement diagram is a pictorial representation of a passive movement (physiological or accessory) that records the relationship of pain, resistance to movement, and muscle spasm (Fig. 13–2).[32–34]

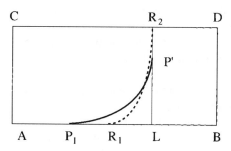

FIGURE 13–2. Movement diagram, depicting the relationship of pain and resistance during a passive movement. *(A)* Starting position from which the movement is taken. *(B)* End of the normal range of movement. *(A-C)* Force of pressure given, as determined by severity, irritability, and nature (e.g., known pathology such as RA) of the disorder. *(L)* Limit of movement available in the specific movement tested (normal range of movement L=B, excessive range L>B, limited range L<B). *(R_1)* Point in range where an increase to resistance is first felt. *(R_2)* Point in range where movement was stopped due to resistance or where the nature of the disorder (e.g., RA, instability) dictated the movement not be taken further. *(P_1)* Point in range where the patient first reports an onset of pain or an increase in resting pain. *(P_2)* (Not illustrated in this figure.) Point in range where the movement was stopped either because of the intensity of pain provoked, or the therapist's assessment of the severity, irritability, and nature of the disorder dictated further movement was not indicated. *(R')* Amount of resistance the therapist judged the movement to be in to when the movement was stopped due to pain P_2 (not illustrated in this figure). *(P')* Amount of pain the patient reports (e.g., 1-10) when the movement was stopped due to resistance R_2.

A full description of movement diagrams can be found elsewhere.[32–34] The steps taken to draw a movement diagram are the following:

1. Find P_1.
2. Move to L and decide what is limiting the movement (R_2 or P_2).
3. Find R_1.
4. Draw the behavior of pain through the movement (either P_1 to P_2 or P_1 to P').
5. Draw behavior of resistance through the movement (either R_1 to R_2 or R_1 to R1').

Grades of Movement

Movement diagrams are also a useful way to visualize the grades of movement available for use in passive treatment. A grade of movement is defined by two parameters, the relationship of the passive movement to resistance and the amplitude of the movement. The grades of movement described by Magarey[32] and Maitland[34] are as follows:

Grade I	A small amplitude movement performed at the beginning of the range
Grade II	A large amplitude movement performed in the resistance-free part of the range
Grade III	A large amplitude movement performed to the point of approximately 50% of the resistance
Grade IV	A small amplitude movement performed to the point of approximately 50% of the resistance (Fig. 13–3)

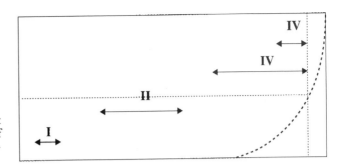

FIGURE 13–3. A movement diagram depicting basic grades of movement in relation to a resistance curve.

In situations in which it is inappropriate to assess the end-range resistance to determine whether it is equivalent to a grade III or IV movement (e.g., in a moderately irritable disorder), 50% of the resistance is estimated.

Pluses (+) and minuses (–) are also used to describe the variations possible within the four definitions given previously (Fig. 13–4). A plus or minus added to a grade I and II refers to an increase or decrease in the amplitude (and hence range) of the passive movement. Large (III) and small (IV) amplitude passive movements are also subclassified according to degrees of resistance as follows:

Grade III^{--} and IV^{--} Movement taken to the point at which resistance is first perceived (R$_1$)

Grade III^{-} and IV^{-} Movement taken to 25% or less of the limit of resistance (R$_2$)

Grade III^{+} and IV^{+} Movement taken to approximately 75% of the limit of resistance

Grade III^{++} and IV^{++} Movement taken to the maximum resistance or limit of the joint range

The reliability and validity of detecting the various components of the movement diagram is limited.[35,36] In each instance, the precision by which the amount of resistance can be determined is limited by the type of movement and the clinical expertise of the examiner. Therefore, mobilization grades are never an exact point in the range. Rather, they represent an estimate of the amount of resistance encountered

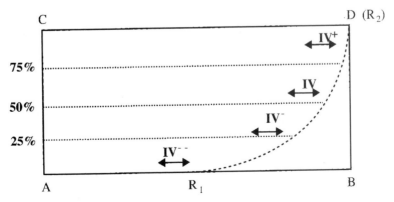

FIGURE 13–4. A movement diagram depicting variations on a grade IV movement (grades IV^{--}, IV^{-}, IV, IV^{++}). Variations on a grade III movement would reach the same points in range as those related to grade IV, but grade III movements are large amplitude.

during the performance of a technique by a single therapist. Therefore, they cannot be used as more than a clinical guide to facilitate communication between therapists.

The remainder of this chapter focuses on selection and application of passive movement techniques for the nociceptive dominant pain state, assuming appropriate precautions are taken for known pathologies, medical conditions, medication use, and surgical repairs. Two patient case studies are compared to illustrate principles of passive movement selection, application, and progression in a clinical context.

CASE STUDY 13–1: PATIENT 1

INFORMATION FROM THE PATIENT INTERVIEW

Patient 1 is a 42-year-old painter whose key symptoms include a constant ache (3-8/10 severity) felt around the whole shoulder and a sharp localized pain felt anteriorly under the acromion (10/10 severity). This is the fourth episode of these symptoms during the past 2 years. The first episode began after a long painting job, which involved a lot of detailed overhead work. Although painting ceilings was not new to him, the intricacy of this particular job required longer periods of sustained shoulder elevation than to which he was accustomed. The first episode settled following a 2-week break from overhead activities and a course of anti-inflammatory medication. Since the initial episode, he has had three other episodes that were also brought on by prolonged overhead painting, something he more recently has tried to delegate to others. In between episodes, his only primary limitation was an inability to sleep on the involved side because of the shoulder aching. This most recent episode, starting 1 week prior to attending physical therapy, was also elicited by an overhead painting job. His local doctor gave him an injection of cortisone and local anesthetic into his subacromial space and provided him with anti-inflammatory medication. After spending the last week off from work without a reduction in symptoms, the patient was referred for physical therapy.

The patient reports that any attempted movement of his arm immediately increases his resting ache and also provokes a severe, sharp pain. All movements seem equally painful to him. His only relief comes from supporting the arm in a sling-like position. He is not sleeping well because of the constant ache. Symptoms are also bad in the mornings, with continued pain and a feeling of stiffness that takes at least an hour to resolve. He has received no previous treatment other than the injection, and anti-inflammatory and analgesic medication. His general health is good, without any apparent contraindications to physical therapy. A recent diagnostic ultrasound (static and dynamic) revealed thickening of the subacromial bursa and buckling of the bursa under the coracoacromial arch on attempted active abduction.

From a diagnostic reasoning perspective, the ultrasound evidence of bursal thickening and subacromial impingement alone is insufficient to guide specific day-to-day treatment. He has already received a trial of anti-inflammatories and a cortisone injection, neither of which produced any significant lasting improvement. Although the pathology detected by ultrasound might truly be the source of his symptoms, other contributing factors exist that maintain the subacromial irritation.

PHYSICAL EXAMINATION

A full physical examination of the patient is not indicated initially because all tests (active, passive, resistive, palpation) are likely to provoke symptoms, which would have added little to their discriminative value. Additionally, these tests probably would only worsen his symptoms. Therefore, a limited examination is performed.[32,37] The assessments and the responses are as follows:

Active shoulder elevation	• 20° before increase in pain; shoulder hitching evident in movement
Cervical clearing tests	• Active movements: full range and pain free
	• Passive accessory movements of each cervical intervertebral level: full range and pain free
Gentle neurodynamic differentiation	• With the arm passively positioned in abduction to the onset of pain (30°), passive wrist and finger extension or cervical contralateral flexion with no alteration in the resting ache or shoulder pain
Glenohumeral and cervicoscapulothoracic soft tissue tone/ mobility	• General tenderness in the subacromial and scapular fossae areas; increased muscle tone/guarding apparent through the scapulothoracic and scapulohumeral muscles on the involved side

The emphasis of the physical examination is to determine the patient's most comfortable resting position and evaluate the effect of several different passive movements. The intent in this case is not to differentially stress specific tissues or movements, but rather to establish whether any physiological or accessory movements can be performed without aggravating his symptoms. Ideally, the examination would also identify movements that decrease his resting ache. The goal of the physical examination is not to further test the ultrasound diagnosis, but to use an impairment-based examination to judge if passive movement should have a place in the management of his problem at this stage. Maitland[34] has recommended an extremely useful strategy to assist this decision, in which the relationship of pain to resistance during passive movement is used to judge which movement is used for treatment and the grade at which it should be performed.

In this case, after careful explanation about finding the most easing position and movement, the therapist, guided by the patient, cautiously maneuvers the patient's shoulder into a combined position of slight elevation in the plane of the scapula with approximately 20° of medial rotation. The arm is securely supported in this position with two pillows and a towel (Fig. 13–5). Although the ache is still present in this position, the symptoms decrease from an intensity of 6/10 to 3/10.

While attempting to find the easing position, the patient's pain response makes it obvious that all physiological movements either provoke his pain or increase his ache. Therefore, the therapist, on the basis of Maitland's[34] strategies for decision making in this context, determines that accessory movements should be the appropriate treatment technique. Treatment is aimed at reducing both the resting ache and the pain with movement.

Several accessory movements, including a glenohumeral posteroanterior glide, an anteroposterior glide, and a lateral and caudal distraction of the

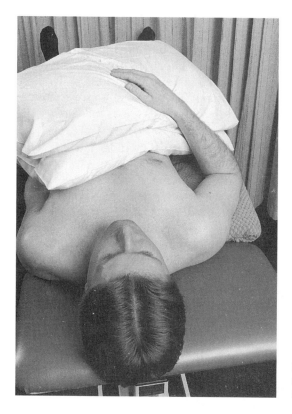

FIGURE 13–5. Positioning for maximal comfort to optimize the effect of pain-easing treatment techniques.

humeral head are performed with careful handling and continual monitoring of symptoms. The physiological movement of gentle rotation is also effective in reducing pain in similar presentations. However, these small movements of rotation increase this patient's symptoms, so this movement is not pursued. If acromioclavicular involvement is suspected, gentle accessory movements of the clavicle and acromion should also be tested. Similarly, in the presence of positive neurodynamic signs, gentle nonprovocative through-range neural mobilizing techniques might be effective.[38] In this particular patient, no supporting evidence exists for involvement of these structures, so a trial of neurodynamic treatment is not evaluated at the first appointment.

When assessing the effect of accessory movements in a nociceptively pain-dominated presentation such as this, determining the relationship of pain to tissue resistance and the amplitude of the accessory movement that is possible before any symptoms are provoked is important. Here, the greatest amplitude of accessory movement without aggravating symptoms is available, with a posteroanterior glide performed slowly and smoothly from the position of relative comfort (Fig. 13–6).

As resistance to the different accessory movements is not encountered before there is an increase of symptoms, the impairment presentation is described as limited by pain. The movement diagram reflecting the findings on posteroanterior glide is illustrated in Figure 13–7.

Maitland[34] espoused the concept of treatment with passive mobilization for relief of pain. The movement with the largest possible range available without

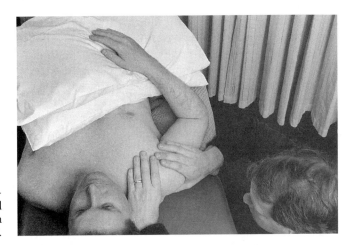

FIGURE 13–6. A postero-anterior glide being performed as a pain-easing technique from a position of maximal comfort.

provocation of symptoms is usually found to be most effective in relieving symptoms when performed through the full available symptom-free range as a slow and smooth oscillation. With this patient, a posteroanterior glide as a grade II decreases his resting ache beyond that achieved by careful positioning. During and after the technique, the ache reduces to 1/10.

Clearly, no prescription exists for the amount of treatment that will be optimal for all patients. Generally, when reassessment within the session is restricted to evaluation of alteration in resting symptoms, the dosage is small (e.g., possibly several applications of the technique of under 2 minutes in the one-treatment session).

A patient presenting with a condition similar to this pattern would appear to have a disorder in the early phases of the inflammation cycle. At this stage in his disorder, the pathobiological mechanisms of tissue healing must be respected. Treatment should, at least, do nothing to disturb these mechanisms and, at best, facilitate them. To prevent aggravation of the inflammatory process, gentle movement is performed through a pain-free range, with no joint compression. Movement performed in this way might facilitate absorption of inflammatory chemicals at the site of tissue damage.[23] Such movement also

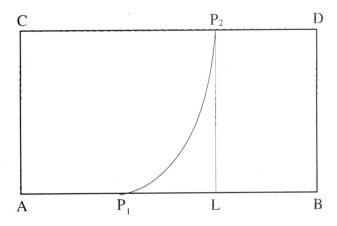

FIGURE 13–7. A movement diagram demonstrating a postero-anterior GH movement performed in a neutral, pain-free position, Patient 1.

might be responsible for alteration of the afferent input from the affected site to the dorsal horn, thereby reducing the sensation of pain.[39]

Following a strategy of relating treatment by passive movement to the relationship between symptoms, tissue resistance, and range, the technique can then be progressed to different grades, different positions, and different movements. For example, this patient obtains significant relief from three treatments performed over 1 week. The first two treatments consist of passive accessory posteroanterior glides, education regarding the nature of the problem, and resting positions to use at home. At the third visit, further examination is possible because the condition is less irritable. Assessment of scapulothoracic movement patterns demonstrate poor awareness and control of scapular position and reduced mobility of the scapula on the thoracic wall. These findings are addressed with scapulothoracic passive and active mobilization (scapular Proprioceptive neuromuscular facilitation (PNF) diagonals performed passively, actively with assistance, and against manual resistance in sidelying, from a position of maximal glenohumeral comfort). This approach completely eases the patient's resting ache and improves active shoulder elevation to 90° before symptoms begin.

The pattern of impairment has changed to one where accessory movements can now be performed into resistance without provocation of symptoms. Further examination at this stage also includes assessment of passive physiological movements that are still limited by pain (Table 13–1). Medial rotation from 45° abduction is the only passive physiological movement in which resistance (R_1) is perceived before further movement is limited by pain (P_2).

With each of these movements, a comparison of the involved to the uninvolved side is made to provide an estimate of normal range for a particular patient. Students will benefit from drawing movement diagrams for each movement to practice communicating what they feel and what the patient reports. With experience, therapists can mentally draw these movement diagrams as they perform the movements.

Several options exist when determining the progression of treatment. A clinician can progress the posteroanterior glide into resistance and slight pain (e.g., a grade IV) or change to a medial rotation technique in which resistance could be treated more directly. The latter approach would be more aggressive and could provoke a small amount of pain (e.g., a grade IV⁻⁻) (Fig. 13–8).

A trial of progressing the posteroanterior glide offers no improvement, as demonstrated by a lack of alteration in the movement diagram of medial

TABLE 13–1 Passive Physiological Movement Testing Findings

Testing	Findings
Lateral rotation from neutral	• P_1 40°, P_2 45° (Left R_2 80°)
Medial rotation from neutral	• P_1 ¼ range P_2 (½ range compared to Left)
Extension	• P_1 10°, P_2 40° (Left R_2 80°)
Abduction	• P_1 45°, P_2 50° (Left R_2 80°)
Lateral rotation from 45° abduction	• P_1 10°, P_2 30° (Left R_2 80°)
Medial rotation from 45° abduction	• P_1 40°, R_1 50°, P_2 and R′ 60° (Left R_2 80°)
Flexion	• P_1 50°, P_2 60°
Quadrant and locking	• Not tested

rotation, and no change in response to reassessment of active movement. Therefore, a medial rotation mobilization is used, comparing a grade IV oscillation to a sustained stretch. Greater improvement is made with the sustained stretch. This response correlates well with improvement gained from posterior scapulohumeral soft-tissue techniques, also directed at improvement of medial rotation range. By improving the range of movement available, this treatment technique is likely to provide more clearance of the greater tuberosity as it passes the acromion during movement. This improved movement pattern might have reduced impingement of subacromial tissues, with a concomitant reduction in inflammation and pain.

After 2 weeks using a combination of passive glenohumeral mobilization, scapulohumeral soft-tissue techniques, and muscle re-education, the passive glenohumeral movements have improved considerably. Elevation increases to 170° with the hand behind the back position movement being most impaired. The patient feels he is almost back to what he considered normal, as long as he avoids sustained elevation or lying on that shoulder.

Examination for this patient, which was not appropriate in the beginning, is included as the symptoms settle. Examination of the quadrant reveals slight restriction of movement with provocation of subacromial pain.[34,40] Treatment at this stage includes the following:

1. Stronger (i.e., IV$^+$) passive mobilization of physiological movement around the quadrant
2. Posteroanterior glenohumeral mobilization, performed at the end range of shoulder elevation with the patient prone
3. Medial rotation
4. Anteroposterior glides performed in a position of hand behind the back

All these techniques are aimed at stretching the capsuloligamentous structures and associated soft tissues around the GH joint. Continued postural and scapular re-education is emphasized. In addition, treatment frequency is reduced to twice a week, and the patient is instructed in self-glenohumeral mobilization and scapular exercises. After a total of 4 weeks of treatment, the

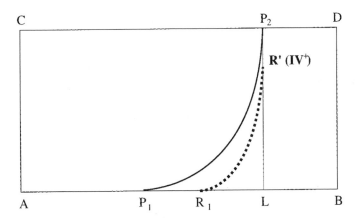

FIGURE 13–8. A movement diagram depicting GH internal rotation from 45° abduction, Patient 1.

patient states he feels "better than 100%," and that he is now able to paint overhead again without trouble (although he has not tested it with any prolonged jobs). The only remaining problem he notes is an inability to sleep on the involved shoulder. His glenohumeral mobility and muscle control has improved significantly, but these gains do not improve his symptoms when lying on the involved side. More advanced differential testing of his glenohumeral quadrant reveals that the patient is still painful at end range. When subacromial compression is added to this position at the point at which pain is initially provoked, the pain increases. Other maneuvers performed from this position, including glenohumeral compression, acromioclavicular accessory movements, and neurodynamic loading, have no effect on the symptoms. However, subacromial distraction applied in this position results in a decrease in symptoms. The findings from these tests, described more fully elsewhere, indicate continued subacromial dysfunction (e.g., chronic bursitis).[34,40,41] More importantly, however, the findings provide further signs of impairment that can be directly addressed in treatment.

Procedures directed at contributing factors to the hypothesized secondary impingement, such as soft-tissue hypomobility and poor neuromuscular control, are ineffective at changing this residual dysfunction of difficulty lying on the involved side. Because the patient's disorder is assessed to be very stable, based on signs of irritability, treatment is progressed to a passive technique in which subacromial compression is added to mobilization of the quadrant into pain (Fig. 13–9). This particular technique might be unfamiliar to, or considered inappropriate by, some therapists because the presumed source of the symptoms, the subacromial tissues, are deliberately compressed during the mobilization. Whereas such a technique is clearly not indicated in an acute inflammatory presentation and might not be required in all patients with similar presentations, it can be very effective in some cases. For this patient, this mobilization appears to be the key technique that will eventually resolve his inability to sleep on that shoulder.

Birnbaum and Lierse[42] demonstrated that, in the normal subacromial bursa, the unattached subdeltoid component folds in on itself and slides under the acromion during abduction, forming a double layer between the coracoacromial arch and the superior surface of the rotator cuff. Any thickening of the bursal walls or adhesions between the two surfaces of the bursa would prevent this normal bursal movement. A technique such as mobilization into the quadrant under subacromial compression might be similar to a form of friction massage of the subacromial tissues. In a chronic stage of the healing process, this technique might be effective by breaking down or stretching the bursal adhesions, perhaps increasing production of synovial fluid. The goal is to restore friction-free bursal movement and, through provoking an acute inflammatory process, to enable normal healing processes to recommence.[23]

Based on this patient's assessment and response to treatment, a likely diagnosis is a secondary subacromial impingement. According to the *Guide to Physical Therapist Practice,* this patient would be included in overlapping practice patterns. He would be classified under practice pattern D because of the primary limitation in movement. This musculoskeletal practice pattern identifies patients with impaired joint mobility, motor function, muscle performance, and ROM-associated capsular restriction and is discussed in Chapter 7. He also had a presentation in which subacromial inflammation and pain were dominant and

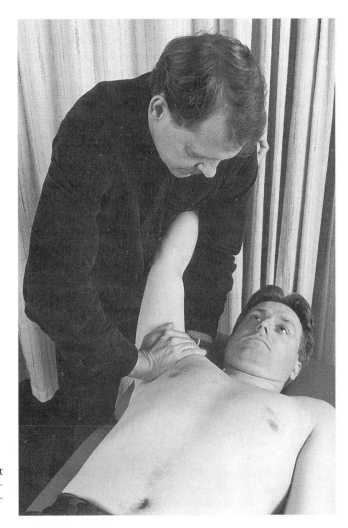

FIGURE 13–9. The treatment technique of GH quadrant performed while maintaining subacromial compression.

significantly influenced the choice of treatment. For this reason, the patient also would be classified under practice pattern F. This practice pattern includes the same impairments listed for practice pattern D, but these impairments are attributed to localized inflammation.

This case study illustrates how the practice patterns can overlap. Techniques must be directed at resolving the impairments in each pattern for treatment to be successful.

CASE STUDY 13–2: PATIENT 2

INFORMATION FROM THE PATIENT INTERVIEW

Patient 2 is an 18-year-old college baseball catcher who presents with complaints of a gradual reduction in throwing power through the course of a game. In addition, he experiences pain of increasing sharpness that is felt inside the shoulder joint at the point of ball release in later innings. He also notes a feeling of stiffness around the back of his shoulder that seems to accompany the feeling of weakness. All symptoms are directly proportional to the number of strong throws he makes. An easy toss of the ball back to the pitcher is not a problem, but after multiple hard throws to a base, the feeling of weakness, stiffness, and eventually sharp pain begins. These symptoms continue to worsen with additional hard throws. The sharp pain diminishes immediately after the throw, but he is left with a general ache inside the shoulder for a couple of hours following a game. He is still able to play through a game, but the symptoms are affecting his performance on the field. Sleeping is not a problem, but the shoulder always feels stiff for an hour the morning after a game. He is not troubled with his shoulder at any other time and has no other musculoskeletal or general health problems.

His shoulder problem first developed 2 months prior to coming for treatment, approximately 1 month into his first season playing at a collegiate level. Initially, he believed that the symptoms of weakness and stiffness were related to the increased training and level of play in college ball. However, his performance had been slipping during the past 4 weeks because of the onset of pain. He has had no previous treatment, and his team doctor had referred him for a physical therapy assessment and a trial of treatment before considering other investigations or surgery. Other than two minor episodes of tendonitis when playing in high school, both of which settled within 2 weeks with physical therapy, he has no past history of shoulder or other musculoskeletal problems.

PHYSICAL EXAMINATION

A full examination can be performed because the symptoms are nonirritable and no aspect of the patient's presentation contraindicates any specific testing.[32,37] He has good symmetrical muscle development. His posture is unremarkable except for bilaterally protracted scapulae and anteriorly displaced humeral heads, which are more pronounced on his involved dominant side. Active movements have no restriction, but pain is reproduced at the end of full elevation and extension, particularly if combined with medial rotation. The position of the hand behind the back is restricted relative to the other side. The medial rotation component of this movement is stiff but pain free, and the extension component is restricted and painful. Medial rotation at 90° abduction reveals marked limitation on the symptomatic side. A similar restriction is noted for horizontal adduction in this position when the scapula is stabilized.

Resisted muscle testing for the rotator cuff is strong and painless. Resisted testing of the long head of the biceps is performed from a position that induces a stretch on the tendon. The resistance is applied in a position of glenohumeral extension-medial rotation, elbow extension, and pronation and is advanced to an inner range position of shoulder flexion-lateral rotation, elbow flexion-supination. This test also reproduces the pain and sensation of weakness he experiences in games.

Passive movement testing highlights excessive lateral rotation and relatively marked restriction of medial rotation, typical of many baseball players.[43] Stability tests are negative for frank instability, although they are consistent with the passive physiological movement tests.[1,44] The posterior glide is clearly more restricted and anterior, and anteroinferior glide tests are proportionally more lax on the involved shoulder. Apprehension and clunk tests combined with horizontal flexion-medial rotation, commonly provocative with both subacromial and subcoracoid impingement, are also negative.[45-48] Tests directed at involvement of the long head of the biceps, including Speed's and Jergason's tests[49] and the isometric test of combined elbow flexion-supination with shoulder flexion, are positive, reproducing his weakness and pain. These positive findings correlate with the painful restriction of active extension and medial rotation. There is no physical evidence of direct spinal or neurodynamic involvement. Posterior deltoid, infraspinatus, and teres minor feel markedly tighter on soft-tissue assessment, but further palpation of the GH joint is unremarkable. Movement testing and palpation of the acromioclavicular, sternoclavicular, and scapulothoracic joints are negative.

The most marked impairment, along with his painful end of range elevation and extension and the resisted shoulder and elbow flexion tests, is the muscular performance of his scapulothoracic upward rotators and stabilizers, particularly his dynamic rotator cuff control from 90° elevation. This control is evaluated using the dynamic rotary stability test (DRST). This test was developed from the premise that, because of the stabilization from the musculocapsular force couples of the rotator cuff, the humeral head should remain centered during resisted isometric, isotonic, and eccentric medial and lateral rotation at varying angles of flexion and abduction (Fig. 13–10).[50-52]

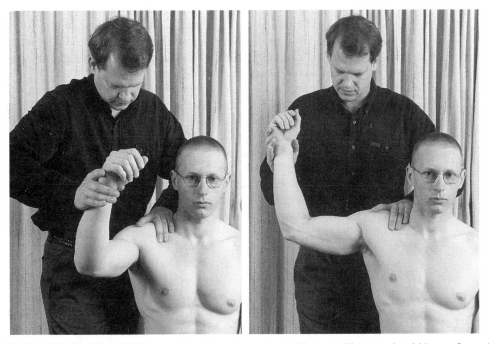

FIGURE 13–10. Two positions of the dynamic rotary stability test. This test should be performed isometrically and isotonically into both internal and external rotation through varying positions of elevation.

When the therapist tests dynamic lateral and medial rotation at 90° of elevation, this patient's humeral head has significantly more anterior and posterior translation than normal. When the patient is then instructed to stabilize his humerus against a distraction force in this position and hold this position while the dynamic rotations were repeated, his dynamic control is markedly improved. This ability to activate the force closure (i.e., dynamic stability) necessary for good functional stability of the GH joint is a sign that is indicative of good prognosis for a muscular re-education and strengthening approach. The poor humeral head centering during the dynamic rotary stability test might be related to an imbalance of anterior and posterior cuff control in the so-called "transverse force couple" in the presence of poor form closure (i.e., structural stability) secondary to increased anteroinferior laxity.[50] This imbalance is likely to include aspects of reduced strength and endurance, as well as altered timing of onset.

Studies from the Shoulder Research Group (Center for Allied Health Research, School of Physiotherapy, University of South Australia)[53] have revealed that, in the normal shoulder, the deep glenohumeral stabilizers are usually activated prior to the more superficial prime movers. Recent pilot work completed by the Shoulder Research Group has shown that timing of onset is dramatically altered in an unstable shoulder. Similarly, during isokinetic rotations, activity was consistently found in all components of the rotator cuff, regardless of the direction or speed of contraction.[53] Contraction in the antagonists occurred at approximately 20% of maximal voluntary contraction, a level identified by Pink et al.[54] as representing a stabilizing function. These findings support the concept of a stabilizing role for the rotator cuff, similar to that provided by transverse abdominis and multifidus for the lumbar spine, as shown by Richardson and Jull[55] and O'Sullivan et al.[56] This role of the rotator cuff demonstrates the importance of improving force closure or dynamic support for the GH joint through muscle re-education and motor programming in patients with similar impairments (see Chap. 14).

This patient has clinical features suggestive of a minor instability with possible labral involvement, associated with insufficient dynamic control and excessive translation. This subtle instability has led to superior labral strain from eccentric biceps activity, used to decelerate the extending elbow during the follow-through phase of throwing. However, clinical diagnosis of labral injury is difficult.[57–59] Although further investigations, such as CT arthrography or MRI, might confirm the diagnosis, surgical repair is generally not a first option, and conservative management might be sufficient to resolve his symptoms.[60–63] If conservative management fails to decrease symptoms and increase function, the improvement in strength and motor control will help expedite recovery if surgery is performed.

Despite the obvious need for a muscle re-education approach in this presentation, this case study is included here to highlight the benefits that might also be achieved from treatment by passive movement. The appropriateness of passive (and active) mobilization in a truly stiff shoulder is obvious. However, therapists should be careful not to prematurely categorize a presentation as either a stiff joint, only focusing on stretching techniques, or conversely as an unstable (static and/or dynamic) joint, only focusing on muscle re-education. Structures restricting medial rotation, whereas more likely a contributing factor than the actual source of his pain, might be a partial cause of the dynamic imbalance or a result of the patient's poor motor control. In this case, it is important not to be too biased by theory that is still evolving and impossible to substantiate on clinical testing alone. Rather, therapists must be prepared to experiment with treatments to address different hypothesized components of the problem and be guided by their reassessments. In some patients, improving medial rotation range will improve dynamic rotation control and stabilization.

Similarly, what role could passive mobilization have for management of this patient's slightly restricted and painful shoulder elevation and extension? If management is solely based on diagnostic reasoning, it could be questioned what passive mobilization could do for a minor instability with an apparent biceps anchor-superior labral lesion. Although being passionate about trying to improve understanding of shoulder diagnostics and the associated clinical patterns, physical therapy will never be an exact science.[1] Therefore, therapists are encouraged to remain open-minded to the benefits of movement (passive and active) in all presentations of shoulder dysfunction.

In this patient, when scapulothoracic and scapulohumeral muscle re-education are combined with active and passive techniques to improve medial rotation, significant improvement is noted in scapular and dynamic glenohumeral rotation control, medial rotation and extension range, and throwing performance. However, shoulder elevation remains slightly restricted and painful, his humeral head remains in an anterior resting position, and symptoms with prolonged strong throwing have not completely resolved. Therefore, passive mobilization into flexion is added, again guided by the relationship of pain to resistance found during this movement. In his case, the limiting factor is resistance (R_2) with pain (P') at end range being 5/10, so flexion is mobilized as a grade IV$^+$. Systematic introduction of different treatments and continual reassessment of all key signs clearly demonstrate that this passive mobilization contributes to his further improvement. The flexion stiffness and pain clear, and the humeral head resumes a more normal position relative to the glenoid, allowing better placement of the axis of rotation of the GH joint. The muscle control also improves both clinically and functionally, with the patient returning to full playing status without problems. Whether passive mobilization can actually help a SLAP lesion, if this diagnosis is in fact correct, or whether other pathology within the subacromial space or GH joint was responsible for the flexion sign that responded to passive treatment, is not known. However, as long as therapists have good clinical reasoning skills, are open minded to the approaches they use, and are disciplined in their assessment and reassessment of impairments, the optimal combination of treatment procedures should be found.

OTHER FACTORS INFLUENCING THE EXECUTION AND SUCCESS OF A TECHNIQUE

As alluded to previously, recognition of pathobiological mechanisms, including the dominant pain mechanisms operating and the stage of tissue healing, is important to judgments regarding the suitability of hands-on treatment. Whether a therapist decides to intentionally stress a structure and perhaps provoke symptoms, as opposed to selecting a less stressful, nonprovocative movement technique, is based on these clinical reasoning skills. For example, continued hands-on treatment by passive movement is not indicated when a dominant, centrally evoked pain mechanism has been established. Similarly, if the aim of treatment is to reduce stiffness in a patient with chronic hypomobility, biological changes to the capsuloligamentous and contractile tissues will be achieved more efficiently through the use of frequent exercise specifically designed to complement the aims and augment the effects of any hands-on treatment.

The neurophysiological mechanisms underlying successful treatment (i.e., reduced impairment, dysfunction, and disability) by passive movement are still poorly understood.[64–66] Local tissue and circulatory effects, along with neural modulation, are the most likely mechanisms activated by manual therapy techniques.[39,66,67] However, why is it that the same or similar techniques in the hands of an expert clinician will more often than not produce more significant improvement than the same technique delivered by a novice? Some skeptics might quickly suggest the confidence of the expert is likely to more successfully activate a neural modulatory placebo response. Although this theory might be true and does not refute simultaneous effects from the other proposed mechanisms, an understanding of the clinical variables that can maximize the success of a technique, regardless of the mechanisms operating, is advantageous to a manual therapist.

Patient Understanding

Perhaps of foremost importance is patient understanding. Skilled, collaborative reasoning will assist patients to develop an accurate, realistic, and healthy understanding of their problems. Research has demonstrated patients' understanding significantly influences pain tolerance, disability, and eventual outcome.[18–20] Greater understanding will increase the involvement and personal responsibility the patient takes in the management process, leading to better compliance and improved self-efficacy.[67] Besides these broader, perhaps central, effects of good collaborative reasoning, skilled communication between therapist and patient before, during, and after delivery of a technique is essential to both therapist and patient for understanding and logical treatment progression. An accurate baseline of resting symptoms and key impairments will increase the sensitivity of both the therapist and patient to detect changes during and after a technique. The aim of the technique should then be explained so the patient can assist the therapist in achieving the desired effect.

For example, if the patient understands that the intent is to ease the resting symptoms best achieved from a position of maximal comfort, the patient is then better able to guide the therapist in finding the most comfortable position and for reporting subtle changes in symptoms. Similarly, if a pain provocation or stretching sensation is sought, clear communication will assist the therapist to achieve this effect and to monitor for any change in this response during execution of the technique. In this way, techniques can be modified during their applications to better achieve the desired results. Appropriate reassessment of the technique movement itself, as well as resting symptoms and key impairments, is critical to establish the treatment effect and to further clarify the relationship between different impairments. For example, the use of passive movement to treat one impairment, such as capsular hypomobility, can simultaneously affect other impairments such as pain, posture, and muscle control.

Patient Comfort and Pain-Relieving Techniques

Patient comfort during treatment is important to achieve maximal relaxation and to avoid aggravation of other problem areas that might exist. Measures such as pillows under the patient's knees when supine or under the abdomen when prone can minimize stress to a symptomatic lumbar spine. The manner in which the patient's arm is held will also affect patient comfort significantly. Essentially, when gentle pain-easing passive movement techniques are performed, the arm should be placed in a position of maximal comfort before commencing the technique. This requires good communication with the patient to find the optimal position at which the arm should be supported to maintain the position with full patient relaxation (Fig. 13–5).

If accessory techniques are used, the therapist's hand placement is important, ensuring that no discomfort is created from the contact itself. Full hand-to-shoulder contact will typically feel more supportive to the patient. When physiological passive movement techniques such as flexion, abduction, or movement around the quadrant are used, the support given to the patient's arm is critical, particularly when pain is a dominant feature. Supporting under the patient's forearm (Fig. 13–11) can help the patient to relax. Similarly, standing above the patient with the therapist's thigh placed to create a block to further movement can also give confidence to the patient that the arm will not be moved too far (Fig. 13–12).

Once appropriate explanation is given and patient comfort is addressed through careful positioning and proper hand placement, the way the technique is performed should also be considered for optimal success. In the very painful shoulder, in which

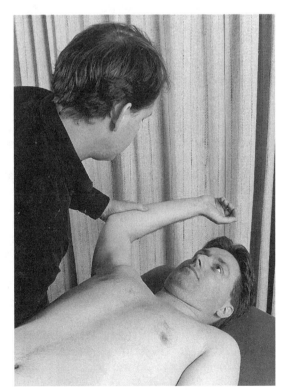

FIGURE 13–11. The GH quadrant being performed as a gentle technique with support under the patient's forearm.

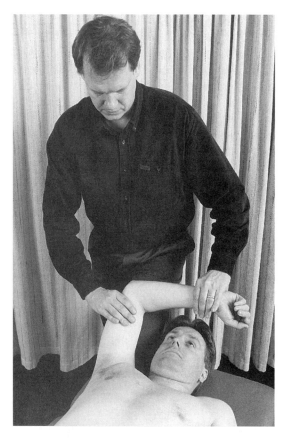

FIGURE 13–12. GH flexion being performed as a large amplitude movement, using the therapist's thigh as a block to end range movement.

any active or passive physiological movement increases symptoms, the largest amplitude pain-free movement usually will be one of the available accessory movements (e.g., posteroanterior or anteroposterior translations and caudal or lateral distractions). Although these mobilizations can be performed with scapular stabilization to create a more localized effect, the stabilization might only result in more discomfort and muscle guarding. In this instance, a better response might be achieved without any fixation (Fig. 13–6).

Skill in creating the passive movement chosen to treat a pain-dominant presentation is critical to its success. When passive movements are performed with a slow and smooth rhythm while avoiding abrupt movement transitions, the patient will be able to relax best. Subsequently, the techniques for pain relief are most effective. The patient should be continually encouraged to "let the shoulder go" (i.e., relax) while various speeds of movement are tried in the search for the most easing application.

Performing gentle pain-easing techniques or techniques that move into controlled amounts of pain and resistance require the greatest skill. The clinician must control the patient's arm, monitor the symptoms during the technique, and make the necessary adjustments to alter the amplitude, speed, and degree of pain and/or resistance challenged. In addition, the patient must be confident in the clinician's handling, to allow the clinician to provoke pain and have the patient still remain relaxed.

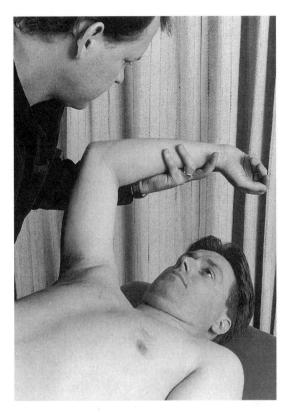

FIGURE 13-13. GH quadrant being performed as a treatment with the scapula supported.

Techniques to Treat Tissue Resistance

When stronger techniques are performed, stabilizing the scapula is important to ensure movement that is more localized to the GH joint. Grip here is still important, and care should be taken to ensure comfortable handling (Fig. 13–13).

Stronger techniques, used when pain is less dominant and the aim is to decrease stiffness to movement, are relatively easier to perform. Although strong techniques might require somewhat less therapist finesse, the large number of movement options requires skilled decision making to establish the optimal techniques to achieve the greatest gains. Movement options range from pure physiological movements to combinations of physiological with accessory movements in various ranges of physiological positions, all with or without the scapula stabilized. Symptom-easing techniques performed after a pain-provocative technique will also maximize the potential improvement by relieving any treatment soreness and muscle guarding that might have been elicited. Clinical experience has shown that passive movement using the same mobilizing technique, but performed short of any pain, is often effective in minimizing treatment soreness. For a pain-dominant presentation, this technique will typically be a smaller amplitude movement than that performed for treatment. In a presentation in which stiffness is greater than pain, a large amplitude movement in a pain-free range, which is performed with an abrupt end point (e.g., a flexion II$^+$ up against the therapist's thigh) (Fig. 13–12), is often most effective.

Generalizations, such as "treatment should not cause any pain" will limit the options available, also possibly limiting the rate of improvement achieved. The strategies outlined in this chapter demonstrate the relationship of pain and resistance to passive movement, along with broader consideration of muscle performance and associated contributing factors (e.g., thoracic mobility, posture, ergonomic issues). Such strategies for technique selection enable therapists to systematically compare different treatments when identifying the most effective approach for any particular stage of the patient's presentation. Optimal results will be made when the therapist continually re-evaluates the patient's status and regularly tries different combinations of passive (i.e., "joint" and soft-tissue mobilization) and active (muscle re-education and exercise) treatment intermixed with goal-specific self-management.

CHAPTER SUMMARY

Throughout this chapter, information focuses on the selection and progression of passive movement, qualifying this emphasis with reference to the importance of other forms of passive (e.g., soft tissue) and active (e.g., muscle re-education) treatment. Two patient case studies described the successful use of passive movement for managing the patient's condition. The chapter also highlights a useful strategy of selecting and progressing passive movement treatment. However, therapists should not consider their hands-on treatment the complete answer to the patient's problems. Assessment findings and past experience will also suggest other procedures that can be equally or, possibly, more effective than passive movement. These procedures should also be used, particularly if the initial attempts at passive movement do not provide relief. For example, if muscle guarding is a dominant finding of the active and passive movements assessed, active or passive scapulothoracic mobilization and soft-tissue techniques can also be very effective. Electrotherapy might also be effective and, like passive movement techniques, might be best for the pain-dominant presentation when delivered from a position of maximal comfort.

Hands-on treatment should be seen as a trial of the benefit of movement and exercise at any particular stage of the patient's presentation. Whereas hands-on treatments clearly produce improvements in their own right, they should also be considered a guide to the selection and progression of the patient's self management. For example, if passive mobilization of the GH joint in a quadrant position is effective for decreasing pain in the subacromial area, a home program of mobilizing exercises should be considered. Self-mobilizations should be performed in the same direction, at the same depth and intensity, and coupled with other mobilizations to ensure dynamic control of any new range gained.

Lastly, key factors are highlighted that influence the execution and success of treatment by passive movement. These include the patient's understanding, patient comfort during a technique, and skill in selecting and performing different techniques.

REFERENCES

1. Magarey, ME, et al: Evaluation of physiotherapy accuracy in shoulder diagnosis: A comparison with orthopaedic clinical and arthroscopic diagnosis (in press for 2001).
2. Jones, MA, et al: Clinical Reasoning in physiotherapy. In Higgs, J, and Jones, MA (eds): Clinical Reasoning in the Health Professions, ed 2. Butterworth Heinemann, Oxford, 2000, 117-127.

3. Higgs, J, and Jones, MA (eds): Clinical Reasoning in the Health Professions, ed 2. Butterworth Heinemann, Oxford, 2000.
4. Jones, MA: The clinical reasoning process in manipulative therapy. In Dalziel, BA, and Snowsill, JC (eds): Proceedings, Fifth Biennial Conference, Manipulative Therapists Association of Australia, 1987, p 62.
5. Gifford, LS: Pain. In Pitt-Brooke, J (ed): Rehabilitation of Movement: Theoretical Basis of Clinical Practice. WB Saunders, London, 1997, p 196.
6. Gifford, L, and Butler, D: The integration of pain sciences into clinical practice. J Hand Ther 10:86, 1997.
7. Jones, MA: Clinical reasoning and pain. Manual Ther 1:17, 1995.
8. World Health Organization: International Classification of Impairments, Disabilities and Handicaps. Geneva, Switzerland, 1980.
9. Gifford, LS: Tissue and input related mechanisms. In Gifford, L (ed): Topical Issues in Pain. Physiotherapy Pain Association Yearbook 1998-1999, NOI Press, Falmouth, 1998a, p 57.
10. Meyer, RA, et al: Peripheral neural mechanisms of nociception. In Wall, P, and Melzack, R (eds): Textbook of Pain, ed 3. Churchill Livingstone, Edinburgh, 1994, p 13.
11. Bennett, GJ: Neuropathic pain. In Wall, P, and Melzack, R (eds): Textbook of Pain, ed 3. Churchill Livingstone, Edinburgh, 1994, p 201.
12. Merskey, H, and Bogduk, N: Classification of Chronic Pain, ed 2. Task Force on Taxonomy of the International Association for the Study of Pain. IASP Press, Seattle, 1994.
13. Gifford, L: The "central" mechanisms. In Gifford, L (ed): Topical Issues in Pain. Physiotherapy Pain Association Yearbook 1998-1999, NOI Press, Falmouth, 1998b, p 67.
14. Fields, HL, and Basbaum, AI: Central nervous system mechanisms of pain modulation. In Wall, P, and Melzack, R: Textbook of Pain, ed 3. Churchill Livingstone, Edinburgh, 1994, p 243.
15. Gifford, L: Output mechanisms. In Gifford, L (ed): Topical Issues in Pain. Physiotherapy Pain Association Yearbook 1998-1999, NOI Press, Falmouth, 1998c, p 81.
16. Goodman, C: The endocrine and metabolic systems. In Goodman, C, and Boissonault, W (eds): Pathology Implications for the Physical Therapist. WB Saunders, Philadelphia, 1998, p 216.
17. Goodman, C, and Snyder, T: The immune system. In Goodman, C, and Boissonault, W (eds): Pathology Implications for the Physical Therapist. WB Saunders, Philadelphia, 1998, p 91.
18. Borkan, JM, et al: Finding meaning after the fall: Injury narratives from elderly hip fracture patients. Soc Sci Med 33:947, 1991.
19. Feuerstein, M, and Beattie, P: Biobehavioural factors affecting pain and disability in low back pain: Mechanisms and assessment. Phys Ther 75:267, 1995.
20. Malt, UF, and Olafson, OM: Psychological appraisal and emotional response to physical injury: A clinical, phenomenological study of 109 adults. Psych Med 10:117, 1995.
21. Cooper, DE, et al: Anatomy, histology and vascularity of the glenoid labrum. J Bone Jt Surg Am 74A:46, 1992.
22. Bigliani, LU, et al: The relationship of acromial architecture to rotator cuff disease. Clin Sports Med 10:823, 1991.
23. van Wingerden, BAM: Connective Tissue in Rehabilitation. Scipro Verlag, Vaduz, 1995.
24. Zusman, M: Instigators of activity intolerance. Manual Ther 2:75, 1997.
25. Zusman, M: Structure-oriented beliefs and disability due to back pain. Aust J Physiother 44:13, 1998.
26. ACC, and the National Health Committee: New Zealand Acute Low Back Pain Guide, Wellington, New Zealand, 1997.
27. Leadbetter, WB: An introduction to sports-induced soft-tissue inflammation. In Leadbetter, WB, et al (eds): Sports-Induced Inflammation. American Orthopaedic Society for Sports Medicine Symposium, American Academy of Orthopaedic Surgeons, Park Ridge, IL, 1990, p 3.
28. Woo, SL, and Buckwalter, JA (eds): Injury and Repair of the Musculoskeletal Soft Tissues. American Academy of Orthopaedic Surgeons Symposium, American Academy of Orthopaedic Surgeons, Park Ridge, IL, 1988.
29. Harryman, DT, et al: Laxity of the normal glenohumeral joint: A quantitative in vivo assessment. J Shoulder Elbow Surg 1:66, 1992.
30. Harryman, DT, et al: The humeral head translates on the glenoid with passive motion. In Post, M, et al (eds): Surgery of the Shoulder. Mosby Year Book, St. Louis, 1990, p 186.
31. Burkhead, WZ: Frozen shoulder syndrome: Frozen shoulder, idiopathic chronic adhesive capsulitis, post-traumatic stiff shoulder and painful stiff shoulder. In Burkhead, WZ (ed): Rotator Cuff Disorders. Williams and Watkins, Baltimore, 1996, p 220.
32. Magarey, ME: The first treatment session. In Grieve, GP (ed): Modern Manual Therapy of the Vertebral Column. Churchill Livingstone, Edinburgh, 1986, p 661.
33. Maitland, GD: Vertebral Manipulation. Butterworth Heinemann, London, 1986.
34. Maitland, GD: Peripheral Manipulation, Butterworth Heinemann, London, 1991.
35. MacDermid, JC, et al: Intra- and inter-rater reliability of goniometric measurement of shoulder passive lateral rotation. J Hand Ther 12:187, 1999.
36. MacDermid, JC, et al: Validity of pain and motion indicators recorded on a movement diagram of shoulder lateral rotation. Aust J Physiother 45:269, 1999.
37. Jones, MA, and Jones, HM: Principles of the physical examination. In Boyling, JD, and Palastanga, N

(eds): Grieve's Modern Manual Therapy: The Vertebral Column, ed 2. Churchill Livingstone, Edinburgh, 1994, p 491.
38. Butler, DS: Mobilisation of the Nervous System. Churchill Livingstone, Melbourne, 1991.
39. Vujnovich, AL: Neural plasticity, muscle spasm and tissue manipulation: A review of the literature. J Manual Manipulative Ther 3:152, 1995.
40. Magarey, ME, and Jones, MA: A clinical note: The shoulder quadrant revisited. Manual Ther (in press for 2001).
41. Magarey, ME, and Jones, MA: Clinical examination and management for minor instability of the shoulder complex. Aust J Physiother 38:260, 1991.
42. Birnbaum, K, and Lierse, W: Anatomy and function of the bursa subacromialis. Acta Anat 145:354, 1992.
43. Brown, LP, et al: Upper extremity range of motion and isokinetic strength of the internal and external shoulder rotators in major league baseball players. Am J Sports Med 16:577, 1988.
44. Gerber, C, and Ganz, R: Clinical assessment of instability of the shoulder, with special reference to anterior and posterior drawer tests. J Bone Jt Surg (Br) 66B:551, 1984.
45. Jobe, CM, et al: Anterior shoulder instability, impingement and rotator cuff tear. In Jobe, FW (ed): Operative Techniques in Upper Extremity Sports Injuries. Mosby, St. Louis, 1996, p 164.
46. Andrews, JR, and Gillogly, S: Physical examination of the shoulder in throwing athletes. In Zarins, B, et al (eds): Injuries to the Throwing Arm. WB Saunders, Philadelphia, 1985.
47. Hawkins, RJ, and Bokor, DJ: Clinical evaluation of shoulder problems. In Rockwood, CA, and Matsen, FA (eds): The Shoulder. WB Saunders, Philadelphia, 1990, p 149.
48. Gerber, C, et al: The subcoracoid space: An anatomic study. Clin Orthop 215:132, 1987.
49. Hawkins, RJ, and Kennedy, JC: Impingement syndrome in athletes. Am J Sports Med 8:151, 1980.
50. Burkhart, SS: A unified biomechanical rationale for the treatment of rotator cuff tears: Debridement versus repair. In Burkhead, WZ (ed): Rotator Cuff Disorders. Williams and Wilkins, Baltimore, 1996, p 293.
51. Guanche, CA, et al: Arthroscopic versus open reconstruction of the shoulder in patients with isolated Bankart lesions. Am J Sports Med 24:144, 1996.
52. Wuelker, N, et al: Passive glenohumeral joint stabilization: A biomechanical study. J Shoulder Elbow Surg 3:129, 1994.
53. David, G, et al: Electromyographic activity of rotator cuff and delto-pectoral muscles during isokinetic glenohumeral joint rotations. Clin Biomech 15:95, 2000.
54. Pink, M, et al: The normal shoulder during freestyle swimming. Am J Sports Med 19:569, 1991.
55. Richardson, C, and Jull, GA: Muscle control—pain control: What exercises would you prescribe? Manual Ther 1:2, 1996.
56. O'Sullivan, PB, et al: Altered abdominal muscle recruitment in patients with chronic back pain following a specific exercise intervention. J Orthop Sports Phys Ther 27:114, 1998.
57. Magarey, ME, et al: Biomedical considerations and clinical patterns related to disorders of the glenoid labrum in the predominantly stable glenohumeral joint. Manual Ther 1:242, 1996.
58. Snyder, SJ, et al: An analysis of 140 injuries to the superior glenoid labrum. J Shoulder Elbow Surg 4:243, 1995.
59. Snyder, SJ, et al: SLAP lesions of the shoulder. Arthroscopy 6:274, 1990.
60. Chandnani, VP, et al: Glenohumeral ligaments and shoulder capsular mechanism: Evaluation with MR arthrography. Radiology 196:27, 1995.
61. Hayes, MG, et al: The shoulder complex: Correlation of clinical examination, computed arthrotomography, magnetic resonance imaging, and arthroscopic evaluation. In Post, M, et al (eds): Surgery of the Shoulder. Mosby Year Book, St. Louis, 1990, p 18.
62. Nelson, MC, et al: Evaluation of the painful shoulder. J Bone Jt Surg Am 73A:707, 1991.
63. Suder, PA, et al: Magnetic resonance imaging evaluation of capsulolabral tears after traumatic primary anterior shoulder dislocation. J Shoulder Elbow Surg 4:419, 1995.
64. Haldeman, S: Manipulation and massage for the relief of back pain. In Melzack, R, and Wall, PD (eds): The Textbook of Pain, ed 3. Churchill Livingstone, Edinburgh, 1994, p 1251.
65. Wright, A: Hypoalgesia post-manipulative therapy: A review of a potential neurophysiological mechanism. Manual Ther 1:11, 1995.
66. Zusman, M: What does manipulation do? The need for basic research. In Boyling, JD, and Palastanga, N (eds): Grieve's Modern Manual Therapy: The Vertebral Column, ed 2. Churchill Livingstone, Edinburgh, 1994, p 651.
67. Strong, J: Self-efficacy and the patient in chronic pain. In Shacklock, M (ed): Moving In On Pain. Butterworth Heinemann, Chatswood, 1995, p 97.

CHAPTER 14

Neuromuscular Re-education Strategies for the Shoulder Girdle

Jenny McConnell, BAppSci (Phty), Grad Dip Man Ther, MBiomedE

INTRODUCTION

The shoulder girdle must balance mobility with stability to provide sufficient flexibility, dexterity, and precision for the upper extremity. However, because of the bony configuration of the humeral head and the glenoid fossa, the shoulder is an inherently unstable joint. Despite the limited stability of this joint (only 25% to 35% of the humeral head is in contact with the glenoid at any time), shoulder kinematics are maintained by the passive (ligaments and joint capsule) and dynamic (muscles) restraints. Therefore, only a few millimeters of translation should occur in any plane during motion.[1] To accommodate the extremes of rotation that occur in multiple planes at the glenohumeral (GH) joint, the capsule must have some degree of laxity. At the same time, sufficient tension in the system is necessary to control excessive translation. This fine balance of movement is attributed to the anatomy of the capsule and the changing role of the various passive and active restraints, which accommodate to the changing positions of the arm.

The shoulder, essentially dependent on the muscles for stability, is prone to chronic overuse injuries. The management of shoulder problems involves analyzing the underlying causes of the symptoms (impairments) and directing treatment to resolve the symptoms, thus preventing reoccurrence. Treatment directed exclusively at the relief of symptoms will only be partially effective because the presenting symptoms are usually the result of a specific impairment as described in Chapter 4. Two common impairments include poor muscle performance and motor control.

Accurate identification of the impairments altering normal function is critical to the success of treatment. When examining the shoulder complex, the physical therapist must consider all muscle attachment sites that contribute to the dynamic stability of the joint. Two of the twelve muscles that span the shoulder joint have remote attachments: the latissimus dorsi from the iliac crest, and the pectoralis major from the anterior ribs along the thorax. The latissimus dorsi and the lower and middle fibers of trapezius have extensive attachments onto the thoracic spine. Through the origin on the ribs, the pectoralis major is also indirectly attached to the thoracic spine. Therefore, the mobility of the thoracic spine through various muscle attachments can affect the mobility and function of the shoulder joint complex. Additionally, the pattern of activation of the various muscles around the shoulder complex affects control and coordination of the shoulder movement. This chapter examines neuro-muscular re-education strategies for the shoulder girdle.

SPECIFICITY OF TRAINING

Before examining the exercise prescription for the patient with shoulder problems, it is necessary to understand different philosophies of strength training. The traditional strength training view suggests evidence of a carry-over in strength gained from nonspecific muscle training to the requirements of performance. For example, whereas the engine (muscles) is built in the strength training room, learning how to turn the engine on (neural control) is acquired on the field.[2] Strength is increased by using the overload principle. This means exercising at least 60% of maximal voluntary contraction (MVC) of a muscle.[3] Muscles around the GH joint are stabilizing muscles that need to be trained for endurance by working at 20% to 30% of MVC for longer durations. A more recent interpretation of how to facilitate strength is based on the premise that the engine (muscles) and how it is turned on (neural control) should both be emphasized during rehabilitation.[2] Training should therefore simulate movement in terms of the following:

1. Anatomical position. Training has been shown to be specific to limb position. As early as 1957, Rasch & Morehouse[4] demonstrated postural specificity to training. In their study examining the training effects of isometric exercises on the elbow flexors in standing position, a significant increase in isometric elbow flexor torque was noted when tested in standing. However, only a slight increase occurred when tested in the sitting position.
2. Pattern of movement. Although training effects have been observed in the nonexercised contralateral limbs in subjects who have undergone unilateral exercise, effects of strength training are largely muscle specific. The most likely explanation for the contralateral strength changes is that subjects learn muscle activation strategies so that they can lift heavier loads. These activation strategies can be utilized by the contralateral limb.[5]
3. Velocity of contraction. If muscles are trained at one velocity, they become stronger at that velocity, and the strength gains at other velocities are less apparent.[6]
4. Type and force of contraction. Although some carry-over exists, training effects are specific to joint angle. If a muscle is trained isometrically at one angle, or dynamically through a limited range, the increases in strength occur in the training range with limited increases at other joint angles.[7,8] Conversely, if the muscle has

been trained isokinetically, there will be an increase in isokinetic strength (one study demonstrating 180% increase after 12 weeks), but only a minimal change in isometric strength (11%).[6]

Thus, training causes changes within the central and peripheral nervous system, allowing an individual to better coordinate the activation of muscle groups.[9] The neuromuscular system will develop improved recruitment strategies for activities that simulate the muscle actions employed in training, but not necessarily for other movement patterns. Both internal and external feedback, an integral part of this training process, must be precise to maximize learning.

External Feedback

External feedback is frequently referred to as knowledge of results, indicating the outcome produced is a consequence of movement.[10,11] For example, when playing the piano, auditory input enables the pianist to determine whether the correct notes have been played. Although external feedback is available only for a very short period of time, it is categorized and coded so it can be remembered later. This process establishes a future reference so that the pianist can recall whether the correct notes are being played or whether the finger position needs to be altered to prevent a mistake. This organized and coded input indicates the level of goal accomplishment.

Internal Feedback

Internal feedback is often referred to as knowledge of performance because it signals how movement is occurring. Information is received in the following four subsystems:

1. The configuration of movement. This involves spatial and temporal features of the environment and body. For example, a car door can be closed slowly and carefully, or it can be slammed. The configuration of the movement is similar, but the rate and/or force can vary.
2. The constraints placed on the timing or force of movement. These constraints dictate that the movement must be performed within a specific time interval (e.g., receiving a tennis serve), at a certain time (e.g., when the traffic light turns red), with reference to external velocity features (e.g., stepping on an escalator), or with appropriate force (e.g., holding a polystyrene cup).[11]
3. The organization of functional movement patterns. This simplifies movement and the processing of sensory feedback. Muscles and joints act in synergy as opposed to moving as separate entities.[11,12] Humans have a variety of functional synergies for stabilization and locomotion. For example, gait has a similar sequence of joint motion occurring at the ankle, knee, and hip regardless of the cadence. Central pattern generators (CPGs), preset units that allow movements to occur automatically, have been identified as the mechanism responsible for this orderly sequence of joint movement. Oscillatory networks of interneurons have been implicated as the neural substrate for the CPGs.[12]
4. Joint torques and muscle forces. These forces are controlled by ongoing modulation

of excitatory and inhibitory states within alpha and gamma motor neuron pools. The recruitment of specific muscles depends on limb orientation relative to gravity, as well as the position of the body segments relative to each other.[11] When a muscle spans more than one joint, the relative position of the body and limb will influence muscle function. The order and pattern of muscle firing is also affected by joint stiffness. To resist perturbation from external forces, cocontraction of muscles surrounding the joint occurs to improve joint stability. Cocontraction is a strategy that is also used when learning a new skill.

During skill acquisition, increasing the mechanical stiffness of a joint through cocontraction of opposing muscle groups decreases the freedom of movement. The result is lack of efficient and coordinated movement.

With adequate training, appropriate muscles can be activated. Sensory information from the periphery is processed centrally to determine limb position and muscle tension, so adjustments can be made before the movement is activated. Sensory setting and feedback can contribute in two ways: preparing for movement and ensuring the programmed relaxation of postural tensions at a joint; and detecting whether a mismatch exists between the intended program and the actual movements and ensuring that appropriate corrections can be made by the CNS.

Feed-Forward System

External feedback involves learning the motor program so that fewer adjustments are needed for movement. Programmed movements can exist without sensory feedback, referred to as a feed-forward or open loop system. The advantage of this system is speed, but the system lacks the fine-tuning offered by feedback. In the feed-forward system, adjustment occurs in a muscle so that it is "set" in advance for a particular activity. The feedback mechanism is too slow to fine tune for any error because by the time the information is received, the muscle is already in a new position. In motor control systems, a combination of feed-forward and feedback occurs.

Adaptive Servo-Assist Theory

In the adaptive servo-assist theory of control, both gamma and alpha motor neurons are involved in volitional movements, whereas the sensitivity of the spindles is modulated according to the program. Programmed muscle spindles acting on a joint can detect mismatches between the actual and the expected movement. Central control of spinal gamma motor neurons is an example of a subprogram, which functions to provide models of the intended movement on the spindles to make them act as error detectors. The spinal alpha motor neurons respond to any mismatch of information by adjusting the length of the muscle. The mismatch messages are relayed to the association cortex. Although movement can be performed continuously, the underlying movement programs are updated intermittently.[13]

When the speed of the movement increases, the movement is more dependent on the inherent muscle properties for stability. Feedback during explosive movements is unlikely because of time delays. Plus, the role of sensory input is limited to signaling the initial position of movement. Small errors in supraspinal input can affect explosive movements, so this input must be finely tuned to the properties of the musculoskeletal system.[13] Many shoulder movements, particularly during sporting activities, are explosive movements involving stability and control of the shoulder muscles. Shoulder muscle training needs to be specific, so the relevant muscles are activated at the right time with the appropriate intensity. For example, certain individuals with postural changes and associated muscle imbalances might require adjustments in the usual patterns of muscle activation. Individuals with forward-sitting shoulders might require changes in the intensity and timing of the scapular stabilizers such as the upper trapezius, lower trapezius, and serratus anterior. Faulty scapular position that occurs in these individuals can result in impingement between the humerus and the acromion during overhead activities. This impingement can cause a reduced range of total shoulder flexion, as well as pain and loss of function.[14,15]

TAPING THE GLENOHUMERAL JOINT

Faulty patterns of movement are difficult to correct because they are usually not apparent to the individual. Any attempt to alter posture is usually resisted because new postures often feel abnormal. To facilitate the change in position, and to decrease symptoms, tape may be applied to the shoulder. The effect of tape on the management of shoulder conditions has not been widely investigated, but some parallels can be drawn from studies involving the use of tape on the patellofemoral joint. Numerous studies have established that taping the patella relieves pain, but the mechanism of the effect is still being debated in the literature.[16–19] Patellar taping of symptomatic individuals has been associated with changes in vastus medialis obliquus activation, increases in loading response knee flexion, and increases in quadriceps muscle torque.

The shoulder can be taped using two different methods: correction of the anteriorly translated humeral head (forward sitting shoulder), which usually contributes to impingement problems; and stabilization of the shoulder with multidirectional instability. Differentiation of the two is required.

Anterior Translation of the Humeral Head

Anterior translation of the humeral head might be atraumatic or posttraumatic. Atraumatic anterior instability is relatively common in overhead athletes. Laxity of the anterior capsule develops over time because of repeated stressing of the static stabilizers at the extremes of motion during activities such as throwing, hitting a volleyball, or swinging a tennis racquet.[20] As a consequence of the anterior translation, the humeral head stabilizers become elongated, altering the balance of the deltoid-rotator cuff force couple. This altered function might cause the humeral head to migrate superiorly with a deltoid contraction, narrowing the subacromial space and increasing the potential for ischemia or inflammation of the tendons. If the presence of instability is not recognized and treated, secondary impingement symptoms will persist. Figure 14–1 summarizes the factors involved in impingement.

Patients with an anteriorly translated humeral head are usually athletes involved in overhead sports who might report pain, discomfort, paraesthesia, numbness, fatigue, or apprehension. Other physical findings include a stiff thoracic spine and atrophy of the rotator cuff and trapezius musculature.

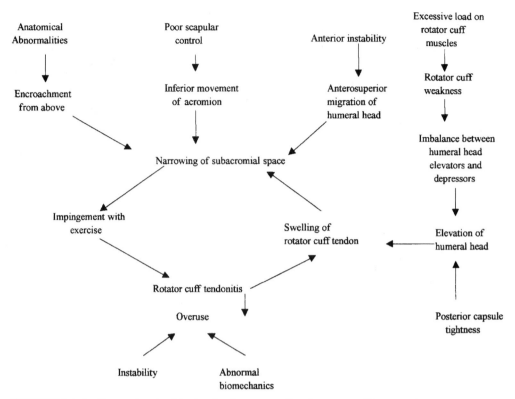

FIGURE 14–1. Factors involved in the development of impingement. (From Brukner, P, and Kahn, K: Clinical Sports Medicine, McGraw Hill, Sydney, 1993, with permission.)

To improve the position of the anteriorly translated humeral head, tape can be anchored on the anterior aspect of the GH joint. The tape is used to lift the head of the humerus superiorly and posteriorly so the head of the humerus is slightly externally rotated (Fig. 14–2). The tape is then pulled diagonally across the scapula, finishing just medially to the inferior border of the scapula. Theoretically, this placement is designed to help stimulate lower trapezius activity by re-establishing its normal length-tension relationship. A second piece of tape is placed anteriorly on the humerus and is pulled over the acromion process where it is anchored lateral to the inferior border of the scapula. Once the patient has been taped, the patient's symptomatic activity must be rechecked. If the symptoms are not relieved immediately by at least 50%, use of tape is inappropriate.

Multidirectional Instability

Patients with multidirectional instability are usually females with diffuse joint laxity (often with genu recurvatum, hyperextended elbows), who present initially during adolescence. The condition is generally bilateral and exacerbated by overhead activities.

The shoulder musculature is poorly developed, so patients will often exhibit subluxation with each movement of their shoulders, usually in a posteroinferior direction. These patients present with flat thoracic spines, abducted scapulae, and

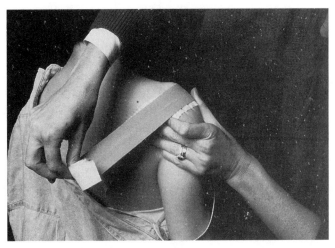

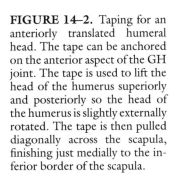

FIGURE 14–2. Taping for an anteriorly translated humeral head. The tape can be anchored on the anterior aspect of the GH joint. The tape is used to lift the head of the humerus superiorly and posteriorly so the head of the humerus is slightly externally rotated. The tape is then pulled diagonally across the scapula, finishing just medially to the inferior border of the scapula.

poor strength of the rotator cuffs, deltoids, rhomboids, and lower trapezius musculature. They also demonstrate positive sulcus signs and posterior laxity. The humeral heads are generally not anteriorly displaced, although they usually have instability in an anterior direction.

In these individuals, the superior glenohumeral and coracohumeral ligaments are stretched, the capsule is lax, and the humeral head is depressed. Here, taping can be used to elevate the humeral head and center it in the glenoid fossa. The patient's arm rests on the table at 45° of abduction. The humeral head is manually placed in neutral position by the therapist. The tape fans the deltoid muscle to pull the humeral head superiorly (Fig. 14–3). The first piece of tape is anchored over the middle deltoid and

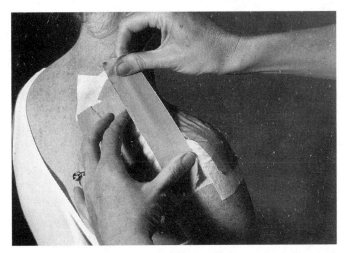

FIGURE 14–3. Taping for multidirectional instability. The goal is to elevate the humeral head and center it in the glenoid fossa. The patient's arm rests on the table at 45° of abduction and the humeral head is manually placed in neutral position by the therapist. The tape fans the deltoid muscle to pull the humeral head superiorly. The first piece of tape is anchored over the middle deltoid and pulled superiorly, attached over the acromion to lift the humeral head. The second piece, beginning anteriorly on the humerus, passes diagonally over the clavicle being anchored on the spine of the scapula, thus elevating the humeral head. The third piece of tape is placed on the posterior deltoid, coursing posteriorly to midway along the upper trapezius. This piece of tape also assists in elevating the humerus, adds posterior stability to the joint, and provides a secure feeling for the patient.

pulled superiorly, attached over the acromion to lift the humeral head. The second piece, beginning anteriorly on the humerus, passes diagonally over the clavicle being anchored on the spine of the scapula, thus elevating the humeral head. The third piece of tape is placed on the posterior deltoid, coursing posteriorly to midway along the upper trapezius. This piece of tape also assists in elevating the humerus, adds posterior stability to the joint, and provides a secure feeling for the patient. Because the arm is already abducted, the therapist does not need to apply a great deal of force on the tape to lift the humeral head.

The tape remains attached for a week, until the patient returns for a subsequent visit. Patients can shower because the tape does not lose its adhesiveness when wet. On the return visit, the therapist needs to remove the tape with care to prevent skin breakdown, particularly on the anterior aspect of the humeral head where there is little soft tissue. Topical skin preparation with a plastic skin or milk of magnesia is essential before the tape is applied. If skin breakdown occurs as a consequence of an allergic reaction to the adhesive, taping is discontinued until the skin is healed. Once the rash has healed, hypoallergenic tape can be applied for short periods, using a plastic skin preparation on the shoulder.

Tape is a useful adjunct in treatment to help train the muscles to maintain the preferred postural alignment. Tape enhances the muscle activation by minimizing the patient's symptoms and enabling the lengthened stabilizing muscles to be shortened.

MUSCLE TRAINING

Muscle training exercises prescribed for the patient should be aimed at correcting any neuromuscular imbalances. Thus, initial training sessions focus more on motor skill acquisition than on strengthening. Strength gains might not be observed because the muscles are trained in a different functional position than that to which they are accustomed, and different muscle synergies are required.[10,21] For example, training of the scapular and glenohumeral stabilizers (the lower trapezius and the rotator cuff muscles), for a swimmer who has shoulder impingement pain during freestyle swimming, should be performed while the patient is prone. However, training in a prone position might not be appropriate for a tennis player with shoulder impingement. Muscle training for the tennis player should simulate tennis positions, incorporating many muscles to improve the efficiency of energy transfer from the ground to the upper extremity.

Training for Multidirectional Instability

Muscle training also needs to be specific to the type of impairment. A volleyball player with a multidirectional instability requires different emphasis in training than a volleyball player with an impingement problem resulting from an anteriorly translated humeral head. In the first example, the emphasis is initially on deltoid training, whereas the patient with the anteriorly translated humeral head begins with scapular stabilizer and rotator cuff exercises. The patient with multidirectional instability might be aggravated by treatment that initially focuses on the rotator cuff, because tension in the rotator cuff musculature causes a depression of the humeral head, further destabilizing the GH joint.

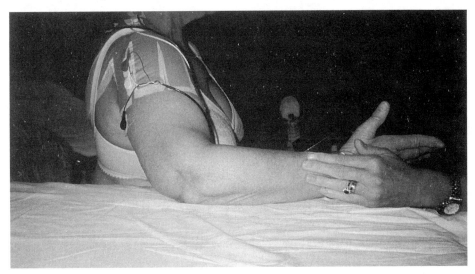

FIGURE 14-4. Training the posterior deltoid to provide posterior stability and vertical displacement of the humeral head. Initially the resistance is applied while the forearm is supported on the table and the arm is abducted 45°, placing the deltoid at a better mechanical advantage. This arm position also ensures minimal upper trapezius activity, which indirectly assists scapular stabilization.

To improve the stability of the shoulder, the posterior deltoid is trained to provide posterior stability and vertical displacement of the humeral head. The posterior deltoid works as a shoulder stabilizer when submaximal resistance is applied to the supinators of the forearm. Initially the resistance is applied while the forearm is supported on the table and the arm is abducted 45°, placing the deltoid at a better mechanical advantage (Fig. 14-4). This arm position also ensures minimal upper trapezius activity, which indirectly assists scapular stabilization. Once the deltoid can be recruited as a stabilizer through the full range of motion, rotator cuff and scapular stabilizing training is initiated. Muscle training is a slow process. Patients must be educated in the importance of perseverance when trying to improve the endurance capacity of this muscle group. Patients who do not have the dedication and are not willing to make the commitment to train their muscles will have a poor treatment outcome.

Muscle training is sometimes facilitated with the use of biofeedback. Dual channel electromyography (EMG) is one biofeedback device that can enhance specificity of training and provide patient motivation through visual or auditory cues about muscle activity (Fig. 14-5).

USE OF BIOFEEDBACK

The value of EMG biofeedback in rehabilitation is currently being challenged in the literature. Confusion exists about the issue of the timing and intensity of the various muscles around the shoulder and whether surface EMG is adequate for rehabilitation. Much of the EMG data available on the shoulder relates to overhead athletes, such as throwers, and might not apply to the nonthrowing population.[22] Some of the exercises used to isolate specific shoulder muscles based on EMG analysis might be unsuitable for a symptomatic individual. For example, the empty can

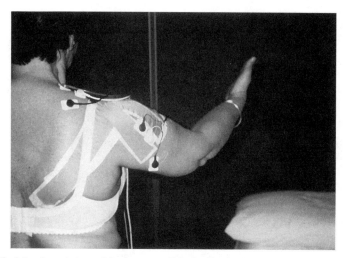

FIGURE 14–5. Muscle training with the use of biofeedback. A dual channel electromyographic is applied to enhance specificity of training and to provide patient motivation through visual and/or auditory cues about muscle activity.

exercise (elevation of the upper extremity in the plane of the scapula, with internal rotation of the shoulder) is one of the most commonly used exercises for strengthening the supraspinatus. When the arm is elevated in this position, impingement of the subacromial space might occur.

Normalization is another issue that affects the EMG interpretation of the relative contribution of various muscles to a movement. This procedure involves the patient performing a normalizing (usually maximal) isometric contraction to be used as a reference value for that muscle, known as the maximum voluntary isometric contraction (MVIC). During movements, the EMG of a muscle is expressed as ratio relative to the MVIC. This analysis enables the therapist to compare the ratio of one muscle relative to another muscle. The normalization procedure could be affected by pain inhibition, which might mask differences when examining the ratio of one muscle relative to another.[23] Some debate about the reliability of using a MVIC for the normalization process has appeared in the literature.[24] Howard and Enoka[25] found considerable variation in the MVIC of the vastus lateralis EMG, even though the force exerted by the quadriceps remained constant. Yang and Winter[24] found that the averaged rectified EMG had a coefficient of variation (SD/mean) of 9.1% in 1 day and 16.4% between days. Therefore, EMG measurements during a MVIC have large internal variation, possibly reflecting variations in neural drive.

Rehabilitation of the Anteriorly Translated Humeral Head

Rehabilitation of the anteriorly translated humeral head requires training of the lower trapezius and rotator cuff muscles. A force couple exists between portions of the upper trapezius muscle and the upper portions of the serratus anterior, lower trapezius, and lower serratus anterior muscles. The force couple causes an upward rotation of the scapula, increasing the bony stability of the shoulder, because more of the glenoid fossa is positioned superiorly. However, an increased thoracic kyphosis and a forward sitting humeral head cause protraction of the scapula and imbalance in the proximal shoulder girdle muscles.[15] An elongated lower trapezius might have less motor activity, which can alter the balance in the scapular force couple, resulting in an earlier onset and increase in the amount of upper trapezius activity. This muscle imbalance or loss of motor control might predispose the individual to an impingement problem.

The aim of training is achievement of greater proximal stability, particularly in the girdle and trunk musculature. Proximal stability can change the entire movement pattern so that scapulohumeral rhythm becomes smoother and more efficient. Restoring the force couple of the deltoid and rotator cuff will resolve the hyperactivity in the upper trapezius because it will no longer be required as a prime mover for abduction. Recruitment of the lower and middle trapezius is needed for upward rotation of the glenoid fossa. This will remove the acromion from the elevating humerus and increase the intrinsic stability of the GH joint, decreasing the amount of tension required in the rotator cuff group to maintain the head of the humerus in the glenoid fossa.

During neuromuscular re-education, the patient needs to be instructed in recruiting the lower trapezius in a manner that matches or exceeds the upper trapezius activity. This recruitment can be achieved by asking the patient to elevate the sternum, maintaining this elevation during movement. This verbal cue is a preferable instruction to "pull your shoulder blades in toward the spine," because the patient might have difficulty moving the scapula. The patient should also concentrate on maintaining shoulder depression, to minimize upper trapezius activity. The use of a dual channel biofeedback considerably enhances the learning process. Figure 14–6 depicts a 17-year-old baseball pitcher training his lower trapezius muscle to minimize his shoulder pain, using a dual channel biofeedback. Tape has been used to reposition the humeral head and minimize his symptoms. A mirror can also be used as feedback,

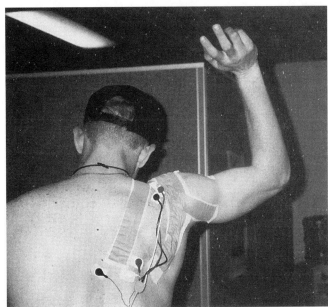

FIGURE 14–6. Training the lower trapezius. A 17-year-old baseball pitcher training his lower trapezius muscle to minimize his shoulder pain, using a dual channel biofeedback. Tape has been used to reposition the humeral head and minimize his symptoms. A mirror can also be used as feedback, allowing the patient to see the upper trapezius activation pattern and make the appropriate changes.

allowing the patient to see the upper trapezius activation pattern and make the appropriate changes. Exercises for the scapular stabilizers should also focus on endurance training.

The lower trapezius and infraspinatus also need to be strengthened, specifically to assist in the repositioning of the humeral head. Elevation of the arm in the first 30° will result in vertical displacement of the humeral head if the pull of the deltoid in not offset. To counter this upward movement, the rotator cuff muscles, particularly the infraspinatus, contract to maintain the humeral head in the glenoid fossa. As the arm continues to elevate, the pull of the deltoid results in less vertical and more compressive forces. Compressive force of the deltoid increases from 14% at 25° elevation to 33% at 75° elevation. Conversely, the compressive force of the rotator cuff decreases from 76% at 30° elevation to 59% at 90° elevation.[26,27] Training of the rotator cuff at 90° elevation should reflect this change in force dominance.

Initial training of the infraspinatus commences in a pain-free range of external rotation with the use of elastic tubing. Increased resistance can be added to the training to enhance recruitment of the infraspinatus. Increased activity of the infraspinatus will help maintain humeral head position by counteracting the upward force exerted by the deltoid. However, when training the infraspinatus at positions close to 90° abduction, emphasis is placed on endurance rather than load because of the narrowing of the subacromial space that occurs in this position. Maximal contractions of the rotator cuff in this position might cause mechanical irritation of the subacromial structures. Biofeedback is used to assess the timing of the muscles and retrain the appropriate motor pattern. A useful home exercise to train the lower trapezius and the infraspinatus in this range is shown in Figure 14–7. The patient

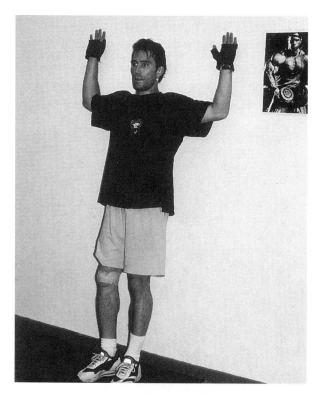

FIGURE 14–7. Training the lower trapezius and the infraspinatus. The patient stands with the back flat against a wall, arms abducted to 70° and the elbows flexed to 90°. The dorsal aspect of the hands are actively pushed back into the wall while the arms are abducted and adducted between 100° and 70°.

stands with the back flat against a wall, arms abducted to 70° and the elbows flexed to 90°. The dorsal aspect of the hands is actively pushed back into the wall while the arms are abducted and adducted between 100° and 70°. Excessive activity of the upper trapezius should not occur during this exercise.

Eccentric muscle training of the subscapularis helps prevent overstretching the joint capsule at the extremes of external rotation by reducing anterior translation of the humeral head.[26]

TRUNK AND GLUTEAL TRAINING

Muscle training should not focus solely on the shoulder complex, because the overhead or throwing athlete must transfer energy from the lower extremity and the ground through the spine to the upper extremity.[27,28] For example, during the pitching motion, the shoulder initiates movement from a position of humeral abduction and maximal external rotation, stressing the internal rotator muscles (latissimus dorsi and pectoralis major). An explosive transition from maximal external rotation to internal rotation ensues as the combined efforts of the trunk and internal rotator muscles result in a peak angular velocity of 7000° per second. The transfer of energy from the gluteus maximus to the latissimus dorsi occurs through the thoracolumbar fascia, a multilayer structure that connects the upper and lower extremities through superficial fibres emerging from the latissimus dorsi and the gluteus maximus. In the lumbar region, the posterior and middle layers of the fascia unite at the lateral margin of erector spinae and at the lateral border of quadratus lumborum. These layers join an anterior layer to form the aponeurotic origin of the transversus abdominis. Hence, gluteal and trunk stability affects the control and power of shoulder movement. During pitching, the gluteus maximus of the throwing side acts as a hip extensor, whereas the contralateral gluteus maximus acts as a stabilizer of the pelvis. Stability of the lumbar spine is also important to shoulder function during overhead activities. During cocking, control of lumbar lordosis is accomplished through eccentric action of the abdominus.[28,29]

The appropriately timed and coordinated activation of muscles influencing spinal motion reduces the need for the shoulder muscles to act as prime movers of the arm. If the muscles from the lower extremity and trunk are unable to transfer energy to the shoulder effectively, the shoulder musculature must generate more tension to maintain the kinetic energy. A professional pitcher utilizes the larger trunk muscles to generate force during the acceleration phase of throwing. During this phase, the subscapularis is the only rotator cuff muscle that is highly active.[29,30] In fact, isokinetic shoulder muscle strength seems to have low correlation with throwing velocity.[31] Although the internal-external rotator strength in pitchers has been shown to be greater than nonpitchers, the tests were performed at one-twentieth the velocity of pitching.[31] The shoulder muscles should therefore be trained for stability and endurance (low load, high repetitions), particularly in a patient with signs of instability. A patient may be trained to use muscles as dynamic stabilizers to compensate for ligamentous laxity and prevent instability. Conversely, the gluteus maximus and latissimus dorsi need to be trained for strength and power (higher load, low repetitions) to enhance explosive force generation. The remaining trunk and pelvic musculature, including the abdominals, spine extensors, and gluteus medius muscles, need to be trained to improve stability so there is efficient transfer of energy from the lower extremity to the upper extremity.

CASE STUDY 14–1

A 19-year-old, elite female volleyball player presents with a gradual onset of right shoulder pain during the past 12 months, which radiates slightly into the deltoid region. The pain has worsened as her frequency of training and playing has increased. A thermal capsular shrinkage surgery, performed 6 months earlier, initially resulted in decreased pain, but the symptoms increased as soon as she returned to volleyball. Although she states she experiences pain when brushing her hair, she continues to play volleyball because she is the star player of the team. Physical examination reveals an arc of pain from 60° to 120° of abduction, pain on resisted external rotation testing, and pain in the empty can position. On ligamentous testing, she has a positive containment test, an increased posterior drawer, and a positive sulcus sign. She also exhibits laxity on ligamentous testing of the left shoulder.

Following the examination, a diagnosis of impingement resulting from a multidirectional instability is made. However, this patient has already received a capsular shrinkage procedure that did not alleviate her symptoms sufficiently to allow a pain-free return to volleyball.

To adequately address this problem, addressing the cause of the patient's symptoms (impairment) is more important than detecting the source of the symptoms (inflamed tissues). In this case, passive instability is the impairment that is contributing to the tissue inflammation. Analysis of the volleyball serve in this individual reveals extremely poor trunk and pelvic stabilization. This suggests that isolated strength training of the shoulder musculature would not improve the patient's symptoms because the reason for the shoulder instability would not be addressed. The shoulder muscles need to be trained for stability and endurance (low load, high repetitions) to compensate for poor ligamentous integrity. The initial muscle training should be directed at the posterior deltoid muscle to improve the centering of the humeral head in the glenoid fossa. As soon as the patient is able to control the humeral head position, rotator cuff muscle training should be incorporated in the rehabilitation program. Training should simulate the volleyball service action, which can be facilitated with biofeedback.

Further progression occurs when gluteal and trunk work is incorporated into the simulated service action. Prior to this, more specific gluteal and trunk training should be practiced to ensure an appropriate recruitment pattern. The posterior gluteus medius is initially trained in weight bearing with the patient standing sideways against a wall (Fig. 14–8). The leg closest to the wall is flexed at the knee approximately 30° to 40° so that the foot is off the ground and the hip is level with the contralateral side. The patient places all the weight on the heel of the stance leg held in slight flexion. The patient externally rotates the stance leg without rotating the foot, the pelvis, or the shoulders. The patient sustains the contraction for 20 seconds, so that a burning can be felt in the gluteus medius region.

Rehabilitation will fail and the symptoms will continue if trunk and gluteal stability training is not incorporated into training. Additionally, to maximize the explosive force generation through the shoulder and decrease the need for local force generation, the gluteus maximus and latissimus dorsi need to be trained

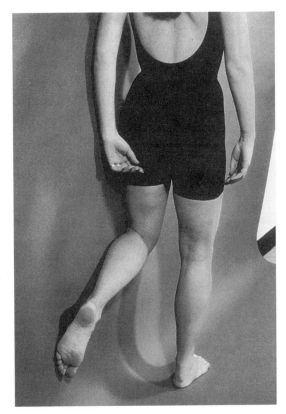

FIGURE 14–8. Training of the posterior gluteus medius. This muscle is initially trained in weight bearing with the patient standing sideways against a wall. The leg closest to the wall is flexed at the knee approximately 30° to 40° so the foot is off the ground and the hip is level with the contralateral side. The patient should place all the weight on the heel of the stance leg held in slight flexion. The patient externally rotates the stance leg without rotating the foot, the pelvis, or the shoulders. The patient should sustain the contraction for 20 seconds, so a burning can be felt in the gluteus medius region.

for strength and power (higher load, low repetitions). The efficiency of the overhead motion might be improved with modification of the serving technique. The technique could be reviewed in consultation with the player's coach.

CASE STUDY 14–2

The following case study is included to highlight the importance of restoring movement so that neuromuscular re-education can occur.

A 70-year-old female with an 18-month history of frozen shoulder presents with a painful and stiff right shoulder. The pain awakens her at night when she is lying on the shoulder. She is unable to fasten her bra from the back, brush her hair using the involved side, or carry a laundry basket. A previous cortisone injection into her shoulder alleviated some of the pain but it did not restore her movement.

During physical examination, assessment of posture reveals an increased thoracic kyphosis. Active range of motion is limited to 100° of abduction and 120° of flexion. Reaching behind her back is limited to the posterior superior illiac spine (PSIS). Poor scapulohumeral rhythm is noted with the upper trapezius initiating the movement. Passive flexion is limited to 140°. Passive accessory movements of the GH joint are slightly restricted when compared to the contralateral side. Considerable hypomobility is noted in thoracic spine accessory motion between T1 to T7. The patient complains of tenderness on palpation of the anterior and posterior aspects of the GH joint.

The neuromuscular recruitment pattern adopted by many patients with adhesive capsulitis results in poor scapulohumeral rhythm. A common recruitment strategy employed in arm elevation is the use of the upper trapezius to initiate and dominate the movement. This recruitment pattern occurs because the deltoid, as well as the rotator cuff and lower and middle trapezius muscles, become inefficient for arm elevation. However, emphasis must be on restoring movement prior to training these muscles. These muscles, which have become elongated, are more difficult to activate. Additionally, the patient's only method of arm elevation (shrugging of the shoulder) should be discouraged during training. The initial focus in rehabilitation should therefore be on improving mobility of the entire shoulder girdle, including the thoracic spine.

Patients with frozen shoulder problems rarely complain of pain or stiffness in their thoracic region. However, gradual diminution of shoulder range often stems from lack of mobility in this area. The thoracic spine is usually overlooked as a contributing factor in decreasing glenohumeral movement. In the older age group, where frozen shoulder conditions are more common, thoracic mobility decreases while thoracic kyphosis increases.[15] A study by Crawford and Jull[15] found that asymptomatic older subjects used almost all their available thoracic extension range of motion when they elevated their arms, whereas younger subjects used only 50% of their available range. In the older age group, the available range of thoracic extension had decreased by 35% and the kyphosis had increased by 36%, but shoulder flexion had only decreased by 9%. Younger subjects with an increased kyphosis did not demonstrate a decrease in shoulder range but did demonstrate an increase in thoracic spine extension during arm elevation when compared with subjects of the same age who had an average thoracic kyphosis. Crawford and Jull felt that individuals with adhesive capsulitis would demonstrate a further decrease in thoracic mobility, which would significantly limit shoulder range. Mobilization of the thoracic region, particularly in the sitting position (Fig. 14–9) can be effective in gaining shoulder range of motion. Mobilization in the sitting position is preferable to the prone position because no counter-resistance is offered by an external object (e.g., the treatment table). This might pose a risk to patients with osteoporosis. Submaximal external rotator resistance may be added when mobilizing the thoracic spine. Doing so helps to improve the centering of the humeral head; the extensibility of the capsule by the intermittent contraction and relaxation of the muscles (many patients with frozen shoulders complain of extreme tenderness on palpation of the GH joint and do not respond favorably to aggressive techniques to the joint, particularly early in the treatment program); and the scapular position.

Some exercises might increase the patient's symptoms. However, avoiding exercises might lead to further complications. The therapist's immediate concern is to choose a treatment strategy to decrease the symptoms during exercise. This goal involves improving the humeral head position and might include unloading the deltoid muscle with the adjunct of tape.

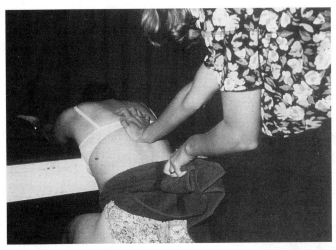

FIGURE 14–9. Mobilization of the thoracic region in the sitting position. Mobilization in the sitting position is preferable to the prone position because no counter resistance is offered by an external object (i.e., the treatment table).

Unloading of the deltoid might decrease shoulder symptoms, particularly night pain, usually the most significant disruption for a patient. The principle of unloading is based on the premise that inflamed soft tissue does not respond well to stretch. Thus, shortening the tissues decreases the tension and therefore the symptoms.

Initial treatment for this patient involves the following:

1. Improving the humeral head position by externally rotating the head (see Fig. 14–2) and unloading the deltoid
2. Mobilizing the thoracic spine in the sitting position
3. Using external rotator exercise, short of pain, in neutral position with a small piece of yellow Thera-Band/tube with the elbows tucked into the side; this should be done twice, three or four times per day
4. Encouraging the patient to think about elevating the sternum whenever the arm is being used; a simple verbal cue for the patient is "thrust the bust" for a female patient or "thrust the chest" for a male patient

The tape remains applied for a week. Showering should not be a problem because the tape dries quickly. On the return visit, the tape is removed carefully to prevent skin damage and the patient's movements are reassessed. The tape is then reapplied and thoracic mobilization is performed with the arm supported on the plinth at a greater flexion range. The patient is taken to the limit of the pain-free range, and the training exercises are continued, perhaps increasing the number of repetitions slightly. A home thoracic stretch program is started if it does not aggravate the symptoms. This stretch involves the patient lying on a rolled towel placed between the scapulae from the base of the neck down the spine. Another rolled towel (perhaps even two, if the patient has a forward head posture and a stiff cervicothoracic junction) is placed under the head while the

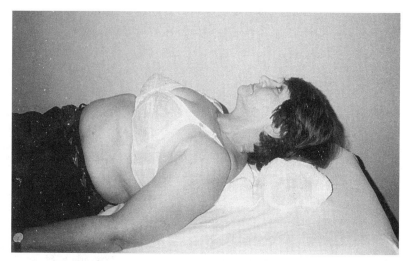

FIGURE 14–10. Stretching the anterior chest musculature. This stretch involves the patient lying on a rolled towel placed between the scapulae from the base of the neck down the spine. Another rolled towel (maybe even two, if the patient has a forward head posture and a stiff cervico-thoracic junction) is placed under the head while the neck is free. A pillow also is placed under the knees. The patient should lie on the towels for 10 minutes. If the shoulder aches in this position, a folded towel is placed under the affected forearm to prevent the humerus from dropping into extension.

neck is free. A pillow also is placed under the knees. The patient should lie on the towels for 10 minutes (Fig. 14–10). If the shoulder aches in this position, a folded towel is placed under the affected forearm to prevent the humerus from dropping into extension. Biofeedback can be added for specific training of the lower trapezius when the symptoms have been reduced and the range of motion is improved. Deltoid training may be added in a position of slight abduction to minimize activity of the upper trapezius. The patient starts with a small range of movement and progresses to a greater range when motor control improves.

CHAPTER SUMMARY

Effective management of shoulder problems requires identification of the impairments leading to the tissue pathology and implementation of an appropriate muscle training program to ensure the desired changes occur. The training must be specific to the limb position and joint angle and the velocity, type, and force of contraction. The aim of training is to promote a motor control program, which minimizes the recurrence of symptoms. As with all training, the success or failure depends on the amount of practice. Therefore, the training must be simple, require minimal equipment so it is readily accessible to the individual, and be amenable to easy and frequent practice. The stabilizing muscles need to be fatigue-resistant for long-term success of treatment, so an appropriate endurance training program should be included. Once the symptoms are resolved, the exercises must become part of the daily routine of many patients (particularly the patients with faulty alignment) so they can remain symptom free.

REFERENCES

1. Bowen, M, and Warren, R: Ligamentous control of shoulder stability based on selective cutting and static translation experiments. Clinics in Sports Medicine 10:757, 1991.
2. Sale, D, and MacDougall, D: Specificity of strength training: A review for coach and athlete. Canadian Journal of Applied Sports Sciences 6(2):87, 1981.
3. Grabiner, M, et al: Neuromechanics of the patellofemoral joint. Med Sci Sports Ex (26)1:10, 1994.
4. Rasch, PJ, and Morehouse, LE: Effect of static and dynamic exercises on muscular strength and hypertrophy. J Appl Physiol 11:29, 1957.
5. Enoka, RM: Muscle strength and its development: New perspectives. Sports Med 6:146, 1988.
6. Moffroid, M, and Whipple, R: Specificity of speed of exercise. Physical Therapy, 50(12):1692, 1970.
7. Kitai, T, and Sale, D: Specificity of joint angle in isometric training. Eur J App Physiol 64:1500, 1989.
8. Thepaut-Mathieu, C, et al: Myoelectric and mechanical changes linked to length specificity during isometric training. J Appl Physiol, 58:744, 1988.
9. Rutherford, O, and Jones, D: The role of learning and co-ordination in strength training. Eur J Appl Physiol 55:100, 1986.
10. Sale, D: Influence of exercise and training on motor unit activation. Exercise & Sports Science Review 5:95, 1987.
11. Brooks, V: Motor control. Phys Ther 63(5):66, 1983.
12. Engelhorn, R: Agonist and antagonist muscle EMG activity pattern changes with skill acquisition. Research Quarterly for Exercise and Sport 54(4):315, 1983.
13. van Soest, AJ, and van Ingen Schenau, GJ: How are explosive movements controlled? In Latash, M (ed): Progress in Motor Control: Bernstein's Traditions in Movement Studies, Vol 1. Human Kinetics, Champaign, IL, 1998.
14. Ayub, E: Posture and the upper quarter. In Donatelli, R (ed): Physical Therapy of the Shoulder. Churchill Livingstone, New York, 1987.
15. Crawford, H, and Jull, G: The influence of thoracic form and movement on ranges of shoulder flexion. Physiotherapy Theory and Practice, 9:143, 1993.
16. Powers, C, et al: The effects of patellar taping on stride characteristics and joint motion in subjects with patellofemoral pain. J Orthop Sports Phys Ther 26(6):286, 1997.
17. Gilleard, W, et al: The effect of patellar taping on the onset of vastus medialis obliquus and vastus lateralis muscle activity in persons with patellofemoral pain. Phys Ther 78(1):25, 1998.
18. Conway, A, et al: Patellar alignment/tracking alteration: Effect on force output and perceived pain. Isokinetics and Exercise Science 2:9, 1992.
19. Cerny, K: Vastus medialis oblique/vastus lateralis muscle activity ratios for selected exercises in persons with and without patellofemoral pain syndrome. Phys Ther (75)8:672, 1995.
20. Brukner, P, and Khan, K: Clinical Sports Medicine. McGraw Hill, Sydney, 1993.
21. Herbert, R: Human strength adaptations: Implications for therapy. In Crosbie, J, and McConnell, J (eds): Key Issues in Musculoskeletal Physiotherapy. Butterworth Heinemann, Oxford, 1993.
22. Townsend, H, et al: Electro-myographic analysis of the glenohumeral muscles during a baseball rehabilitation program. Am J Sports Med 19(3):264, 1991.
23. Souza, D, and Gross, M: Comparison of vastus medialis obliquus: Vastus lateralis muscle integrated electromyographic ratios between healthy subjects and patients with patellofemoral pain. Phys Ther 71:310, 1991.
24. Yang, J, and Winter, D: Electromyography reliability in maximal contractions and submaximal isometric contractions. Archives of Physical Medicine and Rehabilitation, 64:417, 1983.
25. Howard, J, and Enoka, R: Maximum bilateral contractions are modified by neurally mediated interlimb effects. J Appl Physiol 70:306, 1991.
26. Perry, J: Anatomy and biomechanics of the shoulder in throwing, swimming, gymnastics and tennis. Clinics in Sports Medicine 2:247, 1983.
27. Peat, M: Functional anatomy of the shoulder. Phys Ther, 66(12):1855, 1986.
28. Young, C, et al: The influence on the spine on the shoulder in the throwing athlete. J Back and Musculoskeletal Rehabilitation 7:5, 1996.
29. Perry, J, and Glousman, R: Biomechanics of throwing. In Nicholas, and Hershman (eds): The Upper Extremity in Sports Medicine. Mosby, St Louis, 1990, p 725.
30. Bartlet, R, et al: Measurement of upper extremity torque production and its relation to throwing speed in the competitive athlete. Am J Sports Med 17(1):89, 1989.
31. Brown, LP, et al: Upper extremity range of motion and isokinetic strength of the internal and external shoulder rotators in major league baseball players. Am J Sports Med 16(6):577, 1988.

CHAPTER 15

Aquatic Rehabilitation of the Shoulder

Brian J. Tovin, MMSC, PT, SCS, ATC, FAAOMPT

INTRODUCTION

In orthopaedic rehabilitation, specific treatment principles are followed regardless of the diagnosis. As stated in Chapter 4, physical therapists address impairments resulting from injury, surgery, or disease. Common musculoskeletal impairments leading to functional limitations and disability include limited range of motion (ROM), strength, and motor control; and decreased proprioception. When addressing these impairments, a clinician might find that specific tissue pathologies or surgical procedures affect treatment selection by limiting how fast a patient can progress. Excessive loading on healing tissues might compromise surgical fixation or result in inflammation. Some exercises can result in neuromuscular substitution patterns or excessive pain. However, avoiding these exercises might cause muscle atrophy and decreased ROM.

Implementing aquatic exercises might be a solution to this problem. The physical properties of water can reduce compressive and tensile forces on a joint and the thermal properties of water can help increase connective tissue extensibility. Although existing for thousands of years, the use of aquatic exercises in orthopaedics has gained popularity during the past 10 years. This chapter reviews the history and physics of aquatic therapy, discusses the physiological and clinical implications of aquatic exercises, and presents the clinical applications of aquatic therapy for patients with orthopaedic impairments of the shoulder.

HISTORY OF AQUATIC REHABILITATION

The use of water for therapeutic purposes has been documented as early as 2400 BC.[1] It is believed that the early Egyptian, Moslem, and Hindu societies used water for various therapeutic purposes.[2] In 460 to 375 BC, Hippocrates used the thermal properties of water to treat musculoskeletal diseases. This practice continued through the 1600s and 1700s, becoming known as *hydrotherapy*.[3] By the 1800s, some medical doctors were using hydrotherapy as part of their practices.[1] Sebastion Kneipp introduced contrast therapy, the alternating use of hot and cold water, in the mid- to late 1800s.[4] Although the use of hydrotherapy was quite prevalent at this time, no medical research had been done to establish its credibility.

In the mid to late 1800s, a hydrotherapy school and research center was established in Vienna by an Austrian professor named Winterwitz.[5] His research is credited with providing a physiological basis for hydrotherapy. His research and the future work of his students served as a foundation for advancing hydrotherapy beyond a passive modality.

Dr. Simon Baruch,[6] an American studying under Dr. Winterwitz, became the first professor at Columbia University to teach hydrotherapy. He published three texts on the subject outlining treatment guidelines for conditions such as typhoid fever, tuberculosis, rheumatism, gout, and influenza. The introduction of exercises in water was recommended by von Leyden and Goldwater in 1898, being referred to as *hydrogymnastics*.[3,5]

Exercises in water became very popular in the United States in the early 1900s because of the polio epidemic.[7] Patients with poliomyelitis discovered that they could perform movement patterns in water that they could not do on land. Patients experienced a carry-over from the water to land, where improvements in movement patterns performed in the water contributed to improvements performed on land. Some patients progressed from being wheelchair dependant to ambulating with only a cane.

In Europe during the early to mid 1900s, formal water exercise programs were developed. In the 1930s in Bad Ragaz, Switzerland, spas were created for exercising in the water.[8] However, the Bad Ragaz Ring Method, which originated in Germany by Dr. Knupfer, was brought to Switzerland in 1957 by Nele Ipsen. The primary purpose of this exercise program was to promote stabilization of the trunk and extremities. Patients were supported by inner tube "rings" placed at the neck, pelvis, and ankles. Initially, exercises were performed in straight-plane patterns. In 1967, Bridgett Davis incorporated proprioceptive neuromuscular facilitation techniques into this program.[8] Modern techniques use both straight-plane and diagonal movement patterns with added resistance and stabilization. Although Bad Ragaz techniques are most frequently used with neurologically impaired patients, they have also been used with orthopaedic patients.

The Halliwick method, developed in London by James McMillan at the Halliwick School for Girls in 1949, was developed to help patients with disabilities to become independent and safe swimmers.[9] This approach was more recreational than therapeutic. More recently, the Halliwick method has been used therapeutically by physical therapists treating pediatric and adult patients with developmental and neurological disabilities. This program focuses on the patient's abilities in water rather than on their disabilities on land.

During the 1970s and 1980s, hydrotherapy or aquatic rehabilitation began to gain popularity in the treatment of patients with musculoskeletal injuries. The use of water for cardiovascular conditioning was initiated through water aerobics classes and athlete training. Research on the effectiveness of aquatic rehabilitation became more prevalent.[10] Many clinicians have advocated the use of aquatic rehabilitation for patients with upper extremity dysfunction.[11–15] The buoyancy and resistive properties of water make this form of rehabilitation advantageous when compared with traditional rehabilitation. However, aquatic exercises might not be appropriate for every patient.

PHYSICAL PROPERTIES OF WATER AND CLINICAL IMPLICATIONS

When implementing any aquatic program, clinicians should also be familiar with the physical properties of water and how these properties impact the patient's physiological and clinical status.

Hydrostatic Pressure

Hydrostatic pressure refers to the forces exerted on the surface area of an object placed in water.[16] According to Pascal's law, the hydrostatic pressure is directly proportional to the density of the fluid and the depth of immersion of an object. Hydrostatic pressure of water at the surface is 14.7 lbs per square inch, increasing by 0.43 lbs for every foot increase in depth.

Clinically, hydrostatic pressure can be used to reduce effusion and swelling and to increase lymphatic return. Hydrostatic pressure might also prevent further effusion for patients with musculoskeletal dysfunction.[17] Immersion to the neck results in displacement of 700 cm^3 of blood from the extremities into the large veins of the thorax and into the heart.[18] Tovin et al.[17] found reduced knee effusion in a group of patients performing an aquatic rehabilitation program when compared with a group of patients performing a dry-land rehabilitation program following ACL reconstruction.

Buoyancy

According to Archimedes' principle, a body immersed in a fluid environment will experience an upward force (buoyancy) equal to the weight of displaced fluid.[16] Upward force is attributed to increased pressure at the bottom of an object resulting from increased depth (hydrostatic pressure). The body immersed or partially immersed will therefore lose weight equal to the amount of fluid displaced. *Buoyancy* is calculated using specific gravity and is defined as the ratio of an object's weight in a liquid divided by the amount of weight loss in the liquid. An object with a specific gravity greater than 1 will sink, whereas an object with a specific gravity less than 1 will float.

Clinically, buoyancy can be used to provide support and assistance and resistance to movement. Buoyancy can be used to provide support for an object moving parallel to the surface of the water. Using a kickboard to support the upper extremity while a patient performs horizontal adduction and abduction is one example (Fig. 15–1). Objects descending perpendicularly to the surface of the water encounter resistance to movement from the upward thrust of buoyancy. Performing shoulder extension or adduction in a standing position while holding a buoyant device is an example (Fig. 15–2). Objects moving toward the surface of the water are assisted by buoyancy, for example, using a buoyancy device to elevate the upper extremity when standing (Fig. 15–3). Specific uses of buoyancy in aquatic rehabilitation for the shoulder will be discussed in "Clinical Applications."

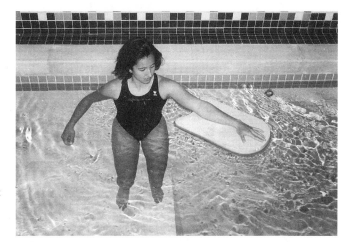

FIGURE 15–1. Using buoyancy as a support. The patient uses a kickboard to provide support for upper extremity horizontal abduction and adduction.

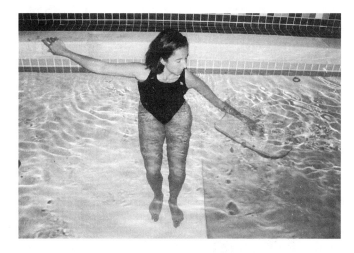

FIGURE 15–2. Using buoyancy as resistance. The patient holds a kickboard under water during upper extremity movements, working against the upward force of buoyancy.

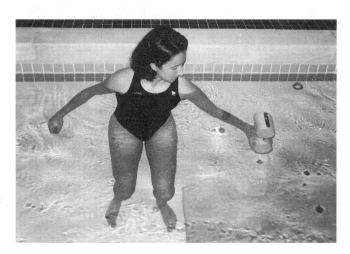

FIGURE 15–3. Using buoyancy as assistance. The patient uses the upward force of buoyancy to facilitate elevation of the upper extremity.

Fluid Dynamics

An object moving through a liquid is influenced by *laminar* (streamline) *flow* and *turbulent flow.*[19] Laminar flow involves molecules that flow parallel to each other at the same speed and do not cross paths. This type of fluid movement creates little resistance. However, minor oscillations can result in uneven flow, forcing the molecules out of a parallel alignment. This type of pattern is referred to as turbulent flow and creates greater resistance to movement. The amount of turbulence and fluid viscosity and the amount of molecular attraction within a fluid (sometimes referred to as *internal friction*) contribute to drag forces acting on an object. The greater the attraction is between layers of molecules in motion, the greater the resistance to movement.

Three different *drag* forces act on an object moving through water.[20] The first drag force is attributed to friction at the interface of the object's surface and the water molecules. Competitive swimmers manipulate this physical property when they remove body hair or "shave down" to decrease drag in preparation for a meet. The second drag force is generated by the shape of the frontal surface area. An object with less frontal surface area will experience less drag than an object with a larger frontal surface area. The third drag force is referred to as *wave drag* and is affected by many variables.

Wave drag is created by the pressure gradient, which develops between the bow wave in front of a moving object and the wake behind it. Water flows from positive pressure in the front of the object to negative pressure in the back, creating turbulent, rotatory movements known as *eddies.* These eddies, which create drag, resist forward movement of an object.

Drag forces are a function of the square of the velocity, so doubling velocity will quadruple the drag forces. An object's drag coefficient is referred to as Reynold's number, which considers an object's geometry and velocity, fluid viscosity, and a gravitational constant.

Clinically, these inertial forces can be used to resist motion or to facilitate motion. Clinicians can increase the drag forces by changing the frontal surface area and geometry of a limb moving though water, often accomplished by using external devices that can be fixed to the moving part (Fig. 15–4). Drag forces can also be

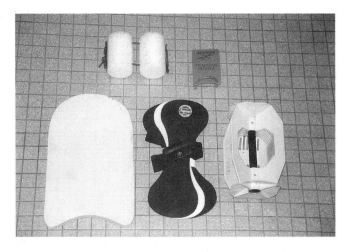

FIGURE 15–4. Increasing resistance to movement. The patient uses an external device to increase the surface area of the moving limb, thereby increasing resistance.

increased by instructing the patient to accelerate faster through the water. Because this type of resistance is self-generating or *accommodating resistance,* it might be safer for the patient. Although an object moving through water will encounter resistance to movement, the inertia generated by the moving water will facilitate movement when the object stops. This additional "push" can stretch the soft-tissue structures, possibly helping to recover range of motion.

Thermodynamics

Water conducts heat 25 times faster than air. Therefore, water temperature must be considered when implementing a hydrotherapy program. Thermal properties of water result in specific physiological changes. The major changes impacting rehabilitation include increased circulation and improved elasticity of soft-tissue structures. If a hydrotherapy program includes cardiovascular exercises, ideal water temperature should be between 82° and 86°F to allow the metabolic heat generated during the exercises to be transferred to the water. A higher water temperature of 98° to 104°F might be more suitable if the primary goal of an aquatic rehabilitation program is to increase ROM and circulation.

Clinical Applications

When deciding whether to use aquatic exercises as part of a rehabilitation program, clinicians must base the decision on several factors. First, a clinician must decide if a patient is willing to enter the water. Patients should be screened for cognitive status, related medical history, and attitude about getting in a pool. Some patients might have a fear of the water and might decline to participate. Other patients might have open wounds or other medical conditions such as epilepsy that prohibit them from getting into the water. Regardless of the potential benefit, these patients might not be suitable for aquatic rehabilitation.

Some patients might be progressing well enough with traditional rehabilitation that aquatic therapy is not necessary. The primary purpose of using aquatic therapy is to supplement the dry-land program, enabling patients to perform exercises that are not possible or are too painful to perform on land. Hydrotherapy is not intended to replace any of the dry-land exercises. This type of rehabilitation is more costly and time-consuming to implement and therefore should be used to meet specific needs. Although the environment and forces are different, specific aquatic exercises are similar to a dry-land rehabilitation program. The key to designing an aquatic exercise program is to use the physical properties of water to address the primary impairments that exist in each practice pattern (Table 15–1). The following section describes how aquatic rehabilitation might benefit patients in each of the practice pattern categories.

PRACTICE PATTERN D

Practice pattern D refers to impaired joint mobility, motor function, muscle performance, and range of motion associated with *capsular restriction.* As reviewed in Chapter 7, capsular restriction of the shoulder can be attributed to different conditions. Although the goal in all of these patients is to restore motion, the level of

TABLE 15–1 Aquatic Exercises for Specific Impairments

Impairment	Benefits of Water	Specific Exercises
Impaired range of motion	Thermal properties Laminar flow of water for facilitation of movement Use of buoyancy for assisted motion	Active or active-assisted motion with buoyancy devices (if needed) in cardinal planes of movement
Impaired muscle performance	Thermal properties Drag forces for resistance Use of buoyancy for resistance	Active range of motion in all planes of movement Resistive devices when needed Reproduction of functional movement patterns
Impaired motor control	Drag forces for resistance Laminar and turbulent flow	Functional movement patterns with quick changes in direction against the flow of water Simultaneous, coordinated movements of the upper extremities to challenge proprioception

irritability and constraints of soft-tissue healing will guide the treatment. Implementing exercises that recruit muscle activity and increase motion in a safe manner is crucial to a successful rehabilitation program.

Aquatic exercises might be beneficial for this population for several reasons. The thermal properties of water might help to increase elasticity of the connective tissues. Buoyancy and fluid movement can help to assist motion, possibly creating a passive stretch. Drag forces can provide resistance to movement for muscle recruitment. This type of resistance might be safer than performing dry-land weight exercises for two reasons. First, the resistance is self-generated, so patients can determine how much or how little resistance they can accommodate. Second, because the resistance is spread over the entire limb rather than at a fixed distal point (e.g., a weight in a hand), the torque at the joint is reduced because of the decreased moment arm.

Specific exercises for patients in this practice pattern focus on using the buoyancy and laminar flow properties of water. Flotation devices applied at the wrists or elbows provide increased buoyancy, assisting in elevation or providing support during movement patterns. Patients can also use the momentum of the water to facilitate ROM. For example, a patient with limited range of motion for shoulder internal rotation can perform internal rotation exercises within an available range. When the motion stops, the laminar flow of the water continues, and the momentum of the water at the end range can provide a "push" or passive stretch to the capsule.

PRACTICE PATTERN E

Practice pattern E refers to impaired joint mobility, muscle performance, and range of motion associated with ligament or other *connective tissue disorders*. As discussed in Chapter 8, patients in this practice pattern usually present with instability of the shoulder. Goals of treatment for the unstable shoulder include enhancing the dynamic stabilizers (muscles), while protecting the static stabilizers (ligaments). If a patient with an unstable shoulder also has secondary impingement, some of the dry-land rehabilitation exercises might be too painful to perform. Patients with instability often have difficulty "setting" the rotator cuff muscles to center the head of the humerus in the glenoid fossa. Additionally, some dry-land exercises might place too much stress on the static stabilizers such as the capsule and ligaments. These patients are ideal candidates for aquatic exercises used to strengthen the rotator cuff and scapular stabilizers. Exercises that are used on land, such as internal-external rotation, abduction-adduction, flexion-extension, and horizontal abduction-adduction, can be performed in the water. Resistance can be progressed by adding hand paddles and other equipment or increasing the speed of movement. Exercises can be progressed from straight, cardinal plane movements to functional movement patterns such as a simulated tennis swing.

PRACTICE PATTERN F

Practice pattern F refers to impaired joint mobility, motor function, muscle performance, and range of motion associated with *localized inflammation*. Patients in this practice pattern usually have some type of impingement syndrome at the shoulder. As reviewed in Chapter 9, impingement syndrome can be attributed to several impairments, including a loss of subacromial space, loss of motor control, or glenohumeral instability. Patients with impingement resulting from instability or poor neuromuscular control often have difficulty with strengthening exercises because of pain. Ideally, exercises in this group of patients focus on proximal stability by strengthening the scapular and rotator cuff musculature. If these muscle groups are not functioning properly, excessive translation of the humeral head might occur, resulting in impingement. The buoyancy property of water might reduce the amount of scapular substitution needed to elevate the upper extremity. This potential improvement in scapulohumeral rhythm might reduce the amount of impingement, thus creating a safer environment for initial stages of strengthening.

Specific aquatic exercises are similar to the program that would be used on land. Emphasis is placed on scapular protraction-retraction, elevation-depression, and glenohumeral internal-external rotation. Hand paddles and other devices can be used as more resistance is needed. The water might also be used as a transitional environment for initiating functional movement patterns such as swinging a tennis racquet.

REFERRED PAIN SYNDROMES: INTEGRATION OF MUSCULOSKELETAL PRACTICE PATTERNS D AND G AND NEUROMUSCULAR PRACTICE PATTERN D

Referred pain syndromes (practice patterns D and G and neuromuscular practice pattern D) refer to impaired joint mobility, motor function, muscle performance, range of motion, or reflex integrity secondary to *spinal disorders*, reflex sympathetic dystrophy, thoracic outlet syndrome, and peripheral entrapment neuropathies. Patients in this category might have shoulder pain because of thoracic outlet syndrome (TOS), adverse neural tension, reflex sympathetic dystrophy (RSD), or referred pain from the cervical spine as described in Chapter 10. Patients with TOS or adverse neural tension might have difficulty holding weights because of excessive traction stress on the brachial plexus. Patients with RSD might not have enough hand strength or might not be able to tolerate the contact of the weight on the skin. For these patients, aquatic rehabilitation can be an ideal environment for ROM and strengthening exercises. No specific aquatic exercises exist for patients in this practice pattern. The clinician must focus on restoring any impaired muscle groups and movement patterns. The use of aquatic rehabilitation for these patients must be made on an individual basis and used only as an alternative rather than as a replacement for dry-land exercises.

PRACTICE PATTERNS H, I, AND J

Practice patterns H, I, and J refer to impaired joint mobility, motor function, muscle performance, and range of motion associated with *fracture, joint arthroplasty,* or *bony or soft-tissue surgical procedures.* Patients in these categories present with similar impairments related to tissue healing. Following disuse or immobilization, patients often have hypomobility, which is treated in a similar manner as for patients in practice pattern D. In addition, patients in this practice pattern also present with impaired motor function and muscle performance. These patients must be careful to avoid overstressing the healing tissues. However, complete avoidance of strengthening exercises will result in disuse atrophy, possibly further delaying recovery time. In an effort to prevent disuse atrophy and adhesive capsulitis, exercises placing minimal stress on the painful tissues should be used. Many clinicians might choose limited range or sub-maximal resistance exercises.

Aquatic exercises might be another choice for patients in these practice patterns. Buoyancy and thermal properties of water can facilitate movement, enabling a patient to exercise through a larger range of motion. Additionally, resistance in the water is self-generated, determined by speed and surface area, so this mode of exercise might be safer than dry-land exercises. Patients can eventually progress to functional movement patterns that simulate a specific activity such as swinging a tennis racquet. Although resistive tubing is sometimes used for this purpose on dry land, tension in the tubing or band increases as it elongates, which inhibits smooth movement patterns. In the water, a patient can focus on fast movement patterns with greater neuromuscular control because the drag forces slow down the movement.

CASE STUDY 15–1

HISTORY

JK, a 20-year-old male collegiate swimmer with a history of instability in the left shoulder, states that his initial dislocation occurred 2 years ago when reaching back to the wall as he finished a backstroke race. Until 6 months ago, he reports that he had only experienced two to three episodes of minor subluxations without functional limitations. During the past 6 months, he has had an additional five episodes of subluxations where he felt the shoulder "came out and popped back in" after 2 to 3 seconds. Because shoulder strengthening was unsuccessful and the symptoms began to limit his ability to swim backstroke, his orthopaedic surgeon recommended a thermal capsular shrinkage procedure to treat the anterior instability. Following the surgery, JK was placed in a sling for 4 weeks and performed daily pendulum exercises, wrist and elbow ROM, and wrist and elbow strengthening. These activities were done in the training room under the supervision of the team athletic trainer. He has now been referred for physical therapy.

PHYSICAL EXAMINATION

Assessment reveals a forward head posture with rounded shoulders and increased thoracic kyphosis. Slight scapular winging and protraction is also noted. The surgical incision is benign. Atrophy is noted in the areas of the upper trapezius, deltoid, and suprascapular region. Passive ROM is limited to 110° of flexion, 85° of abduction, and 15° of external rotation in a neutral position. Modified resisted isometric testing in a neutral position reveals good muscle contractions with generalized weakness because of pain inhibition. No muscle testing grades are given because of the patient's postsurgical status.

EVALUATION AND DIAGNOSIS

Although the primary impairments include limited joint mobility, ROM, motor function, and muscle performance resulting from a soft-tissue surgical procedure (practice pattern J), JK also has impaired posture (practice pattern B), which also needs to be addressed. Because of soft-tissue healing constraints, the initial impairments requiring treatment are limited ROM and joint mobility.

PROGNOSIS

Given JK's age and activity level, and the procedure performed, a full recovery of JK's previous level of function is expected within five to seven months. Short-term and long-term goals include the following:

1. Educating the patient in a home exercise program for ROM and isometrics within two to three sessions
2. Restoring full elevation ROM within four to six weeks and full external rotation ROM within eight weeks
3. Achieving normal strength within three to four months
4. Returning to short-distance, low-intensity swimming in four months
5. Returning to full swimming activity by six months

TREATMENT PLAN

Weeks Four to Eight

When addressing ROM, treatment must avoid overstressing the anterior capsule for the initial six to eight weeks. In addition to the traditional dry-land exercises that are done at this time (pendulum swings, active-assistive ROM with a wand or pulleys, isometrics for the shoulder musculature, and strengthening of the wrist and elbow musculature), many aquatic exercises are implemented. Active-assistive ROM for flexion and abduction is performed using a kickboard

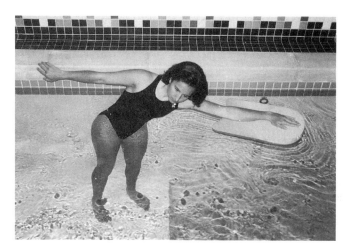

FIGURE 15–5. Using buoyancy as a support for active-assistive range of motion. The patient uses a kickboard to support the upper extremity while sidebending toward and away from the limb, to increase range of motion.

to facilitate motion parallel to the surface of the water (Fig. 15–5). Active ROM for flexion-extension, abduction-adduction, internal-external rotation, and horizontal-abduction-adduction is also added.

Weeks Eight to Twelve

At this time in the rehabilitation program, light dumbbell exercises are added in cardinal plane movements. However, JK begins to experience some soreness after two sessions of dry-land exercises, so resistance exercises in the water are substituted. A hand paddle is added to increase resistance while JK performs flexion-extension, abduction-adduction, internal-external rotation, and horizontal-abduction-adduction exercises. He is instructed to perform 30 repetitions at a speed that is fast enough to generate resistance but not so fast that he experiences pain. JK does experience some discomfort at the end range of external rotation on the transition to internal rotation, which is most likely because of a stretch of the anterior capsule. The ROM is modified so that no symptoms are present. Additionally, as JK progresses, a hand paddle (Fig. 15–6)

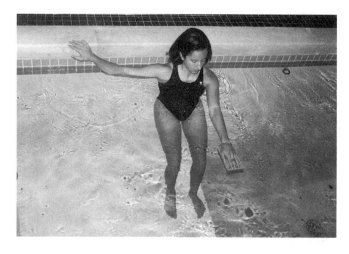

FIGURE 15–6. Use of a hand paddle to increase resistance to upper extremity movement.

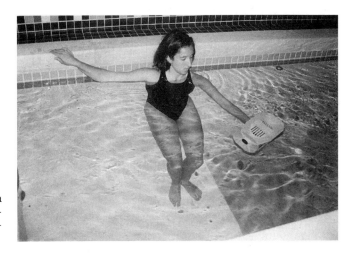

FIGURE 15–7. Use of a Hydrotone Bell to further increase resistance to upper extremity movement.

does not provide enough resistance for flexion-extension. Therefore the Hydrotone Bell (Fig. 15–7) is used because this device provides more resistance from its larger surface area.

Weeks Twelve to Sixteen

By three months, JK has no more symptoms performing cardinal plane movements using free weights and stack weight equipment on dry land. At this time, he is ready to be progressed to functional movement patterns. The goal is to simulate the movement pattern used for freestyle and breaststroke swimming. JK avoids simulated backstroke swimming until the fourth month because this movement is the most stressful to the anterior capsule. Exercises consist of JK standing in four feet of water and bending over at the waist so that his face is in the water. He holds on to the wall with the right arm while simulating a freestyle swimming stroke with his left upper extremity. After one to two weeks of this progression without symptoms, JK performs the same drill using both upper extremities to simulate a low resistance swimming stroke.

Weeks Sixteen to Twenty-Four

At four months, JK returns to modified swimming activities with specific provisions. Swim fins are used during the first month so that the stress imparted to the shoulder is minimized. No backstroke or butterfly is done until six months. During the first week, the workout is limited to fewer than 500 yards for three sessions, progressing to an additional 500 to 1000 yards per week providing there are no symptoms. By the seventh month, JK is back to performing a full workout without any modifications.

CHAPTER SUMMARY

Aquatic therapy can be beneficial for many impairments, including hypomobility, pain and inflammation, and decreased strength. These impairments are found in most of the diagnostic categories discussed previously. The advantages of using aquatic rehabilitation include reduced compressive and torque stress on the joints, increased circulation secondary to water's thermal properties, assisted movement via buoyancy, and strengthening resulting from self-accommodating resistance. The disadvantages include the cost of developing and maintaining a hydrotherapy area, increased time commitment, and patient apprehension of water. If an aquatic therapy environment is present, the goal is to determine what activities in water that cannot be performed on dry land can be beneficial to the patient.

REFERENCES

1. Krizek, V: History of balneotherapy. In Licht, S (ed): Medical Hydrology. Waverly Press, Baltimore, 1963, p 132.
2. Finnerty, GB, and Corbitt, T: Hydrotherapy. Frederick Unger, New York, 1960, p 1.
3. Wyman, JF, and Glazer, O (eds): Hydrotherapy in Medical Physics I. Yearbook Publishers, Chicago, 1944, p 619.
4. Franke, K: Kneipp treatment. In Licht, S, (ed): Medical Hydrology. Waverly Press, Baltimore, 1963, p 321.
5. Campion, MR: Adult Hydrotherapy: A Practical Approach. Heinemann Medical Books, Oxford, England, 1990, p 199.
6. Baruch, S: An Epitome of Hydrotherapy. WB Saunders, Philadelphia, 1920, p 151.
7. Kamenetz, HL: History of American spas and hydrotherapy. In Licht, S (ed): Medical Hydrology. Waverly Press, Baltimore, 1963, p 160.
8. Cunningham, J: Applying Bad Ragaz method to the orthopedic client. Orthopaedic Physical Therapy Clinics in North America (2)251, June 1994.
9. Martin, J: The Halliwick method. Physiotherapy 67(10):288, 1981.
10. Basmajian, JV: Therapeutic Exercise, ed 3. Williams and Wilkins, Baltimore, 1978, p 275.
11. Abidini, MR, et al: A new hydrofitness device for strengthening muscles of the upper extremity. J Burn Care Rehab 9: 402, 1988.
12. Abidini, MR, et al: Hydrofitness devices for strengthening upper extremity muscles. J Burn Care Rehab 9:198, 1988.
13. Speer, KP, et al: A role for hydrotherapy in shoulder rehabilitation. Am J Sport Med 21:850, 1993.
14. Law, LAF, and Smidt, GL: Underwater forces produced by the Hydro-Tone Bell. J Orthop Sports Med 23: 267, 1996.
15. Thein, LM, and Brody, LT: Aquatic-based rehabilitation and training for the elite athlete. J Orthop Sports Phys Ther 27:32, 1998.
16. Edlich, RF, et al: Bioengineering principles of hydrotherapy. J Burn Care Rehab 8:580, 1987.
17. Tovin, BJ, et al: Comparison of the effects of exercise in water and on land on the rehabilitation of patients with intra-articular anterior cruciate ligament reconstructions. Phys Ther 74:710, 1994.
18. Aborelius, M, et al: Hemodynamic changes in man during immersion with the head above water. Aerospace Medicine 43:592, 1972.
19. Becker, BE: Aquatic physics. In Ruoti, RG, et al (eds): Aquatic Rehabilitation. Lippincott, Philadelphia, 1997, p 15.
20. Martin, RB: Swimming: Forces on aquatic animals and humans. In Vaughan, CL (ed): Biomechanics of Sport. CRC Press, Boca Raton, FL, 1989, p 35.

CHAPTER 16

Therapeutic Exercise and Functional Progression of the Shoulder

Terese L. Chmielewski, MA, PT, SCS
Lynn Snyder-Mackler, ScD, PT, ATC, SCS

INTRODUCTION

The need to develop treatment guidelines that improve functional outcomes is imperative in the field of physical therapy. Successful treatment outcomes can no longer be equated with the resolution of impairments, such as restricted range of motion or weakness. Pressure from third party payers to demonstrate improvements in function to receive reimbursement is becoming more common. The American Physical Therapy Association has recently published *The Guide to Physical Therapist Practice*,[1] which describes interventions that integrate the resolution of impairments (deficits at a local level) and disability (the deficit in function resulting from the impairments). Although therapists continue to treat impairments, the ultimate goal of rehabilitation is to improve function. Therapeutic exercise that prepares the shoulder complex to withstand the specific forces and motions experienced during activities must be incorporated into the rehabilitation program to improve function. This chapter discusses various issues involved in incorporating therapeutic exercise for the shoulder into a function-focused rehabilitation program including identifying treatment goals, individualizing treatment, progressing treatment within and between protocol phases, and measuring function. Guidelines for decisions regarding these issues are provided.

DEVELOPING GOALS FOR THE REHABILITATION PROGRAM

The activity level of the patient must be determined to develop a therapeutic exercise program aimed at restoring shoulder function. Information about current and desired activity levels can be obtained from the patient via history and self-report questionnaires. Self-report functional questionnaires can also be administered at various times throughout the course of treatment to measure and document changes in functional levels. Several self-report functional questionnaires have been reported in the literature, each with a slightly different approach to measuring function. The usefulness of the various questionnaires will be critically assessed later in this chapter.[2–10]

Once the functional level and goals of the patient are determined, impairments that need to be resolved to regain full function must be identified. Through the physical examination, various impairments are identified, and their relationships to the shoulder dysfunction must be clearly drawn. Not all impairments adversely affect function. For instance, in the baseball pitcher, an impairment of decreased shoulder external rotation range of motion is more deleterious to function than an impairment involving internal rotation. During the cocking phase of pitching, external rotation of the shoulder can reach a maximum of 180°.[11] Internal rotation of the shoulder is less extreme, with the shoulder returning to neutral rotation or slight internal rotation during the deceleration and follow-through phases of pitching.[12] A range of motion impairment in internal rotation might not prohibit the pitcher from returning to competition. An impairment in external rotation, however, could be career limiting. Each impairment identified during physical examination needs to be analyzed for its effect on functional activities.

A task analysis, performed to ensure that goals regarding resolution of impairments are sufficient to allow for a return to functional activities, involves collecting and analyzing data and applying the information to the target system.[13] Data collected on the task might include range of motion, flexibility, strength, speed of movement, endurance, or neuromuscular demands. A task analysis need not be performed for every task that a patient performs. Rather, a task analysis should be performed on the most challenging task faced by the patient during the day or on a composite of the tasks performed throughout the day. Doing so provides more meaningful information about the maximum requirements for each component of the task or tasks. Range of motion should be analyzed for the greatest range required in any cardinal plane. Strength can be analyzed in a number of ways, such as noting the largest weight that the patient must lift or analyzing the amount of force muscles must generate to overcome forces that can sublux or distract the glenohumeral (GH) joint. Additionally, the type of contraction, such as isometric, concentric, or eccentric, needed to perform the activity should be ascertained. The general speed of movement should be examined, noting if greater than average speeds must be attained. The duration of the activity or the number of repetitions should be identified to determine the endurance component. Finally, neuromuscular control, the coordination of muscle firing, should be assessed, particularly in those activities that produce high forces very quickly or require excessive range of motion.

The history, self-report functional questionnaire, physical examination, and task analysis generate information to assist the clinician in formulating appropriate treatment goals. The history helps identify activities to which the patient wishes to return. The self-report functional questionnaire gives insight into the patient's current level of function. Physical examination measurements identify and quantify the impairments. Physical examination also gives insight into the acuteness of the impairments. The task analysis indicates which impairments interfere with function and the level of impairment resolution that must occur for the patient to return to the desired activity. Once the clinician has assimilated this information, appropriate treatment goals and strategies are readily developed, and the targeted therapeutic exercises can be implemented.

TREATMENT PROTOCOLS

Many treatment protocols have been developed for nonoperative rehabilitation of shoulder pathologies or rehabilitation following shoulder surgery. In recent years, shoulder rehabilitation has become more progressive. Rather than incorporating a prolonged period of immobilization, safe therapeutic exercise is initiated as soon as possible.[14] Initiating therapeutic exercise earlier in the rehabilitation process complements a functional approach in which the primary goal is to return the patient to full function as quickly and safely as possible. Commonly, current shoulder rehabilitation protocols are criteria-based, requiring patients to meet certain criteria before advancing to the next phase.[14] The exact focus of the protocol, number of phases, time frames, and recommended exercises depend on the specific shoulder pathology or type of surgical procedure performed.

Criteria-based protocols set guidelines that assist in treatment decision making for the progression toward full function. Typically, criteria-based shoulder protocols are divided into three (relative rest, resolution of impairments, functional progression) or four (also includes return to activity) phases (Table 16–1). In most protocols involving the shoulder, the relative rest phase focuses on control of inflammation and pain. Shoulder range of motion exercises are performed in a safe and pain-free range. The resolution of impairments phase of rehabilitation focuses on identified deficits in strength, endurance, and neuromuscular control. In the functional progression phase of rehabilitation, the patient prepares for a return to activity either through activity-specific exercise or by increasing the amount of time performing an activity, or both. The return to activity phase includes a controlled, progressive, measured return to all activity. Most individuals will not be receiving formal therapy at this stage.

Individualizing Protocols

The rehabilitation protocol forms the skeleton of the treatment program, outlining the strategies used during each phase and the criteria needed to progress to the next

TABLE 16–1 Phases of Rehabilitation

Phase	Goal
Relative rest	Reduction in pain and inflammation
Resolution of impairments	Rehabilitation of critical impairment
Functional progression	Initiation of sport- or function-specific activity
Return to activity	Gradual progression to unrestricted activity

phase. Often specific exercises, the purveyors of each program used to achieve the criteria, are included. In some cases, best-demonstrated treatment methods for specific impairments exist. In most cases, however, the exercises are a template, based on a clinician's experience and patient needs. The use of a medical diagnosis (e.g., rotator cuff tendonitis) to guide rehabilitation is problematic. The patient with rounded shoulders, weak scapular stabilizers, and a forward head posture who develops rotator cuff tendonitis after increased activity performed above shoulder height likely needs a different therapeutic exercise program than that of a patient with shoulder instability who develops rotator cuff tendonitis from overuse. In both cases the rotator cuff is likely to be irritated and weak, and an early treatment focus in both cases might be to decrease inflammation. In the first case, however, the impairments are likely to include GH joint capsular tightness, contracture of the pectoralis minor, and weakness of the scapular musculature. In the second case, impairments will likely include GH joint laxity, poor neuromuscular control at the GH joint, and weakness of the scapular musculature. Clearly, the same treatment program should not be used to treat these two patients.

Each exercise prescribed or administered during rehabilitation should either address an impairment that must be resolved to improve function, or mimic the functional activity that is to be restored. Exercises that meet these criteria allow the patient to progress toward full function. Insisting that every exercise in the rehabilitation program exactly simulate the functional activity is unrealistic. Exercises that isolate and address the impairment often map directly to function. Treiber et al.[15] demonstrated that a group of healthy tennis players who performed dumbbell and elastic resistance exercises for the rotator cuff had higher peak and average serve speeds as compared to controls. These results suggest that carryover can occur from isolating exercise to function. In addition, exercises that mimic function are not always appropriate, particularly in the early stages of rehabilitation. During this period of rehabilitation, stronger muscles can substitute for weaker muscles, allowing activities to be accomplished while weak muscles remain weak.

However, exercises that mimic function are a crucial part of the rehabilitation program, especially when the functional activity to which the patient will return involves high forces, extremes of range of motion, or great endurance. Resolving impairments in range of motion and strength through passive range of motion and dumbbell exercises will not entirely prepare an overhead athlete for the speeds that must be generated during sports. Nor will these activities give a laborer, such as a construction worker, the endurance to work for extended periods with the arms overhead. Sport- or function-specific exercise must be included and must be tailored to the needs of the patient.

The bridge between isolating exercise and functional activity is addressed in the functional progression phase. Once a patient enters the functional progression phase, therapeutic exercises become more specific to the activity to which the patient will eventually return. When patients cannot be categorized as athletes or laborers, or when their functional activity level does not seem particularly demanding, the bridge between isolating exercise and functional activity is often overlooked. In these patients, the bridge should be their functional activities, performed in progressively increasing lengths of time or repetitions. For instance, a patient who is recovering from a shoulder injury and wishes to return to painting might be advised to paint for a half hour at a time, assess how the shoulder is responding, and then proceed as indicated. The patient could also be instructed to rest the shoulder from the overhead position after every 10 minutes of work. Either way, the idea is to increase the stresses imparted on the shoulder complex gradually. This concept is similar to progressive resistance exercise, but the emphasis is placed on progression of the functional activity. Specific ideas regarding decisions about progression of exercise within a phase will be discussed later.[16]

Gradual progression to full function is equally important for the athlete or laborer. For the athlete, this progression will include sport-specific exercise like plyometrics and agility drills in the functional progression phase. The athlete then moves into the return to activity phase, in which activity or playing time are closely monitored and carefully increased through an interval sport program. Training continues until the athlete has reached the volume and intensity necessary for competition. For the laborer, the progression might include the functional progression phase via a work hardening program, and the return to activity phase consisting of a return to work at half days or spending part of a day at light duty until full-duty status is reached.

Critical impairments identified during the physical examination and task analysis must be adequately addressed prior to the initiation of the functional progression phase of rehabilitation. A patient who begins the functional progression phase without an adequate resolution of impairments is at risk for a return of symptoms or the development of a new pathology. For example, if range of motion has not been restored in the shoulder, a compensatory motion from the scapulothoracic (ST) joint or the thoracic spine might occur to carry out the functional activity. Over time, this substitution could lead to overuse injury or dysfunction at these joints. Before a functional progression is initiated, full, pain-free active range of motion must be restored, strength deficits should be sufficiently resolved, and appropriate neuromuscular control via normalization of the scapulohumeral rhythm must be present. Specific exercises for muscle performance, motor control, and range of motion (ROM), which are characterized by practice patterns, are discussed in Chapters 7 to 12. Additionally, Chapters 14, 15, and 17 present comprehensive strategies for motor control, whereas Chapter 13 discusses manual therapy techniques for the shoulder. Successful progression through the functional progression phase will depend partly on appropriate initiation of exercises.

Progressing Between Protocol Phases

Decisions regarding treatment progression are difficult unless guidelines have been established to direct the decision making process. Although the inflammatory and healing processes move through specific stages, the time frame for healing differs among individuals.[17] Because of these differences, decisions regarding progression cannot be solely based on time from injury or surgery. Criteria-based protocols offer structure for decisions regarding progression between phases of rehabilitation.

In most protocols, criteria involve a set range of motion or level of strength that must be achieved prior to beginning the next phase. Criteria can also include the absence of pain, a certain outcome on clinical examination or the ability to complete a specific task. Many different criteria based on pathology, whether the treatment is nonoperative or operative, and whether the protocol is developed for a specific population of patients (e.g., baseball pitchers or swimmers), can be used. The criteria for progression should describe a level of resolution of the most critical impairments necessary to attain the safe performance of the exercises and activities in the next phase.

Using Strength as a Criterion for Progression

Strength is routinely used as a criterion for progression. However, controversy exists about how strength should be measured. Currently no method of strength testing has been proven to be most valid or to provide the best inferences to function.[18] Shoulder strength is measured by techniques including manual muscle testing, isometric muscle testing performed with a hand-held dynamometer or an isokinetic dynamometer, or dynamic muscle testing on an isokinetic dynamometer. Each type of muscle strength testing has potential problems associated with the collection of data.

Manual muscle testing provides only ordinal data and may be of little value unless there is a debilitating amount of weakness.[18] The inability to discriminate at higher levels of strength was demonstrated in a study where strength deficits were revealed during isokinetic testing of the knee in a population whose strength was graded 5/5 and equal bilaterally during manual muscle testing.[19] Clinicians might also base the strength rating on their own perceived effort during testing rather than the peak or average force of the patient.[18]

Isometric testing can potentially generate more useful information, provided adequate stabilization is given. Test-retest reliability has been shown to be good to excellent in this method of strength testing. The use of a hand-held dynamometer or isokinetic dynamometer during isometric testing allows objective data to be generated, thus removing the subjectivity of manual muscle testing.

Dynamic muscle testing on an isokinetic dynamometer also generates objective data. Good correlation has been found between isokinetic and isometric testing. The reliability of isokinetic testing can be enhanced with a standardized protocol.[20] Results generated in a particular test position (supine, seated, standing, 90° of abduction, scapular plane) or at a particular speed cannot, however, be directly compared to other test positions or speeds.[20,21] Several other issues must be considered when using strength measures as criteria for progression. First, no level of strength has been proven to be predictive of injury or necessary for a return to competition.[18,21] Second, strength criteria are often based on bilateral comparisons that might not be valid if the uninvolved side has been previously injured or subjected to disuse atrophy. Finally, strength patterns might be particular to a subpopulation. This information must be known to interpret strength test results properly.[22] For example, the age of the athlete, the skill level of the athlete, and the sport in which an athlete participates all can affect isokinetic muscular performance.[22] Thus, the method of strength testing and the level of strength chosen as progression criteria in a protocol must be thoughtfully considered.

Progressing Within a Protocol Phase

Progression within a phase of rehabilitation is most often dictated by the patient's response to a particular treatment. Most patients will experience some postexercise soreness the day following a more challenging exercise routine. These symptoms are

---

BOX 16–1 Exercise Progression Guidelines Based on Soreness

If no soreness is present from previous exercise, progress exercise by modifying one variable. If soreness is present from previous exercise, but recedes with warm-up, stay at the same level. If soreness is present from previous exercise, but does not recede with warm-up, decrease exercise to the level prior to progression. Consider taking the day off if soreness is still present with reduced level of exercise. When exercise is resumed, it should be at the reduced level.

---

expected secondary to delayed-onset muscle soreness or from increased stress applied to the shoulder joint. The amount and behavior of the soreness have been reported as criteria for continued progression both in a weight lifting program and in an interval throwing program.[23–25] These rules can also apply to progression within a rehabilitation phase and will be summarized here.

Box 16–1 outlines how a patient's response might dictate progression in rehabilitation. When soreness is experienced the day following a progression in exercise, but the soreness recedes following warm-up, the rehabilitation program remains the same. If a patient experiences an exacerbation of symptoms during exercise, or if the soreness from the previous workout does not diminish with warm-up, the rehabilitation program will need to be decreased to the preceding level.[17] The patient might also need to take a day off from exercising if the soreness is severe enough.[24,25] The therapist should review the progression in a similar fashion to that of advancing two levels on a step-wise progression to ensure that the progression was not too vigorous. Possibly more than one variable was progressed simultaneously, for instance, increasing both speed and repetitions of an exercise. If this has occurred, an intermediate step, an exercise that is slightly less aggressive or that only increases one variable compared to that of the previous exercise level, should be inserted. If a patient does not experience soreness or other symptoms, progression in the rehabilitation program can continue.

Progressing the Difficulty of Therapeutic Exercise

Another aspect of treatment decision making involves selecting exercises that are progressively more challenging or modifying a particular exercise to become more challenging. The shoulder impairments present, and the functional activity to which the patient wishes to return will largely dictate, which exercises are selected and what modifications will constitute progression. A few aspects of shoulder exercises that can be modified to increase or decrease the difficulty of the exercise will be discussed here.

In treating shoulder injuries, the range of motion, specifically the amount of abduction and external rotation, used when performing the exercise is an important consideration. The demands on the rotator cuff to centralize the humeral head are greater in lower degrees of abduction and decrease as 90° of abduction is approached.[26] Rhythmic stabilization prescribed for a patient with a partial rotator cuff tear or a patient undergoing rehabilitation after a rotator cuff repair may begin at 90° of abduction and progress by moving to 60°, then 45° of abduction. When abduction is combined with external rotation, a patient with anterior instability is predisposed to subluxation. Consequently, 90° of abduction and external rotation is used as a testing position for apprehension.[27] External rotation strengthening may

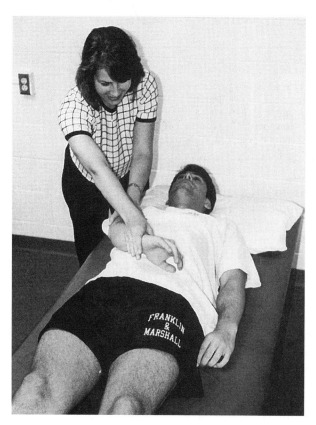

FIGURE 16–1. PNF D2 pattern start position.

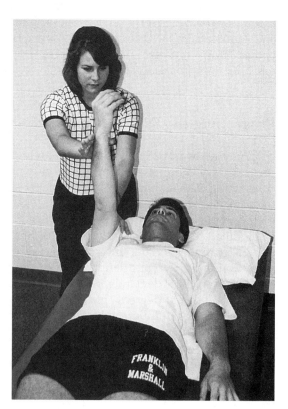

FIGURE 16–2. PNF D2 pattern stopping at 90° of flexion, 0° of abduction, and neutral rotation.

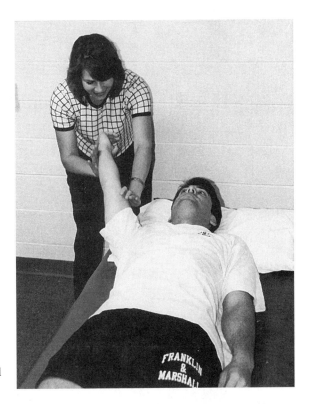

FIGURE 16–3. PNF D2 pattern at end range.

initially be prescribed at 0° of abduction and then gradually progressed to 45° of abduction and finally 90° of abduction. Or a manually resisted PNF D2 pattern may begin in a shortened range (Fig. 16–1), stopping at 90° of flexion, neutral rotation and 0° of abduction (Fig. 16–2), eventually progressing through full range (Fig. 16–3).

The effect of gravity can also change the aggressiveness of an activity. A patient might need to begin an exercise in a gravity-reduced position until adequate strength or neuromuscular control is acquired to do the exercise against gravity. For example, rhythmic stabilization is performed in the supine position at 90° where work against gravity is minimized (Fig. 16–4), progressing to a seated position where work against

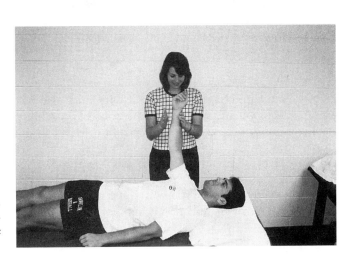

FIGURE 16–4. Rhythmic stabilization performed in the supine position, minimizing the effects of gravity.

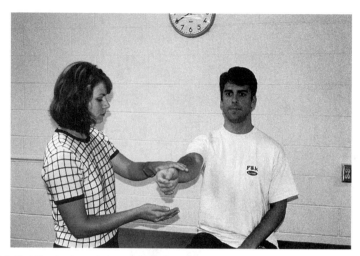

FIGURE 16–5. Rhythmic stabilization performed in a seated position, maximizing the effects of gravity.

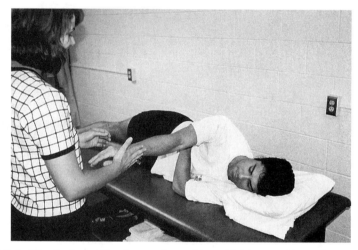

FIGURE 16–6. Rhythmic stabilization performed in a sidelying position, allowing gravity to assist in compressing the humeral head in the glenoid fossa.

gravity is maximized (Fig. 16–5). Gravity may also be used to assist an exercise; for example, a patient with multidirectional instability may perform a rhythmic stabilization exercise in sidelying position to aid in glenohumeral compression (Fig. 16–6).

The level of proximal stabilization required to perform an activity is another important consideration in progressing the difficulty of an exercise. A patient may begin plyometric external rotation in the supine position (Fig. 16–7), progress to sitting on a chair (Fig. 16–8), and finally move to a standing position (Fig. 16–9). Starting in

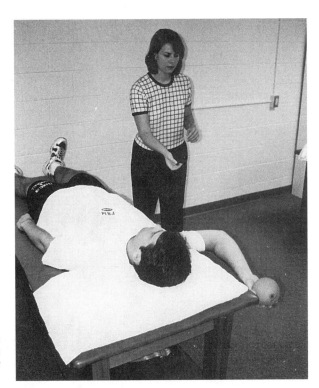

FIGURE 16–7. External rotation plyometric performed in the supine position. The scapula is stabilized by the table in this position.

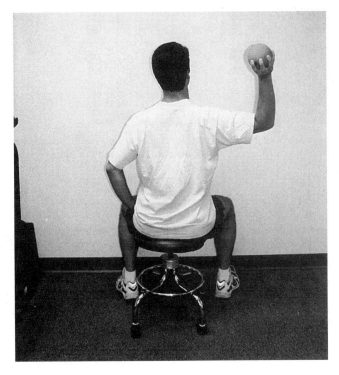

FIGURE 16–8. External rotation plyometric performed in a seated position. In this position there are increased demands for stabilization of the trunk and scapula.

389

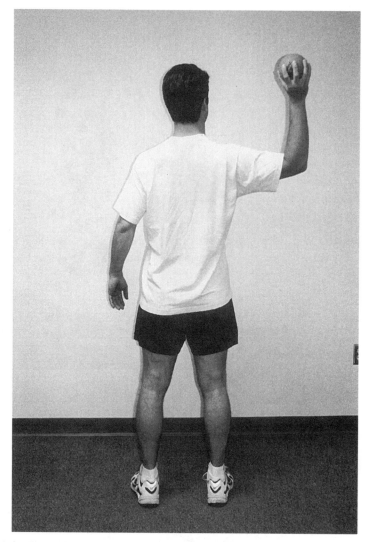

FIGURE 16–9. External rotation plyometric performed in a standing position. The demands for stabilization at the GH joint, scapula, and trunk approach the demands encountered during overhead sport activities.

the supine position reduces the neuromuscular control and stabilization demands on the scapular stabilizers. Moving into sitting increases the challenge to the scapular stabilizers while minimizing trunk stability requirements. Once the patient is in the standing position, the challenge to the scapula and trunk is maximized, beginning to simulate the challenge experienced during overhead activities.

Many other ways are available to vary the level of difficulty of an exercise, including increasing the resistance, speed, and number of repetitions. Regardless of how the exercises are progressed, the patient's response should always be assessed to determine the appropriateness of the progression.

Using Interval Sport Programs

Most patients will meet the requirements to perform their daily activities and be discharged sometime during the functional progression phase. Athletes, however, need a final step to ensure that they are ready to withstand the demands of their sports. The return to activity phase, the final phase, includes an interval sport program designed to gradually increase the amount of effort and difficulty of technique required. For example, the interval program for a racquet sport would dictate the number of strokes needed, the distance the ball travels, and the type of stroke used. Many interval sport programs have been developed. However, few have been tested for their effectiveness or have used actual game statistics to enhance the program development. Without a structured interval sport program or with a poorly constructed interval sport program, the demands to the shoulder joint can inadvertently be progressed too quickly.

In one of the few interval sport programs to be based on actual data, Axe et al.[25] presented a model for the development and implementation of an interval-throwing program for young baseball pitchers. The timing and repetition parameters of the conventional short and long toss interval throwing program were developed from data collected during 400 innings of Little League and Babe Ruth baseball during a single season. Data involving maximal distance and speed measurements were recorded from 852 boys ages 8 to 14 who participated in organized baseball. Game data included mean pitch counts, ranges for pitches per inning, ranges for seconds between pitches, mean innings per outing, and mean number of pitches per outing. Little League rules for field dimensions were also used to shape the short toss portion of the program. A mathematical model was developed from these data to predict maximal throwing distance from maximal throwing speed. This study resulted in a data-based, age-specific, speed-dependent, distance-based, functional, practical, progressive interval throwing program for Little League-age athletes. Interval programs developed for various sports can be enhanced if they are constructed using a model like the model described previously.

When the athlete has successfully completed the interval sport program, a gradual return to competition is allowed. Often the athlete is first cleared to participate in practices. Then, if no symptoms are experienced, the athlete is allowed to begin competition.

Progressing Rehabilitation for In-Season Athletes

Although the rehabilitation progression framework outlined in this chapter is sequential, sometimes an ideal progression through the rehabilitation process cannot be followed, particularly with an athlete who is in the midst of the competitive season. Often, athletes with shoulder injuries are unable to modify their activities during the season, especially if a pending competitive event is significant. In these situations, the traditional rehabilitation approach might need to be altered. Russ[28] reported on a case study of a swimmer with shoulder pathology during the competitive season treated with modalities and therapeutic exercise to address impairments. The athlete was only allowed to perform kickboard workouts during practice, but was allowed to compete without restriction. Through this approach, the athlete was able to minimize symptoms and still participate in competition.

This approach will not work for an athlete with an acute injury, because participation in competition will continue to exacerbate symptoms and prevent injured tissue from healing. Athletes must also understand that whereas this approach allows them to finish the season, off-season rehabilitation aimed at improving impairments is crucial. A team approach among the physician, physical therapist, and athletic trainer can help to ensure that a progression back to full function occurs even when the ideal rehabilitation program cannot be followed.

MEASURING SHOULDER FUNCTION

To document the effectiveness of a rehabilitation program, or to document an improvement in function, a reliable, valid, and responsive measure is needed for assessing function. Self-report questionnaires and health status indices that combine questionnaire and physical examination findings are commonly used to assess functional outcome. A shoulder index can be used at the initial evaluation to determine a base level of function. Then, at discharge, the index can be administered again, allowing measurement of the change in function resulting from the rehabilitation process. The process of gathering and analyzing these data is called *outcomes research.* Outcomes research compares the initial and final functional level achieved by patients to determine the effectiveness of a rehabilitation program. Outcomes research can also be used to compare different rehabilitation programs and to determine if one program is superior to another. This section relates the clinical aspects of functional outcome measures as they relate to functional progression. Chapter 6 presents a comprehensive overview of functional outcome measures for the shoulder.

Unfortunately, the measurement of shoulder function is clouded with controversy. Many shoulder health status indices have been reported in the literature, including Hospital for Special Surgery Questionnaire, Constant-Murley Questionnaire, Shoulder Disability Questionnaire, Simple Shoulder Test, American Shoulder and Elbow Surgeons Form, Shoulder Pain Score, Subjective Shoulder Rating Scale, Shoulder Severity Index, and Shoulder Pain and Disability Index.[2–10] This list is not all-inclusive, and even with the many questionnaires listed here, no gold standard for shoulder outcomes indices exists. Each instrument differs in the design for measuring shoulder function. Specific advantages and disadvantages are inherent in every design. Clinicians should understand how the design of a health status index can affect the results. They also need to know the issues relating to the development of a questionnaire. This information will allow clinicians to make better-informed decisions when choosing an instrument to assist them in evaluating the effectiveness of their shoulder rehabilitation programs.

Key Factors for Choosing a Shoulder Index

One way that the shoulder indices can be distinguished is by the categories or domains in which function is measured. All indices include questions regarding the presence of shoulder pain. The questionnaires differ in whether pain is assessed during rest, during activity, at night, at the usual level, at the worst intensity, or in various combinations. Most instruments also contain questions regarding function, and some include questions regarding strength, motion, or shoulder stability.[2,3,5,6,8–10] Because the various instruments use different categories to assess function, outcomes cannot be easily compared when different shoulder indices are used.

The categories that are included in a shoulder index can greatly affect the final result, possibly causing the patient's functional level to be overestimated or underestimated. The inclusion of physical examination findings in an index can be particularly problematic. Consider, for example, the Hospital for Special Surgery instrument that subtracts points for every 20° of motion deficit in any plane.[26] Because baseball pitchers typically have excessive external rotation as compared to other adults, a 20° loss of motion in the pitching shoulder would be scored as normal, although a 20° loss of motion could be career-ending for the athlete. Furthermore, motion deficits exist in shoulders that are not painful, and range of motion has been found to decrease with age.[29,30] Thus, an elderly person might score poorly because of deficits (when compared to healthy young adults) in range of motion yet be able to complete all activities of daily living without complication.

Similarly, the amount of strength and what muscles must be strong to restore function differs from person to person and activity to activity. The same criteria might not appropriately measure function for all patients. Being aware of the potential influences of physical examination findings on the shoulder index score can assist the clinician in making better choices in the tool used to measure function in a particular population.

The shoulder indices also vary in their methods of scoring. Because the scoring methods are not consistent among indices, the results cannot be compared to each other. Different scoring methods can give different results for the same individual, which might result in function being overestimated or underestimated. The Subjective Shoulder Rating Scale, for example, includes a stability category.[8] Because of the way the categories are weighted, simply by lacking instability a patient would be more likely to score higher on the questionnaire.

Many other issues have to be considered when determining the usefulness of a shoulder index. One is responsiveness to functional change. A ceiling effect might be inherent in an index; for example, a patient is able to achieve a high score very early in the rehabilitation process, but the instrument is insensitive to further functional gains. If the index has functional intervals that are too large, it might not capture the improvements that occur in function. The wording of function questions could also interfere with the responsiveness of a questionnaire. Kinematic analysis has shown that the arm is adaptable, with different strategies being used to perform activities of daily living.[31] If the wording of a question is not specific to reveal shoulder function, a patient might be able to score at a higher functional level because activities are performed with substitutions in motion made at other joints, interfering with the measurement of true shoulder function change.

Another issue to consider is whether the questionnaire is sensitive to disability. A questionnaire that simply asks questions about pain and the ability to perform activities of daily living would not identify the true disability experienced by an athlete or, possibly, a manual laborer. Finally, the utility of the questionnaire should be considered. That is, will the questionnaire be used to measure function, or will it be used for diagnostic purposes?

Generic Questionnaires Versus Site-Specific Questionnaires

The acute version of the Short Form 36 (SF–36) is a generic questionnaire that has been shown to be a reliable and valid measure of the health of patients with musculoskeletal conditions.[32] This generic index offers a way to measure other aspects of function besides those that directly relate to the shoulder joint. A complete description of this scale is presented in Chapter 6. Beaton and Richards[33] compared the results from 90 subjects with shoulder pathologies who completed the Shoulder Pain and Disability Index, the Simple Shoulder Test, the Subjective Shoulder Rating Scale, The American Shoulder and Elbow Surgeons questionnaire, the Shoulder Severity Index, and the SF–36. The shoulder questionnaires performed differently from the SF–36 and did not discriminate between levels of overall health. Gartsman et al.[34] reported the results from the administration of the SF–36 to patients with five shoulder conditions including glenohumeral instability, complete reparable rotator cuff tear, adhesive capsulitis, glenohumeral osteoarthritis, and impingement. The results revealed that these patients had significant decreases in their health in several areas, and that the severity ranked with major medical conditions including depression and diabetes mellitus. This suggests that both disease-specific and generic health status questionnaires should be administered to capture the true impact of the shoulder dysfunction.

An Integrated Approach to Measuring Function

No single existing self-report functional questionnaire has the ability to capture the functional level of all patients and all shoulder pathologies. The fact that so many questionnaires have been developed demonstrates the lack of agreement about what aspects of shoulder function are important. The same problems were faced in creating a questionnaire to evaluate knee function. Through a collaborative effort headed by Irrgang[35] at the University of Pittsburgh, some of these problems have been overcome. The Irrgang format could serve as a model for evaluating shoulder functional outcome. The self-report functional questionnaire that has been developed consists of three parts. The first part is the activities of daily living score that includes pain and function questions. The second part, used when applicable, is a sports activity score. The last part is a global rating score.

In addition to the shoulder functional questionnaire, the acute form of the SF–36 is administered. This format has been demonstrated to be useful in capturing the functional level of patients with a variety of activity levels and knee pathologies. Several aspects of this format make it superior to using a single questionnaire to assess function. By assessing activities of daily living and sports activity separately, the ability to function during high-demand sports is evaluated. However, the questions do not result in an underestimation of activity level for those patients who are not involved in sports. By documenting, but not scoring, objective measurements, tester bias in the score and having to create different forms for different subpopulations are not concerns. By including a general health rating, the SF–36 form, psychological and well-being aspects of function are tested, aspects that might be missed in a site-specific questionnaire. Therefore, measurement of shoulder function could become more accurate if a multifaceted approach is used.

CASE STUDY 16–1

EXAMINATION

History

A 12-year-old male baseball pitcher developed pain in his throwing shoulder and a reduction in pitching speed over the course of a Little League season. At the time of physical therapy evaluation, his primary complaint was posterior right shoulder pain during the deceleration phase of pitching. His pain increased as pitching activity increased. When the pain was severe, he also had difficulty during the follow-through phase of batting. The patient was in-season at the time of initial evaluation, reduced to playing only first or second base to decrease his frequency of throwing.

Tests and Measures

Physical examination reveals reduced active and passive internal rotation and horizontal abduction. Resisted isometric abduction and external rotation are strong and painful. Manual muscle testing reveals 4/5 strength for external rotators and supraspinatus and 4+/5 strength for internal rotators and middle/lower trapezius on the right (involved) side. Scapular winging is present during a press-up from the sitting position. All other muscle groups of the shoulder girdle are graded 5/5. The relocation test is positive for pain. He has no specific tenderness to palpation of the rotator cuff tendons.

EVALUATION

The history, review of systems, and tests and measures indicate that this patient should be classified in practice pattern E: impaired joint mobility, muscle performance, and ROM, associated with ligament or other connective tissue disorders.

DIAGNOSIS

The history suggests that the patient's shoulder pain is occurring because his rotator cuff is not able to overcome the distraction forces that occur during the deceleration phase of pitching and the follow-through phase of batting. The physical examination reveals a positive relocation test, possibly implicating subtle anterior subluxation of the humerus. Anterior subluxation would increase the demand on the posterior rotator cuff. In addition, the weakness noted in the external rotators could result from microtrauma suffered from these demands. In turn, this weakness would prevent him from being able to overcome the forces, resulting in further microtrauma. The impairment in horizontal adduction range of motion suggests tightness of the posterior capsule. A lack of flexibility in the posterior capsule could cause migration of the humerus anteriorly, again increasing the stabilization demands on the posterior rotator cuff. Finally, weakness of the scapular stabilizers and winging of the scapula suggest that the patient might not have had a stable base from which the rotator cuff could work. The impairments addressed to return the patient to pitching include (1) weakness of the rotator cuff muscles, (2) weakness of the scapular musculature, (3) tightness of the posterior capsule, and (4) poor neuromuscular control at the GH and ST joints.

INTERVENTION

The patient is given a home program consisting of isotonic exercise for the internal-external rotators, serratus anterior, and middle trapezius and stretches for the posterior capsule. Physical therapy treatments include posterior capsule mobilizations and stretches, rhythmic stabilization for the GH and ST joints, and electrical stimulation to the posterior rotator cuff insertion for pain control.

The patient is seen for 15 visits after initial evaluation over a 6-week period. He continues to play infield positions, but is not allowed to throw harder than 75% effort during practices. The patient is progressed to performing supine external rotation at 90° of shoulder abduction and external rotation after 2 weeks of treatment. The 90/90 position is a functional position for a pitcher. However, because of weak scapular musculature, this patient begins the exercise in the supine position. A week later, the patient is progressed to performing the exercise in a standing position. The patient fatigues quickly when performing strengthening in this position, and his scapula begins to abduct when the he becomes fatigued. The patient is slowly progressed in this exercise with an emphasis on repetitions to increase endurance. Within 1 month, the patient is reporting no pain with throwing while playing infield positions. He demonstrates increased posterior capsular flexibility and an overall improvement in strength. The patient is allowed to begin an interval-throwing program with modifications made for long-toss throwing. These modifications are made because the patient had been playing on a Little League field. It is felt that progressing to larger field dimensions would be too aggressive. Physical therapy visits are decreased to one time per week.

The patient is contacted via phone approximately 2 weeks after initiation of the interval throwing program and 1 week after his last physical therapy treatment. He reports no pain or difficulty performing his interval-throwing program. The patient is consequently discharged from physical therapy.

CHAPTER SUMMARY

In this chapter, an outline of the process to implement therapeutic exercise into a functional approach is presented. The process integrates self-report information gained from the patient and through questionnaires, physical examination findings from various forms of testing, and activity information gained through task analysis. This information sets measurable impairment-resolution and functional goals. Criteria-based treatment guidelines are then used to guide the patient's treatment toward these goals. Obviously, many steps in this process still require refinement and support from research. For instance, there is a need to develop a standard for strength testing of the shoulder and specific strength criteria for return to sport activity. Also, interval sport programs based on data need to be developed. Shoulder indices and the process of measuring shoulder function must be improved to allow function to be more accurately measured. This will increase the precision of assessing the effectiveness of shoulder rehabilitation programs through outcomes research. Once areas such as these become refined, superior functional outcomes in shoulder rehabilitation should result.

REFERENCES

1. Guide to Physical Therapist Practice. Part One: Description of patient/client management and Part Two: Preferred practice patterns. Phys Ther 77:1163, 1998.
2. Altchek, DW, et al: Arthroscopic acromioplasty: technique and results. J Bone Jt Surg 72A:1198, 1990.
3. Constant, CR, and Murley, AHG: A clinical method of functional assessment of the shoulder. Clin Orthop Rel Res 214:161, 1987.
4. Van der Windt, DAWM, et al: The responsiveness of the shoulder disability questionnaire. Ann Rheum Dis 57:82, 1998.
5. Lippitt, SB, et al: A practical tool for evaluating function: the simple shoulder test. In Matsen III, FA, et al (eds): The shoulder: a balance of mobility and stability. American Academy of Orthopaedic Surgeons, Chicago, IL, 1993, p 501.
6. Richards, RR, et al: A standardized method for the assessment of shoulder function. J Shoulder Elbow Surg 3:347, 1994.
7. Winters, JC, et al: A shoulder pain score: a comprehensive questionnaire for assessing pain in patients with shoulder complaints. Scand J Rehab Med 28:163, 1996.
8. L'Insalata, JC, et al: A self-administered questionnaire for assessment of symptoms and function of shoulder. J Bone Jt Surg 79A:738, 1997.
9. Patte, D: Directions for the use of the index severity for painful and/or chronically disabled shoulders. Abstracts of the First Open Congress of the European Society of Surgery of the Shoulder and Elbow. Paris, 1987, p 36.
10. Roach, KE, et al: Development of a shoulder pain and disability index. Arthrit Care and Res 4:143, 1991.
11. Fleisig, GS, et al: Biomechanics of the shoulder during throwing. In Andrews, JR, and Wilk, KE (eds): The Athlete's Shoulder. Churchill Livingstone, New York, 1994, p 359.
12. Dillman, CJ, et al: Biomechanics of the shoulder in sports. Throwing activities. Postgrad Adv Sports Med Forum Medicum, Berryville, VA, 1991.
13. Stammers, RB: Factors limiting the development of task analysis. Ergonomics 38:588, 1995.
14. Wilk, KE: Current concepts in the rehabilitation of athletic shoulder injuries. In Andrews, JR, and Wilk, KE (eds): The Athlete's Shoulder. Churchill Livingstone, New York, 1994, p 335.
15. Treiber, FA, et al: Effects of Theraband and lightweight dumbbell training on shoulder rotation torque and serve performance in college tennis players. Am J Sports Med 26: 510, 1998.
16. DeLorme, T, and Watkins, A: Techniques of progressive resistance exercise. Arch Phys Med Rehabil 29:263, 1948.
17. Curwin, S, and Stanish, WD: Tendinitis: Its Etiology and Treatment. DC Heath, Lexington, MA, 1984.
18. Sapega, AA: Current concepts review. Muscle performance evaluation in orthopedic practice. J Bone Jt Surg 72A:1562, 1990.
19. Wilk, KE, et al: A comparison of manual muscle test results to isokinetic peak torque results in 100 ACL reconstructed knees. Presented at APTA, Denver, CO, 1992.
20. Wilk, KE, et al: Standardized isokinetic testing protocol for the throwing shoulder: the thrower's series. Isokin Exerc Sci 1:22, 1991.
21. Rothstein, JM, et al: Clinical uses of isokinetic measurements. Phys Ther 67:1840, 1987.
22. Wilk, KE, and Arrigo, CA: Isokinetic exercise and testing for the shoulder. In Andrews, JR, and Wilk, KE (eds): The Athlete's Shoulder. Churchill Livingstone, New York, 1997, p 523.
23. Ebbeling, CB, and Clarkson, PM: Exercise-induced muscle damage and adaptation. Sports Med 7: 207, 1989.
24. Fees, M, et al: Upper extremity weight-training modifications for the injured athlete. A clinical perspective. Am J Sports Med 26: 732, 1998.
25. Axe, MJ, et al: Development of a distance-based interval throwing program for Little League aged athletes. Am J Sports Med 24:594, 1996.
26. Poppen, NK, and Walker, PS: Forces at the glenohumeral joint in abduction. Clin Orthop 135:165, 1978.
27. Zarins, B, and Rowe, CR: Current concepts in the diagnosis and treatment of shoulder instability in athletes. Med Sci Sports Exerc 16:444, 1984.

28. Russ, DW: In-season management of shoulder pain in a collegiate swimmer: a team approach. J Orthop Phys Ther: 371, 1998.
29. Pope, DP, et al: The frequency of restricted range of movement in individuals with self-reported shoulder pain: results from a population-based surgery. Br J Rheumatol 35: 1137, 1996.
30. Chakravarty, K, and Webley, M: Shoulder joint movement and its relationship to disability in the elderly. J Rheumatol 20:1359, 1993.
31. Buckley, MA, et al: Dynamics of the upper limb during performance of the tasks of everyday living: A review of the current knowledge base. Proc Instn Mech Engrs 110: 241, 1996.
32. Ware II, JE, et al: SF–36 health survey: manual and interpretation guide. The Health Institute, Boston, 1993.
33. Beaton, DE, and Richards, RR: Measuring function of the shoulder: a cross-sectional comparison of five questionnaires. J Bone Jt Surg 78A:882, 1996.
34. Gartsman, GM, et al: Self-assessment of general health status in patients with five common shoulder conditions. J Shoulder Elbow Surg 7:228, 1998.
35. Irrgang, JJ, et al: Development of a patient-reported measure of function of the knee. J Bone Jt Surg 80A (8):1132, 1998.

CHAPTER 17

Open and Closed Chain Exercises for the Shoulder

Beven P. Livingston, MS, PT, ATC

INTRODUCTION

Physical rehabilitation is now at a crossroads due to the economic pressures from insurance companies demanding the most cost-effective care for patients. As a result, some of the previous methods of rehabilitation based on anecdotal outcomes and treatment of the patient's symptoms must be re-examined. A more scientific basis for rehabilitation should be established focusing on the process of disablement, which is the impact of the patient's impairment on function.[1] Re-examination of the disablement process has led to greater focus on functional rehabilitation.

Functional rehabilitation emphasizes restoring functional capacity while resolving symptoms.[2] This involves restoring the movements of joints and limbs in a coordinated way to perform a specific task, whether it is a work, a recreational, or an athletic task. With this in mind, it is important to understand how the joints and limbs of the body are interconnected and how they function together as a unit to achieve the desired functional task.

This chapter discusses the development of the kinematic and kinetic chain terminology, reviews the characteristics that describe open and closed kinetic chain exercises, and discusses the rationale for the use of closed kinetic chain exercises in upper extremity rehabilitation. It presents the most current research on upper extremity closed kinetic chain exercises and incorporates this information into a suggested shoulder rehabilitation program and case study.

KINEMATIC AND KINETIC CHAIN TERMINOLOGY

In the late nineteenth century, a mechanical engineer named Reuleaux[3] coined the term *kinematic chain*. A kinematic chain is mechanically defined as rigid, overlapping segments connected in a series via pin joints. The system is considered closed if both ends are fixed and immovable. Movement at one joint produces predictable movement at the other joints in the series.

Brunnstrom[4] applied this concept of *kinematic chain* to human movement; that is, successive joints linked together in the upper and lower extremities create an open kinematic chain. A continuous path such as the ribs connecting the sternum with the thoracic vertebrae is a closed kinematic chain.

Open and Closed Kinetic Chain Activities

Steindler[5] used the notion of a *closed kinematic chain* and linked segment motion for engineering systems and adapted it to describe human movement. He also changed the terminology to *kinetic chain.* Although the human extremities can be thought of as rigid, overlapping segments in a series, physiologically, a true closed kinematic chain system does not exist. In human extremities, the end segments such as the hand and the shoulder or the foot and the hip are never both fixed and immovable. Thus, Steindler proposed that two types of kinetic chains, open and closed, exist under different limb loading conditions in the human body. He defined the closed kinetic chain (CKC) condition as one in which the foot or the hand meets considerable resistance. This resistance prohibits or restrains free motion, requiring muscles to fire consecutively in a distal to proximal direction.[6] The open kinetic chain (OKC) condition involves a combination of links in which the terminal segment, the foot or the hand, is completely free to move. The goal is to attain large accelerations of distal segment through sequential activation of muscles from proximal to distal.[6] According to his classification system, some examples of OKC activities of the upper extremity include waving a hand, throwing a baseball, hitting a tennis ball, or putting a shot-put. CKC activities include chin-ups, push-ups, rowing, and boxing. Steindler and others[6–10] stated that classifying functional activities as either *open* or *closed* is difficult because some activities are a combination of the two or the activities occur somewhere along a continuum or as a transition between the two types of kinetic chains. For example, with a leg press, the feet are fixed on the plate but the plate is moving with the exercise.

Others have added to Steindler's definition of open and closed kinetic chain activities. Gray defines an OKC as a system in which the distal segment is free. The motion is isolated and occurs usually in a single plane. CKC activities occur if the distal segment is fixed, and motion takes place in multiple planes.[11,12] Gray states that a CKC results if either set of limbs is supporting the body's weight.

In an attempt to classify various strength training exercises, Panariello[7] defined a CKC activity as one in which the foot is in contact with the ground. Conversely, he describes an OKC activity as one in which the foot is not in contact with the ground. He agrees with Gray[11,12] that body weight must be supported for a CKC to exist. He suggests the existence of a transition area between an open and a closed kinetic chain. This *transition area* was defined as something between the two absolute points on a continuum. These two absolute points are described as exercises that support body weight and the end segment is fixed (CKC), such as a squat, and those in which the distal segment is free to move (OKC), such as a leg extension. As a result, an attempt was made to classify lower extremity exercises that use free weights as CKC versus those that use machines as OKC. However, Panariello did not consistently use this transition area to describe all exercises. For example, he classified exercises that use machines, such as the leg press (in which the end segment is fixed to a plate but the plate is free to move), as OKC. He justified this classification because the biomechanics of the machines used in these types of exercises eliminate the effects of body weight and balance.

Because operational definitions of OKC and CKC differ, categorizing activities or exercises as an open or a closed kinetic chain is problematic.[8] In general, exercises can be considered as falling within a continuum, with open and closed kinetic chain being the extremes. Dillman and colleagues[9] attempted to clarify this confusion with an alternative classification system based on the mechanics of the activity. They considered the following two points in their system: the boundary condition (defining the limits of the distal segment) and the external load encountered at the distal segment. The boundary condition of the distal segment might be either fixed or movable, whereas the external load might or might not be present at the distal segment. According to this classification system, the conditions include the following: (1) a fixed boundary with an external load (FEL), such as a push-up, (2) a movable boundary with an external load (MEL), such as a standard bench press, and (3) a movable boundary with no external load (MNL), such as a bench press movement pattern without resistance.

Confusion in kinematic and kinetic chain terminology partly results from the application of mechanical engineering terms to the human body. Biological tissue rarely behaves in the manner described by engineers. For example, the definition of closed kinematic chain describes a series of pin joints producing joint rotational movement with 1° of freedom. However, many of the joints within the human body, such as the glenohumeral (GH) joint, produce rotational movements in several planes with more than 1° of freedom. Furthermore, as stated previously, the extremities in the human body are not fixed at both ends. Unique characteristics of human movement, such as joint compression and muscle cocontraction, occur when one end segment is fixed in space (supporting body weight) versus when the end segment is free to move in space. Differences between machines and biological systems warrant maintaining the use of the general terminology (*open kinetic chain* versus *closed kinetic chain*) with a more inclusive definition that applies to the human joint movement. The author proposes that a CKC is defined as a successive combination of joints in which the distal segment is immovable. Translation of the joint centers occurs in a predictable manner that is secondary to the distribution of body weight (gravity) through a base of support. An OKC is defined as a successive combination of joints in which the distal segment is free to move. Translation of the joint centers occurs in a less predictable manner than in a CKC that is secondary to the planned motor program. Finally, OKC and CKC activities are not independent entities, but rather two extremes of the same spectrum.

Characteristics of Open and Closed Kinetic Chain Exercises

Both open and closed chain activities are used in rehabilitation because each type of activity or exercise demonstrates different characteristics. The primary characteristics associated with CKC exercises include large resistance forces and small accelerations at the end segment, greater joint compressive forces and congruency with decreased shear stress, stimulation of joint proprioception, and enhanced dynamic stabilization through muscle coactivation.[2,6,9,11,13] The characteristics of OKC exercises include large accelerations and small resistance forces at the end segment of the extremity. As a result of these large distal segment accelerations, the joints undergo greater distraction forces, and the muscles around the joints produce large torques. During OKC exercises, it is important to establish a stable proximal base of support, such as the scapulothoracic (ST) joint, or the sacroiliac and hip joint, so that distal joint motions of the wrist and ankle can occur with appropriate timing and force. The joint mechanoreceptors are facilitated through stimulation occurring at the extremes of joint ROM, such as throwing a baseball or performing various plyometric medicine ball exercises with the shoulder. Finally, concentric acceleration and eccentric deceleration that occur in OKC exercises simulate some functional activities mentioned previously.[6,9,11]

Gray listed some comparisons of the characteristics of open versus closed kinetic chain exercises (Table 17–1). However, it is important to note some of the limitations of these comparisons. First, this chart was originally done to compare and contrast the characteristics of OKC and CKC exercises for the lower extremity. Therefore, analogies to the upper extremity should be made cautiously. Furthermore, generalizations are presented that are not supported by research. For example, isolated joint movement and isolated muscle contraction proposed with OKC exercises rarely occur. When an individual attempts to isolate voluntary movement at one joint, a change occurs in the body's center of gravity that results in a compensatory reflex muscle contraction to control and maintain an upright posture.[14,15]

Other areas also need to be considered when applying this comparison. Various force couples exist in the human body, allowing joint movement to occur via two muscles working concurrently, for example, the deltoid-supraspinatus force couple at the shoulder.[2] Loads that are very similar to normal loads can be applied, such as those OKC activities of kicking a soccer ball or a football. Also, velocities of movement, such as using different speeds on isokinetic testing and exercise equipment (OKC), or changing the speed or power with which one performs a squat or power clean exercise (CKC), can vary during both OKC or CKC exercises. Stresses and strains might vary in either OKC or CKC, depending on which joint in the kinetic chain is being considered, the range of motion (ROM) that the joint is experiencing, or the muscle length and moment arm of the muscles that cross that particular joint.

TABLE 17–1 Characteristics of Open vs. Closed Kinetic Chain Exercises

Characteristic	Open	Closed
End Segment	Free	Not Free
Axis of Motion	Motion distal to the axis of the joint	Motion both distal and proximal to the joint
Muscle Contraction	Primarily concentric	All types
Movement	Usually isolated	Certain muscle groups
Loads	Artificial and abnormal	Normal
Velocity	Predetermined	Variable
Stress/Strain	Inconsistent	Consistent
Stabilization	Artificial	Postural
Planes	Occurs in one of the cardinal planes	Combination of motion in all three
Proprioception	Foreign, erroneous	Normal
Techniques	Limited to equipment, done to failure	Unlimited, done to substitution
Reaction	More of an action, isolated	Both reaction and action, integrated
Muscle-firing Patterns	Agonist/antagonist	Coactivation

Stabilization is not always artificial in OKC exercises. Artificial stabilization refers to various exercise machines, such as a leg extension machine, which tend to allow movement of one joint in one direction without requiring other joints to provide balance and stabilization, as in a free-weight squat. Many times it is necessary to use machines to work on specific weaknesses in muscle groups such as the quadriceps, which could be compensated for by other muscles such as the gluteus maximus in such CKC exercises as the squat.[16] Finally, functional joint motion rarely occurs in the cardinal planes; very few joint axes lie in the cardinal planes.

Therefore, a clear definition of kinetic chain terminology is important to understand and examine OKC and CKC exercise characteristics precisely. To date, scientific research has delineated some differences and rationale for using CKC versus OKC exercises.

Rationale for Use of Closed Kinetic Chain Exercises

The scientific and clinical rationales for using CKC exercises in the lower extremity are well established.[17–24] It has been suggested that CKC exercises at the knee are safer because weight-bearing forces cross the tibiofemoral joint. These forces cause an increase in agonist-antagonist muscle coactivation, a decrease in joint shear forces, and a minimization of the amount of joint displacement and ACL strain.[24–27] Gray[11] stated that CKC exercises facilitate proprioceptive feedback mechanisms that occur because of the mechanics specific to CKC exercises. Davies and Dickoff-Hoffman[13] stated that:

> When we perform kinesthetic rehabilitation techniques, we usually begin with closed kinetic chain exercises. Although there is limited research, the closed kinetic chain exercises cause axial loading and compression in the joint, therefore, increasing noncontractile stability. This causes cocontraction of the agonist/antagonist muscle groups, thereby creating increased dynamic joint stability. (p 453)

Rowe[28] also agrees that axial loading and compression facilitate dynamic joint stability. Steindler[5] described the *concurrent shift* of the biarticular muscles that occurs during simultaneous movement of the hip, knee, and ankle in rising from the squat exercise. He emphasized the same muscle undergoing an eccentric action at one joint and a concentric action at the other; this is the hallmark of CKC exercises. He further emphasized that biarticular muscles play an important role in joint stabilization, resulting in great efficiency when paired with uniarticular muscles.

Whereas the rationale for using CKC exercises for the lower extremity appears obvious, the scientific rationale for using CKC exercises in the upper extremity is less clear. Kibler[2] has offered several theories about the benefits of CKC exercises in upper extremity rehabilitation. First, the shoulder functions as a funnel, transferring forces from the trunk and lower extremities through the shoulder and finally out through the wrist and hand in a predictable way, as in hitting a tennis serve. Similarly, CKC exercises can transfer forces through the shoulder in a predictable way. Second, as suggested in the lower extremity and for the upper extremities, CKC exercises promote coactivation of the force couples around the scapula and GH joint through joint compression, thereby enhancing their stabilizing role. Third, by fixing the hand in various exercises such as the push-up, press-up, or chin-up, the scapular muscles might be more highly activated than in OKC exercises such as the bench press or the overhead press. Fourth, by providing joint compression and coactivation of muscles about the GH joint in 90° of abduction, tensile stresses on the capsular ligaments and the rotator cuff decrease. Fifth, proprioceptive activity is enhanced by emphasis on coactivation and stability.[29–32] Finally, CKC activities result in muscle loads and activation that are safe to use in the early phases of rehabilitation.[33,34] However, the use of upper extremity CKC exercises poses a distinct disadvantage. Most upper extremity functional activities are done as an OKC task, such as throwing a baseball, lifting a box, or painting a fence. Thus, the use of CKC upper extremity exercises should probably be used early in the rehabilitation process, whereas OKC exercises should be used later when return to functional upper extremity tasks is the goal.

Closed Kinetic Chain Research

Currently, little scientific research has been done comparing the effects of CKC and OKC exercises for the upper extremity on muscle activation, joint forces, and joint movement, or providing an explanation about the relevance to functional rehabilitation. However, one area, the quantitative comparisons of muscle activity between OCK and CKC upper extremity exercises, has received more research attention. Townsend and colleagues[35] recorded the intramuscular electromyographic (EMG) activity of seven glenohumeral muscles (pectoralis major, latissimus dorsi, deltoid, supraspinatus, infraspinatus, teres minor, and subscapularis) in 15 subjects while performing seventeen OKC and CKC shoulder exercises (exercises used by professional baseball teams). A comparison of these exercises is listed in Table 17–2. Of the 17 exercises, the press-up exercise (CKC), defined as lifting oneself from a chair while seated, was found to be the most effective at producing high levels of EMG activity in the pectoralis major and the latissimus dorsi muscles. The standard push-up (CKC) with a wide hand placement was the second-best exercise for activating the pectoralis major. The military press (OKC) was found to be the most effective to activate the supraspinatus, whereas the bench press (OKC) elicited the lowest EMG activity in all the seven muscles tested.

A similar study, by Moseley and colleagues,[36] analyzed the EMG activity in eight muscles (upper, middle, and lower trapezius; middle and lower serratus anterior; rhomboids; levator scapula; and pectoralis minor) about the ST joint in nine subjects performing 16 OKC and CKC exercises (Table 17–2). The press-up (CKC) elicited the highest EMG activity in the pectoralis minor. The push-up (CKC) and the push-up with a plus (protraction at the top of the movement) elicited the second highest EMG activity on the pectoralis minor, the fourth highest of the lower serratus anterior, and the fifth highest of the middle serratus anterior. The military press (OKC) elicited the second highest EMG activity in the upper trapezius and the fourth highest EMG activity in the middle serratus anterior. Again, it was concluded that the bench press (OKC) did not elicit a high level of EMG activity for any of the eight scapular muscles evaluated.

Both of these studies support the use of CKC exercises to elicit high levels of muscle activation across both the GH and ST joints. They also support that CKC exercises are comparable to OKC exercises. Furthermore, this increased muscle activity might facilitate improved glenohumeral proprioception through feedback from the muscle afferents.[29–32]

TABLE 17–2 Comparison of the Optimal OKC or CKC Exercise
for the Glenohumeral and Scapulothoracic Joint Musculature
on the Basis of % Manual Muscle Test

	Townsend et al. (35)			Moseley et al. (36)	
	OKC	CKC		OKC	CKC
Pectoralis major		Press-up-84% Push-up-64%	Upper trapezius	Rowing-112%	
Latissimus dorsi		Press-up-55%	Middle trapezius	Horizontal Abd. (neutral)-108%	
Anterior deltoid	Scaption/ IR 72%		Lower trapezius	Abduction-68%	
Middle deltoid	Scaption/ IR 83%		Middle Serratus Anterior	Flexion/ Abduction 96%	Push-up-80%
Posterior deltoid	Horizontal Abd. (IR)-93%		Lower Serratus Anterior	Scaption-84%	Push-up-72%
Supraspinatus	Military Press 80%		Rhomboids	Horizontal Abd. (neutral)-66%	
Infraspinatus	Horizontal Abd. (ER)-88%	Push-up (hands in)-54%	Levator Scapulae	Rowing-114%	
Teres Minor	External Rot. 80%		Pectoralis Minor		Press-up-89%
Subscapularis	Scaption/ IR 62%				Push-up-58%

Adapted from Townsend, H, et al: Electromyographical analysis of the glenohumeral muscles during a baseball rehabilitation program. Am J Sports Med 19:264, 1991; and Moseley, JB, et al: EMG analysis of the scapular muscles during a shoulder rehabilitation program. Am J Sports Med 20(2):128, 1992.

One of two published studies to date specifically designed to compare open versus closed chain upper extremity exercises was performed by Dillman and colleagues.[9] This case study compared the mean EMG amplitude for each phase of movement represented as a percentage of maximum voluntary contraction in six muscles (supraspinatus, infraspinatus, deltoid, pectoralis major, triceps, and biceps). The comparisons of EMG amplitude were made across the following conditions: one unloaded bench press condition (MNL), three various loaded bench press conditions (MEL), five various loaded push-up conditions (FEL), and one loaded dumbbell press condition (MEL). Two phases occur during the exercises, the *force phase*, defined as the portion of the movement where the distance between the distal segment and the body increases (the up phase of the push-up, concentric muscle contraction); and the *absorption phase*, defined as the portion of the movement when the distance between the distal segment and the body decreases (the down phase in the bench press, eccentric muscle contraction), characterized each condition. Results showed that muscle activity was considerably greater in the force phase (concentric muscle contraction) and less in the absorption phase (eccentric muscle contraction). Although no statistical comparisons were made, the average EMG amplitude increased from the MNL condition (OKC) to the progressively greater resistance MEL conditions (OKC). Specifically, for the supraspinatus, the average EMG activity for the FEL conditions (push-up, CKC) was less than that for all the other exercise conditions. This finding contradicts the findings of Townsend and colleagues,[35] and Moseley and colleagues,[36] who found the bench press exercise (OKC) to produce less EMG activity of the supraspinatus as compared to the push-up exercise (CKC). This contradiction might be the result of differences in the loads (resistance) used in the three studies or the normalization of muscle activity (percentage of MVC versus percentage of MMT). This contradiction points out the importance of using the same load (resistance) when making EMG comparisons or recognizing that the load differences in the activity or exercise might explain the EMG activity differences. However, all the previously mentioned studies indicate that CKC exercises challenge the proximal glenohumeral and scapular musculature, which facilitates their use in upper extremity rehabilitation.

Recently, Blackard and colleagues[37] published a study using EMG analysis to challenge the kinetic chain terminology, and the importance of the boundary condition (hand fixed or hand free). Blackard and colleagues recorded the EMG activity of the pectoralis major and the long head of the triceps in 10 subjects performing push-ups, bench presses with loads that were equal to the loads of the push-ups, and bench presses with no loads. No significant differences between the equivalent loaded exercises with different boundary conditions (bench press-free distal boundary and the push-up-fixed distal boundary) were identified. However, there was statistical significance ($p < 0.05$) between the equivalent boundary condition with different loads (the bench press loaded and the bench press no load) and the different load with different boundary conditions (the push-up and the bench press with no load). As a result, the conclusion of this study suggests that the external load is more important than the boundary condition in describing human activity. However, this statement should only be considered with respect to quantitative muscle activity (%MVC) about two prime movers, the pectoralis major and the long head of the triceps. Other factors such a joint forces and timing of muscle activation in this study were not compared.

At the American College of Sports Medicine 1998 annual meeting, Murray and Hawkins[38] presented a follow-up to Dillman's study, and for the first time attempted to look at the differences in GH joint forces between OKC and CKC exercises. Specifically, the compressive (long axis of the humerus) and the anterior-posterior forces at the GH joint and the EMG activity of the same six muscles were compared across four load matched OKC and CKC exercises. The results indicated that there were no significant differences between the matched exercises (the 135-lb bench press and the push-up) in compressive or shear forces at the GH joint. There were also no significant differences in percentage of MVC in the EMG activity of the six muscles across the matched exercises. Care should be taken when interpreting these results because each subject performed a 135-lb bench press instead of having the loads based on a percentage of the subject's body weight, which would ensure the load matched conditions. However, the GH joint compressive and shear forces are comparable across both OKC and CKC exercises.

Livingston[39] performed a study comparing OKC and CKC exercises for the shoulder. The interest of the study was to examine Steindler's definition that OKC activities promote sequential activation of muscles from proximal to distal and that, in CKC activities, the muscles fire consecutively from a distal to proximal direction. The goal was to evaluate the timing of muscle activation rather than the percentage of maximal muscle activation. The study compared muscle onset times and duration in load and matched bench press (OKC), and push-up (CKC) exercises of the supraspinatus, infraspinatus, anterior deltoid, pectoralis major, biceps brachii, triceps brachii, wrist extensors, and wrist flexors.[39] These muscles transcend the length of the upper extremity from proximal to distal and are considered prime movers during upper extremity exercises. Significant differences ($p < 0.01$) were found in the onset time of all eight muscles in the bench press (OKC) exercises, whereas no significant differences were found in the onset time of the eight muscles in the push-up (CKC) exercise. These findings support the idea that CKC exercises promote muscular cocontraction, and therefore, increased stiffness and joint stability. The findings refute Steindler's definition of CKC activities, which suggested that the muscles would fire consecutively from distal to proximal. Specifically in post-hoc analysis, there was no significant difference in the onset times of the supraspinatus ($p = 0.13$), infraspinatus ($p = 0.18$), and anterior deltoid ($p = 0.07$) times across both OKC and CKC exercises. These results support the notion that the deltoid-rotator cuff force couple acts as the primary agonist initiating these similar joint movement tasks in the bench press and the push-up. A *force couple*, as described by Speer and Garrett,[40] is two groups of muscles contracting synchronously, enabling a specific motion to occur. This force couple of the shoulder girdle also helps maintain the congruent relationship between the glenoid and the humeral head, which again is pivotal for joint stability.

In an attempt to evaluate the safety and progression of various CKC exercises, an unpublished study of normal volunteers was performed by Dr. Ben Kibler (Lexington Sport Medicine Center, Lexington, Kentucky, 1996). Kibler demonstrated that specific upper extremity CKC exercises could be done with muscle activation in the range of 10% to 40% of maximum. These activation levels as a percentage of MVC are well within the safety limits for utilization early in upper extremity rehabilitation programs for such pathologies as rotator cuff and capsular repair (Table 17–3).

TABLE 17–3 Muscle Firing as a Percentage of the Maximal Muscle Activity for Different Closed Chain Exercises

Activity	Serratus Anterior	Supra Spinatus	Infra Spinatus	Rhomboid	Upper Traps	Lower Traps	Ant. Deltoid	Post. Deltoid
Standing weight-shift	<10	<10	<10	<10	<10	<10	<10	<10
Standing rocking board	<10	<10	<10	<10	<10	<10	<10	<10
Four-pt. weight-shift	30	<10	<10	<10	<10	<10	30	<10
Four-pt. rocking board	30	<10	<10	<10	<10	<10	30	<10
Clock Flexion	20	20	20	20	20	<10	20	<10
Clock Scaption	20	20	20	40	20	<10	20	<10
Standard Push-up	25	20	20	35	35	10	70	30
Modified Push-up	25	20	20	35	35	10	45	30

In summary, closed kinetic chain exercises should be used in upper extremity shoulder rehabilitation because they stimulate and enhance one of the most important functions of the shoulder joint, proximal stability, through the promotion of dynamic joint stability (muscle cocontraction), joint compression, and facilitation of joint proprioception. Furthermore, CKC exercises are safe to use in early rehabilitation.

SUGGESTED SHOULDER PROGRAM DESIGN

Rehabilitation must progress in a logical manner. It begins with an accurate medical diagnosis and continues through examination and evaluation. The physical therapist determines the interrelationship among impairments, functional limitations, and disability for a specific diagnostic group and implements a functional intervention based on the evaluation and anticipated goals to achieve a productive outcome.[1] A functional shoulder rehabilitation program should be based on sound scientific research. Closed kinetic chain exercises are only one component of this program. According to the author, there are five progressions in CKC exercises. These progressions are as follows:

1. Weight or load distribution (minimum to maximum)
2. Stable to unstable surface
3. Eyes open to eyes closed (variation in proprioceptive inputs)
4. Manual or external resistance (intensity and work/rest ratio)
5. Static to dynamic movement (balance to movement)

Each of these will be described within the framework of the three stages of rehabilitation that are based on clinical reactivity and healing constraints.

Acute Phase

The acute phase begins with the onset of clinical symptoms such as pain, soreness, limited motion, or weakness of the shoulder. The general goals in this phase of rehabilitation are to resolve the clinical symptoms or tissue injury, to promote conditions for healing, to reduce pain and inflammation, to re-establish nonpainful ROM, to retard muscle atrophy, to obtain neuromuscular control of the scapula in a glenohumeral neutral position, and to maintain fitness of the rest of the body.[2]

CKC exercises begin with static, lightweight loads distributed in a loose-pack shoulder position, with the patient's eyes open, thereby aiding in proprioception, with minimum resistance and intensity (Fig. 17–1). Next, the patient progresses to dynamic movement on uneven surfaces with eyes closed, thereby challenging the muscle proprioceptors by removing the visual inputs. Then, the program progresses by adding greater resistance, intensity, and ROM (Fig. 17–2). The work/rest ratio is usually 3:1 in this phase of the program, thus challenging the aerobic energy system, which is important to re-establish in the early phases of rehabilitation.

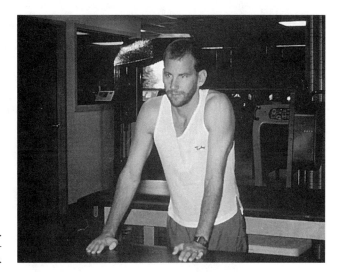

FIGURE 17-1. Acute Phase. Stabilization with weight distributed through hands to shoulder.

Recovery Phase

During the recovery phase, work continues to address the clinical symptoms and tissue injury while progressing to more functional deficits such as strength, power, endurance, and flexibility. The general goals in this phase of rehabilitation are to regain and improve upper extremity muscle flexibility, strength, balance, power, and endurance and to improve neuromuscular control of the scapulohumeral rhythm and normal arthrokinematics of the shoulder.

Use of CKC exercises can continue throughout this phase of rehabilitation, depending on the goals of the patient and the functional task to which the patient would like to return, such as sports or work. The patient begins with an increase in load distributed through axial compression at the shoulder in a more closed-packed

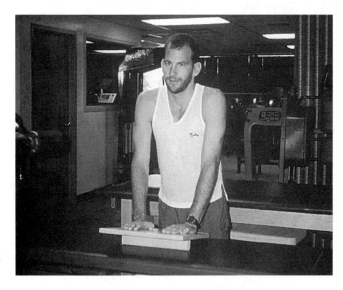

FIGURE 17-2. Acute Phase. Standing weight-shift with hands on tilt board.

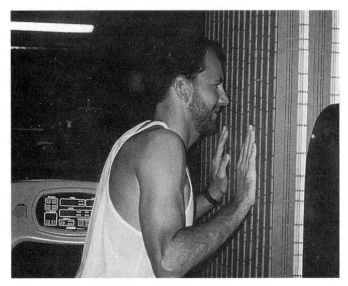

FIGURE 17–3. Recovery Phase. Wall push-up exercise.

position, such as a wall push-up (Fig. 17–3). Then the patient progresses to the scapular clock exercise (moving the scapula through the position along a hypothetical face of a clock with the hand fixed) with the eyes closed (Fig. 17–4). Dynamic movements, which promote proprioception and scapulohumeral stability, are performed in various postures. The load distribution through the shoulder is increased by progressing from quadruped (Fig. 17–5) to biped (Fig. 17–6), and, finally, to using complete body weight in the press-up exercise (Fig. 17–7). The work/rest ratio in this phase is 1:1. These CKC exercises are very useful in the early part of the recovery phase when neuromuscular training is important, along with establishing a stable scapular base for distal movements. At the same time, tension and shear across healing joints and tissues are minimized.

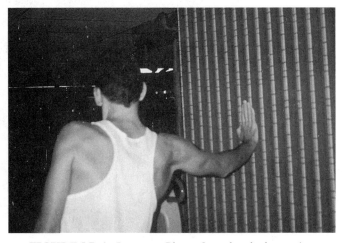

FIGURE 17–4. Recovery Phase. Scapular clock exercise.

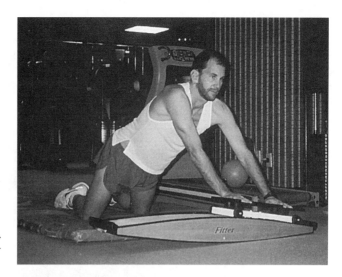

FIGURE 17–5. Recovery Phase. Quadruped stabilization and dynamic weight-shift exercises.

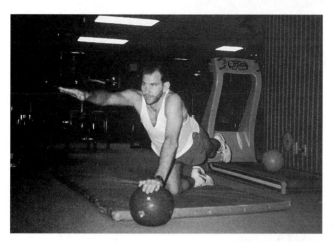

FIGURE 17–6. Recovery Phase. Biped stabilization exercise.

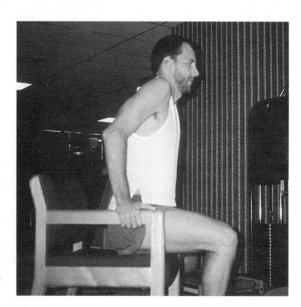

FIGURE 17–7. Recovery Phase. Press-up exercise.

411

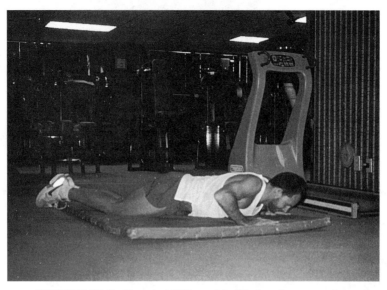

FIGURE 17–8. Functional Phase. Modified push-up exercise.

Functional Phase

The functional phase addresses any of the remaining functional deficits while gradually progressing through a return to competition or work program. Both the task and the energy system demands are simulated. The general goals of this phase are to increase the power and neuromuscular control of the shoulder in all functional planes of motion and to return to the sport or to activity-specific tasks. Outside of the lineman in football or the gymnast, CKC exercises in this phase are probably of little benefit because most uses of the upper extremity in sports or work have a larger OKC component. Some of these advanced CKC exercises include push-ups (Fig. 17–8), dips (Fig. 17–9), and plyometric exercises on the total gym (Fig. 17–10). The work/rest ratio

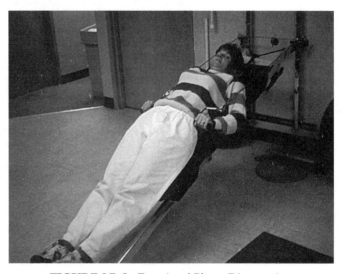

FIGURE 17–9. Functional Phase. Dip exercise.

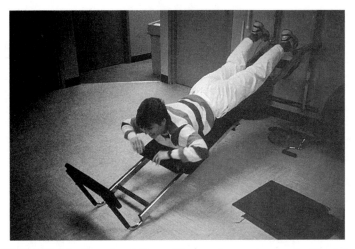

FIGURE 17–10. Functional Phase. Plyometric exercises on the Total Gym.

in this phase is 1:3, thereby facilitating the development of anaerobic power in the cardiovascular and muscular systems.

CASE STUDY 17–1

HISTORY

A 54-year-old female master's swimmer is 1 week post shoulder arthroscopy for an anterior-superior glenoid labrum repair and rotator cuff debridement of the right shoulder. At the time of her physical therapy evaluation, she reported that preoperative pain developed gradually around her superior-anterior right shoulder during her preparation for the National Master's Swimming Competition. One incident she noted was that while she was doing the breaststroke, she experienced a pop on the pull phase of the stroke and was unable to continue. She decreased her yardage and intensity and tried other strokes, experiencing similar sharp pain in the recovery phase of the freestyle stroke. She was forced to discontinue swimming completely. The shoulder pain progressed to pain at night as well as at rest. She expressed that she had a lot of difficulty during overhead activities. Her description of pain was 7 out of 10 on a linear analog pain scale at the time of her initial evaluation.

EXAMINATION

Physical exam reveals a diminutively built female, right-hand dominant, presenting with her right upper extremity in a sling and swathe. She has minimal swelling and ecchymosis around the healing portal incisions. Postural exam reveals a forward and elevated right shoulder compared with the left. She has painful active and passive ROM in all directions, as expected following surgery.

DIAGNOSIS

The patient is classified according to the *Guide to Physical Therapist Practice*[1] as practice pattern J: impaired joint mobility, motor function, muscle performance, and range of motion associated with bony or soft tissue surgical procedures. Evaluation suggests that this patient developed shoulder pathology secondary to glenohumeral hypermobility (common in swimmers) along with having a poorly developed musculoskeletal base, particularly in the scapular muscles and the rotator cuff.

PROGNOSIS

The patient is expected to return to competition, with some possible limitations in her times during competition, in approximately 6 months. The problems to be addressed in order to return the patient to competitive swimming include the following: (1) poor neuromuscular control of the glenohumeral and ST joints, (2) reduced and painful active and passive ROM with improper scapulohumeral rhythm and deltoid-rotator cuff and trapezius-serratus anterior force couples, (3) weakness of the scapular and rotator cuff muscles, and (4) poor training progressions.

INTERVENTION

The patient is given a home exercise program consisting of isotonic exercises for the muscles of the right wrist and left shoulder complex that include the wrist flexors and extensors, the pronators and supinators, the internal and external rotators, the rhomboids, the serratus anterior, and the lower trapezius. She is also given postural exercises of scapular pinches (while sitting or standing, shoulder blades are pinched together) and weight shift on the table (Fig.17–1) at home. Physical therapy treatments include passive ROM of shoulder flexion and scaption (abduction in the scapular plane) to 90° and internal and external rotation at 45° of abduction. Rhythmic stabilization is used for the GH joint and proprioceptive neuromuscular facilitation (PNF) for the ST joint. Modalities and ice are used for pain control.

RE-EVALUATION

The patient is seen twice a week over a 6-week period. She progresses from with-gravity and assisted short-lever arm exercises (elbow bent) and the acute phase CKC exercises to standing against-gravity, longer-lever arm exercises (elbow extended) and the recovery CKC exercises. In the early phases, she works on repetition and endurance with rest upon muscular fatigue or improper arthrokinematics (inability to perform the exercises correctly). In the late stages, she is told to increase the resistance and allow a 1:1 work/rest ratio. Proper scapulohumeral rhythm in movement and proper force couple balance, avoiding the excess trapezius and deltoid overactivation, is emphasized. Finally, a gradual return to her swimming program is outlined, with emphasis on increasing yardage before intensity. Furthermore, importance is placed on good mechanics so that her stroke is pain free.

OUTCOMES

The patient competed the following year and registered several top-10 finishes.

CHAPTER SUMMARY

This chapter reviews the terminology, characteristics, rationale, and current research for using closed kinetic chain exercises in upper extremity rehabilitation. Although a great debate still remains over the true definitions of OKC and CKC, some differences are known. OKC upper extremity exercises, which allow the hand to move freely, differ from CKC exercises in which the hand is fixed to the ground (as in a push-up) or to the bar (as in a pull-up), thus allowing movement to occur at the proximal joints. Analysis of these differences clearly indicates that CKC exercises facilitate dynamic cocontraction of muscles around the shoulder, promoting glenohumeral stability and decreased tensile stress on the capsule and rotator cuff while facilitating the muscle proprioceptors. These are important factors to develop early in a shoulder rehabilitation program so that the distal, function mobility tasks can be performed later. Therefore, upper extremity rehabilitation should include CKC training as one component of the functional rehabilitation program.

REFERENCES

1. Guide to Physical Therapist Practice. American Physical Therapy Association. Alexandria, Virginia, 1997.
2. Kibler, WB: Rehabilitation of the shoulder. In Kibler, WB, et al (eds): Functional Rehabilitation of Sports and Musculoskeletal Injuries. Aspen Publishers, Gaithersburg, MD, 1998, p 149.
3. Reuleaux, F: The Kinematics of Machinery: Outline of a Theory of Machines. Kennedy, ABW (trans, ed). MacMillan, London, 1876.
4. Brunnstrom, S: Clinical Kinesiology. Dickinson, R (ed). FA Davis, Philadelphia, 1972.
5. Steindler, A: Kinesiology of the Human Body under Normal and Pathological Conditions. Charles C. Thomas, Springfield, IL, 1977.
6. Steindler, A: Kinesiology of the Human Body. Charles C. Thomas, Springfield, IL, 1955.
7. Panariello, RA: The closed kinetic chain in strength training. National Strength and Conditioning Journal 8(5):28, 1991.
8. Smidt, GL: Current open and closed kinetic chain concepts: Clarifying or confusing? (editorial). J Orthop Sports Phys Ther 20:235, 1994.
9. Dillman, CJ, et al: Biomechanical differences of open and closed chain exercises with respect to the shoulder. J Sport Rehab 3:228, 1994.
10. Greenfield, B, and Bennett, JG: The application of kinetic chain rehabilitation in the lower extremities. In Donatelli, RA (ed): The Biomechanics of the Foot and Ankle. FA Davis, Philadelphia, PA, 1990, p 324.
11. Gray, GW: Chain Reaction: Successful Strategies for Closed Chain Testing and Rehabilitation. Wynn Marketing, Adrain, MI, 1989.
12. Gray, GW, et al: Closed chain sense. Fitness Management, April:31, 1992.
13. Davies, GJ, and Dickoff-Hoffman, S: Neuromuscular testing and rehabilitation of the shoulder complex. J Orthop Sports Phys Ther 18(2):449, 1993.
14. Bennett, DJ, et al: Gain of the triceps surae stretch reflex in decerebrate and spinal cats during postural and locomotor activities. J Physiol 496:837, 1996.
15. Stein, RB, et al: Modification of reflexes in normal and abnormal movements. Progress in Brain Research 97:189, 1993.

16. Snyder-Mackler, L: Scientific rationale and physiological basis for the use of closed kinetic chain exercise in the lower extremity. J Sport Rehab 5:2, 1996.
17. Anderson, AF, and Lipscomb, AB: Analysis of rehabilitation techniques after anterior cruciate reconstruction. Am J Sports Med 17(2);154, 1989.
18. Fu, FH, et al: Current concepts for rehabilitation following anterior cruciate ligament reconstruction. J Orthop Sports Phys Ther 15:27, 1992.
19. DePalma, BF, and Zelko, RR: Knee rehabilitation after anterior cruciate ligament injury or surgery. Athletic Training, Fall, 1986.
20. Giove, TP, et al: Non-operative treatment of the torn anterior cruciate ligament. J Bone and Jt Surg 65A:184, 1983.
21. Shelbourne, KD, and Nitz, P: Accelerated rehabilitation after anterior cruciate ligament reconstruction. Am J Sports Med 18:292, 1990.
22. Wilk, KE, et al: The biomechanical and electromyographical analysis of open and closed kinetic chain exercises for the lower extremity. Athletic Training: Sports Health Care Perspective 1(4):336, 1995.
23. Yack, HJ, et al: Comparison of closed and open kinetic chain exercises in the anterior cruciate ligament-deficient knee. Am J Sports Med 21(1):49, 1993.
24. Lutz, GE, et al: Comparison of tibiofemoral joint forces during open-kinetic-chain and closed-kinetic-chain exercises. J Bone and Jt Surg 75-A(5):732, 1993.
25. Mangine, RE, and Noyes, FR: Rehabilitation of the Allograft reconstruction. J Orthop Sports Phys Ther 15:294, 1992.
26. Palmitier, R, et al: Kinetic chain exercises in knee rehabilitation. Sports Med 11(6):402, 1991.
27. Wilk KE, and Andrews, JR: Current concepts in the treatment of anterior cruciate disruption. J Orthop Sports Phys Ther 15:279, 1993.
28. Rowe, CR: The Shoulder. Churchill Livingstone, New York, 1989.
29. Borsa, PA, et al: Functional assessment and rehabilitation of shoulder proprioception for the glenohumeral instability. J Sport Rehab 3:84, 1994.
30. Lephart, SM, et al: Proprioception following ACL reconstruction. J Sport Rehab 1:188, 1992.
31. Lephart, SM, and Kocher, MS: The role of exercise in the prevention of shoulder disorders. In Matsen, FA, et al (eds): The Shoulder: A Balance of Mobility and Stability. American Academy of Orthopaedic Surgeons, Rosemont, IL, 1993, p 597.
32. Lephart, SM, et al: Proprioception of the shoulder in normal, unstable, and post-surgical injuries. J Shoulder and Elbow Surg 3:371, 1994.
33. Lephart, SM, and Henry, TJ: The physiological basis for open and closed kinetic chain rehabilitation for the upper extremity. J Sport Rehab 5:71, 1996.
34. Wilk, KE, et al: Closed and open kinetic chain exercises for the upper extremity. J Sport Rehab 5:88, 1996.
35. Townsend, H, et al: Electromyographical analysis of the glenohumeral muscles during a baseball rehabilitation program. Am J Sports Med 19:264, 1991.
36. Moseley, JB, et al: EMG analysis of the scapular muscles during a shoulder rehabilitation program. Am J Sports Med 20(2):128, 1992.
37. Blackard, DO, et al: Use of EMG analysis in challenging kinetic chain terminology. Med Sci in Sports and Exer 31(3):443, 1999.
38. Murray, TA, and Hawkins, R.J: Kinetic and EMG Comparisons of Matched Open and Closed Chain Shoulder Exercises. Paper presented at the meeting of the American College of Sports Medicine, Orlando, FL, June 1998.
39. Livingston, BP: Biomechanical and EMG Comparisons of Open and Closed Kinetic Chain Shoulder Exercises. Master's thesis, University of Kentucky, Lexington, August 1998.
40. Speer, KP, and Garrett, WE: Muscular control of motion and stability about the pectoral girdle. In Matsen, FA, et al (eds): The Shoulder: A Balance of Mobility and Stability. American Academy of Orthopaedic Surgeons, Rosemont, IL, 1993.

Index

An "f" following a page number indicates a figure; a "t" indicates a table.